Sport-Related Skin Conditions

Keyvan Nouri
Editor

Sport-Related Skin Conditions

A Guide for Clinicians

Springer

Editor
Keyvan Nouri
Dr. Phillip Frost Department of Dermatology
and Cutaneous Surgery
University of Miami Health System
Miami, FL, USA

ISBN 978-3-031-90443-1 ISBN 978-3-031-90444-8 (eBook)
https://doi.org/10.1007/978-3-031-90444-8

This Springer imprint is published by the registered company Springer Nature Switzerland AG
The registered company address is: Gewerbestrasse 11, 6330 Cham, Switzerland

Preface

The popularity and diversity of sports present physicians and trainees with challenges of identifying, diagnosing, and treating a multitude of health conditions for athletic patients. Sports-induced dermatoses represent a plethora of skin conditions caused by equipment, the environment, and other athletes. This textbook summarizes different mechanisms of skin conditions caused by different sports, while providing recommendations for prevention, diagnosis, and management. This book is organized based on sport-type to help the reader gain an overview of the dermatological conditions associated with specific sports without necessitating reading through the entire text. This book is written for medical students, residents, and general practitioners that would like to learn more about dermatological concerns for various sports.

Miami, FL, USA Keyvan Nouri

Contents

Contributors

Rahul Aggarwal Dr. Phillip Frost Department of Dermatology and Cutaneous Surgery, University of Miami, Miami, FL, USA

Sarah Antonevich Dr. Phillip Frost Department of Dermatology and Cutaneous Surgery, University of Miami, Miami, FL, USA

Samuel San Antonio Dr. Phillip Frost Department of Dermatology and Cutaneous Surgery, University of Miami, Miami, FL, USA

Kristiana Barbato Dr. Phillip Frost Department of Dermatology and Cutaneous Surgery, University of Miami, Miami, FL, USA

Christina Barrett Dr. Phillip Frost Department of Dermatology and Cutaneous Surgery, University of Miami, Miami, FL, USA

Sophie Bilik Dr. Phillip Frost Department of Dermatology and Cutaneous Surgery, University of Miami, Miami, FL, USA

Edward Brotgandel Dr. Phillip Frost Department of Dermatology and Cutaneous Surgery, University of Miami, Miami, FL, USA

Sophie Cilivio Dr. Phillip Frost Department of Dermatology and Cutaneous Surgery, University of Miami, Miami, FL, USA

Rachel Cohen Dr. Phillip Frost Department of Dermatology and Cutaneous Surgery, University of Miami, Miami, FL, USA

Ricardo Cooke Dr. Phillip Frost Department of Dermatology and Cutaneous Surgery, University of Miami, Miami, FL, USA

Kristen Dean Dr. Phillip Frost Department of Dermatology and Cutaneous Surgery, University of Miami, Miami, FL, USA

Lauren Dender Dr. Phillip Frost Department of Dermatology and Cutaneous Surgery, University of Miami, Miami, FL, USA

Garrett D. Forman Dr. Phillip Frost Department of Dermatology and Cutaneous Surgery, University of Miami, Miami, FL, USA

Daniel Green Dr. Phillip Frost Department of Dermatology and Cutaneous Surgery, University of Miami, Miami, FL, USA

Isabella Guanche Dr. Phillip Frost Department of Dermatology and Cutaneous Surgery, University of Miami, Miami, FL, USA

Eran Gwillim Dr. Phillip Frost Department of Dermatology and Cutaneous Surgery, University of Miami, Miami, FL, USA

Philippe Jean-Pierre Dr. Phillip Frost Department of Dermatology and Cutaneous Surgery, University of Miami, Miami, FL, USA

Eli Kasheri Dr. Phillip Frost Department of Dermatology and Cutaneous Surgery, University of Miami, Miami, FL, USA

Kayla Mashoudy Dr. Phillip Frost Department of Dermatology and Cutaneous Surgery, University of Miami, Miami, FL, USA

Hannah Metheny Dr. Phillip Frost Department of Dermatology and Cutaneous Surgery, University of Miami, Miami, FL, USA

Yasmine Mohseni Dr. Phillip Frost Department of Dermatology and Cutaneous Surgery, University of Miami, Miami, FL, USA

Carlos Lange Nava Dr. Phillip Frost Department of Dermatology and Cutaneous Surgery, University of Miami, Miami, FL, USA

Keyvan Nouri Dr. Phillip Frost Department of Dermatology and Cutaneous Surgery, University of Miami, Miami, FL, USA

Rachel Papavasilopoulos Dr. Phillip Frost Department of Dermatology and Cutaneous Surgery, University of Miami, Miami, FL, USA

Anika Pulumati Dr. Phillip Frost Department of Dermatology and Cutaneous Surgery, University of Miami, Miami, FL, USA

Stefania Radici Dr. Phillip Frost Department of Dermatology and Cutaneous Surgery, University of Miami, Miami, FL, USA

Isabel Rodriguez Dr. Phillip Frost Department of Dermatology and Cutaneous Surgery, University of Miami, Miami, FL, USA

Ryan Scheinkman Dr. Phillip Frost Department of Dermatology and Cutaneous Surgery, University of Miami, Miami, FL, USA

Sheila Sharifi Dr. Phillip Frost Department of Dermatology and Cutaneous Surgery, University of Miami, Miami, FL, USA

Rachel Summers Dr. Phillip Frost Department of Dermatology and Cutaneous Surgery, University of Miami, Miami, FL, USA

Lea Tordjman Dr. Phillip Frost Department of Dermatology and Cutaneous Surgery, University of Miami, Miami, FL, USA

Peter Velthuis Department of Dermatology, Erasmus University, Rotterdam, The Netherlands

Alexia Vignau Dr. Phillip Frost Department of Dermatology and Cutaneous Surgery, University of Miami, Miami, FL, USA

Chapter 1
Introduction

Ryan Scheinkman, Alexia Vignau, and Keyvan Nouri

Sports can be broadly defined as physical activities requiring skill that can be performed individually or as part of a team [1]. Sports are a near cultural universal with 206 national Olympic committees at the time of the writing of the textbook and sports not even being confined to Earth after Alan Shepard played golf on the Moon during the Apollo 14 mission in 1971 [2, 3]. Sports can potentially be traced back 15,000 to 17,000 years ago to cave paintings in France that appear to depict wresting [4]. Sports have historically and traditionally served many cultural purposes such as training for martial activities, ritualistic expression, economics, politics, and entertainment. The Olmec, Maya, Aztec, and Toltec played the Mesoamerican ballgame (a sport with variations involving partial scoring through passing a rubber ball through masonry rings) as part of ritualistic ceremonies and as a potential tool to as a proxy to prevent conflict (Fig. 1.1) [5]. The Birdman religion in Rapa Nui involved a ritualistic swimming event to obtain Sooty Tern Eggs by the swimmers (hopu) from a neighboring island [6]. Each swimmer had a sponsor and the sponsor with the swimmer that obtained the first egg received exclusive rights for eggs and fledglings for the succeeding season [6].

Sports currently provide opportunities for socialization, entertainment, cultural expression, physical fitness, and benefits to health. However, the sporting environment presents unique challenges to the dermatological health of its participants. Sports present its participants with environmental challenges, such as exposure to solar ultraviolet radiation in outdoor sports linked to skin carcinogenesis with inadequate protection, extremes of cold linked to frostbite, and marine environments linked to unique marine pathogens that can contaminate wounds. Equipment used in sports can be a source of cutaneous injury or hypersensitivity reactions, such as blisters induced by ill-fitting climbing shoes or contact dermatitis from swim

R. Scheinkman (✉) · A. Vignau · K. Nouri
Dr. Phillip Frost Department of Dermatology and Cutaneous Surgery, University of Miami, Miami, FL, USA
e-mail: scheinkman@med.miami.edu; axv200@med.miami.edu; knouri@med.miami.edu

K. Nouri (ed.), *Sport-Related Skin Conditions*,
https://doi.org/10.1007/978-3-031-90444-8_1

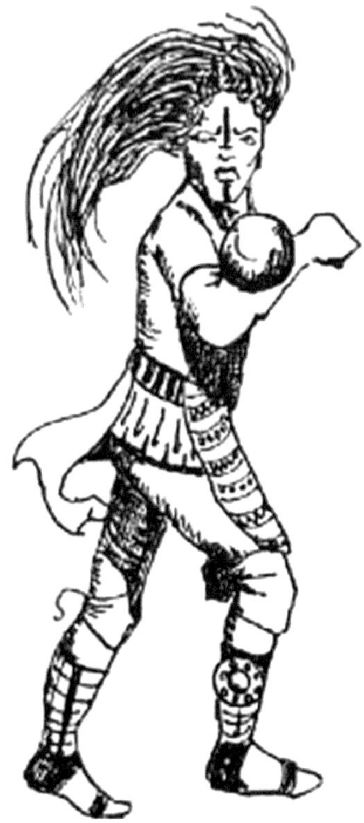

Fig. 1.1 Mesoamerican Ball Player

goggles. Sports expose participants to unique physiological stressors that can induce dermatological conditions ranging from traction alopecia in breakdancers to talon noir caused by traumatic intraepidermal hemorrhages from shearing forces on the feet experienced by racquet sport players. The Spaniard Diego Durán described, roughly half a millennia ago, the large hematomas that Mesoamerican ball players would obtain playing their sport, that would be treated with lancing highlighting the long history of identification and treatment of cutaneous and dermatological conditions [7].

This textbook seeks to provide an overview of skin conditions associated with a variety of sports grouped together as aquatic sports, track & field sports, winter sports, mountaineering sports, racket sports, volleyball bat-and-ball sports, cycling, basketball, football, dance, gymnastics, weightlifting, martial arts, wrestling, and cycling. Each chapter is designed to provide self-contained information about sports dermatoses associated with the physical conditions, environment, and equipment associated with the sports discussed in the chapter to provide an overview for the reader to familiarize themselves with the dermatological challenges of the sport. The chapters highlight many of the overlapping skin conditions associated with sports, such as fungal dermatophyte infections of the head (Tinea Capitis) and the feet (Tinea Pedis), friction-induced acne mechanica, or superficial wound infections to name a few can have different etiologies unique to the equipment, environment, and mechanics of the sports. Unique diseases specific to sporting types, such as cutaneous decompression sickness present in scuba divers or pointe-shoe trauma seen in dancers, are highlighted to provide context for the unique dermatological challenges associated with some sports. The reader is thus encouraged to use this textbook as a starting point for learning about skin conditions associated with different types of sports. To help visualize the clinical presentation of many of the diseases in the text, we recommend that the reader consult *Fitzpatrick's Color Atlas and Synopsis of Clinical Dermatology, Ninth Edition*, which provides images of many common dermatoses. Considering the popularity of sports, healthcare professionals can not only serve a role in identifying and treating skin dermatoses, but can console athletes on preventative practices (e.g. adopting sun protective measures) that can benefit patients overall health.

References

1. Giesbrecht GG, Wilkerson JA. Hypothermia, frostbite and other cold injuries: prevention, survival, rescue, and treatment. The Mountaineers Books; 2006.
2. https://olympics.com/ioc/national-olympic-committees: Olympics; National Olympic Committees.
3. Apollo 14: National Air and Space Museum; [Available from: https://airandspace.si.edu/explore/stories/apollo-missions/apollo-14#:~:text=Golf%20Club%2C%20Apollo%2014%2C%20Replica,the%20museum's%20collection%20in%201975].
4. Madigan T, Delaney T. Sociology of sports: an introduction. McFarland Publishing. Jefferson, North Carolina, USA. 2009.
5. Santley RS, Berman MJ, Alexander RT, Scarborough VL, Wilcox DR. The politicization of the Mesoamerican ballgame and its implications for the interpretation of the distribution of ballcourts in central Mexico. In: The Mesoamerican Ballgame. University of Arizona Press; 1991. p. 3–24.
6. Routledge S. The mystery of Easter Island: the story of an expedition. London and Aylesbury; 1920.
7. Blanchard K. The anthropology of sport. Bergin & Garvey; 2005.

Chapter 2
Aquatic Sports

Sheila Sharifi, Christina Barrett, Ryan Scheinkman, Carlos Lange Nava, Alexia Vignau, Rachel Cohen, Samuel San Antonio, Eran Gwillim, and Keyvan Nouri

2.1 Introduction

Aquatic athletes spend time in pool, fresh, and saltwater present risks for unique dermatoses associated with these environments. These sports include competitive swimming and diving, water polo, scuba, snorkeling, and paddle and board sports. Organisms unique to aquatic environments, including marine bacteria, aquatic vertebrates and invertebrates, and cnidarians pose challenges to the skin health of aquatic sports participants. Common to all aquatic environments is the risk of UV radiation, given participants in these sports often spend significant amounts of time in the sun. Exposure to UV radiation is a known risk factor for skin cancer, which continues to proliferate worldwide. Other environmental factors such as wind exposure render athletes more susceptible to UV-induced skin damage [1]. Previous studies have shown that approximately half of aquatic sports participants, including surfers and sailors, do not use adequate photoprotective measures [2]. Hence, endorsement of appropriate sun protection measures including sunscreen and protective clothing is paramount.

Sheila Sharifi, Christina Barrett, Eran Gwillim and Keyvan Nouri contributed equally with all other contributors.

S. Sharifi · C. Barrett · R. Scheinkman (✉) · C. L. Nava · A. Vignau · R. Cohen · S. S. Antonio
E. Gwillim · K. Nouri
Dr. Phillip Frost Department of Dermatology and Cutaneous Surgery, University of Miami, Miami, FL, USA
e-mail: ss4647@georgetown.edu; christina.barrett@miami.edu; scheinkman@med.miami.edu; cxl1033@med.miami.edu; axv200@med.miami.edu; rachelcohen@med.miami.edu; sxs3273@miami.edu; knouri@med.miami.edu

K. Nouri (ed.), *Sport-Related Skin Conditions*,
https://doi.org/10.1007/978-3-031-90444-8_2

2.2 Infectious and Dermatophyte Diseases Associated with Pool-Based Sports

2.2.1 Swimming Pool Granuloma

Swimmers are at risk for Swimming pool granuloma, or fish tank granuloma, which presents as indurated erythematous or hyperpigmented nodules primarily on the knees, elbows, or dorsum of the hands and feet approximately six weeks following exposure to *Mycobacterium marinum* or Mycobacterium scrofulaceum. Although symptoms are often minimal, these lesions can be pruritic, painful, and may ulcerate [3, 4]. Rarely, serious complications may arise in the form of osteomyelitis, arthritis, bursitis, tenosynovitis, and carpal tunnel syndrome [4]. The current first-line treatment for swimming pool granuloma consists of oral clarithromycin 500 mg twice a day for 6 weeks. Oral minocycline at the same frequency can also prove effective, but resistant mycobacteria have been reported [3, 4]. Continuing antibiotic therapy for 4–6 weeks after resolution is recommended [3]. Warm water soaks to the affected areas for approximately 5–10 minutes three to four times per day is also recommended [4]. Infectious diseases associated with pool-based are summarized in Table 2.1.

2.2.2 Acute Otitis Externa (Swimmer's Ear)

One of the most common aquatic dermatoses, acute otitis externa (AOE), also known as swimmer's ear, is an inflammation of the external auditory canal that often results from bacterial infections [5, 6]. Given the anatomy of the ear canal, it is prone to moisture retention, providing an environment well-suited for bacterial growth that may lead to swelling, erythema, pain, pruritus, discharge, and possible hearing impairment [5, 7]. Among the most common causative pathogens of AOE are *Pseudomonas aeruginosa* and *Staphylococcus aureus* [8]. When treating AOE, antibiotic eardrops used for approximately one week serve as the primary form of therapy, including gentamycin, neomycin, gramicidin, polymyxin B, and ciprofloxacin. These drops often also contain a steroid to alleviate inflammation and pain in the ear canal [5, 9]. Pain management is critical and is often achieved with the use of nonsteroidal anti-inflammatory drugs (NSAIDs) or acetaminophen used either by themselves or in combination with an opioid [5]. Preventing the onset of AOE is done by limiting exposure to predisposing factors. This is done by minimizing moisture retention in the ear canal by using well-fitting earplugs or swim caps. Once out of the water, swimmers should tilt their heads while gently pulling on the ear to drain any water left in the ear canal. A hairdryer on its lowest temperature setting can be used to dry the ear—acidifying drops inside the ear like acetic acid can also be used as a drying agent following exposure to water [9, 10].

Table 2.1 Infectious and Dermatophyte Diseases Associated with Pool-Based Sports

Disease/Condition	Symptoms and physical exam findings	Treatment recommendations
Swimming pool granuloma	Indurated erythematous or hyperpigmented nodules on knees, elbows, or dorsum of hands/feet	Oral clarithromycin 500 mg 2x/day for 6 weeks
Acute otitis external	Inflammation of the external auditory canal	Antibiotic eardrops for 1 week and NSAIDs
Hot tub folliculitis	Follicular, macular, vesicular, or pustular lesions in regions in contact with contaminated water	Topical polymyxin B, topical gentamicin, or warm compress of 2% acetic acid
Bikini bottom	Firm, inflamed, deep nodules in inferior gluteal creases	10-day course of systemic antibiotic therapy
Pseudomonas hot-foot syndrome	Painful nodules in hands and feet	Cold compresses, analgesic agents, and elevation of feet. Antibiotics if needed
Molluscum contagiosum	Small, firm, rounded pearly umbilicated papules that are pink or skin-colored	Usually resolves on its own in 6–12 months
Interdigital tinea pedis	Pruritic erythematous macerations, white scaling, and peeling in webbing between toes	Topical antifungals twice daily for 4 weeks
Hyperkeratotic tinea pedis	Chronic, erythematous, hyperkeratotic, scaling plaques	Topical antifungals twice daily for 4 weeks
Vestibullous tinea pedis	Severely pruritic, painful vesicles/bullae with background erythema	Topical antifungals twice daily for 4 weeks
Verruca	Well-defined, papillomatous or verrucous plaque with a rough surface	Topical salicylic acid-containing compounds and other modalities
Pitted keratolysis	Distinctive small pits or depressions on the soles of the feet and toes	Topical antibacterial agents for at least 10 days and antimicrobial washes

2.2.3 *Hot Tub Folliculitis*

Among the most common skin infections associated with hot tubs and swimming pools is hot tub folliculitis, otherwise known as *Pseudomonas aeruginosa* folliculitis [11]. It is an acquired skin infection from the bacterial colonization of *Pseudomonas aeruginosa* found in unchlorinated or untreated public bodies of water [12]. Estimates show that approximately 67% of hot tubs and 63% of swimming pools are contaminated by *P. aeruginosa* at any given time [13] . Patients usually present with follicular, macular, vesicular, or pustular lesions in regions that came in contact with contaminated waters with a high concentration of the bacterium that arises within 8–48 hours and resolves within 1–2 weeks [14]. Nodular lesions can less commonly arise in the palms and soles [12]. Prevention, particularly in immunocompromised individuals, consists of minimizing exposure to *P. aeruginosa* by avoiding swimming in pools, whirlpools, or hot tubs that are contaminated or lack proper chlorination or treatment [15]. Treatment for symptomatic relief consists of using topical polymixin B, topical gentamicin, or warm compresses of 2% acetic acid [14].

2.2.4 Bikini Bottom

Bikini bottom is a form of deep bacterial folliculitis that can occur in athletes who participate in water sports, particularly after prolonged wear of damp, tight-fitting swimwear [4, 16]. This condition is commonly caused by Streptococcus or Staphylococcus aureus, and presents as firm, inflamed, deep nodules in the inferior gluteal creases [4, 16]. Treatment and prevention involve a ten-day course of systemic antibiotic therapy with adequate skin flora coverage, such as Cephalexin, as well as prompt removal of wet swimwear after exposure to the water, respectively [16].

2.2.5 Pseudomonas Hot-Foot Syndrome

Similar in etiology to hot tub folliculitis, pseudomonas hot-foot syndrome is characterized by the acute onset of very painful nodules in the hands and feet with a benign, self-limiting course. Inoculation of *P. aeruginosa* onto the skin of the palms and soles may arise from trauma to these areas as a result of the abrasive surfaces these areas of the body are often exposed to in swimming pools [17]. Prevention and treatment follow similar guidelines to that of hot tub folliculitis. Hot water, high pH, and low chlorination of pools make them susceptible to infection by *P. aeruginosa*—proper maintenance must be ensured prior to exposure. Moreover, reducing the abrasiveness of pool and hot tub floors can also reduce the risk of infection [12]. Symptomatic relief consists of cold compresses, analgesic agents, and elevation of the feet. Antibiotics with *Pseudomonas* coverage, such as fluoroquinolones like Ciprofloxacin, can aid in resolution, however, antibiotic therapy is not required [17].

2.2.6 Molluscum Contagiosum

Molluscum contagiosum is a common, self-limited, infectious dermatosis transmitted primarily by direct contact with infected skin, frequently seen in the pediatric population, sexually active adults, and the immunocompromised [18]. Transmitted by the poxvirus molluscum contagiosum virus (MCV), it presents as small firm rounded pearly umbilicated papules that are pink or skin-colored; lesions can be single, multiple, or clustered, occasionally with an erythematous halo [18]. Molluscum contagiosum is mostly asymptomatic but may present with pain, itching, redness, or occasionally bacterial superinfection [19]. Outbreaks of molluscum contagiosum are often associated with exposure to swimming pools and associated eczema [19]. Resolution typically occurs in a period of 6–12 months, therefore, the need for therapy and a consensus on the best therapy is not well established [18, 19]. Cryotherapy with liquid nitrogen is commonly utilized but carries the risk of blistering, post-inflammatory hyperpigmentation, and scarring [18, 19]. Other mechanical forms of therapy include curettage, and pulse dye laser (PDL) [18]. Chemical methods involve the destruction of the skin lesion through an inflammatory response. Among the most effective are Cantharidin, a phosphodiesterase inhibitor, and potassium hydroxide, a keratin-dissolving alkaline compound [18]. Prevention of molluscum contagiosum, given its method of transmission, would be through avoiding skin-to-skin contact with individuals known to have lesions. Additional measures include not sharing fomites and avoiding swimming pools associated with molluscum contagiosum outbreaks [19].

2.2.7 Tinea Pedis (Athletes Foot)

Tinea pedis, often referred to as "athlete's foot," is an incredibly common cutaneous infection that's easily transmissible through swimming pools, pool decks, and shower floors [4, 20]. Tinea pedis has three main clinical forms: interdigital tinea pedis, which presents with pruritic erythematous macerations, white scaling, and peeling in the webbing between the fourth and fifth toes; hyperkeratotic (moccasin-type) tinea pedis presents with chronic, erythematous, hyperkeratotic, scaling plaques that typically spare the dorsum of the foot and tend to be asymptomatic; vestibullous (inflammatory) tinea pedis is commonly acquired zoonotically and presents with severely pruritic, often painful vesicles and/or bullae with background erythema [21]. First-line treatments of tinea pedis include the application of topical antifungals like azoles, tolnaftate, or allylamines, twice daily for approximately 4 weeks [20, 21]. In the case of extensive, recurrent, chronic, or resistant-to-topical-treatment tinea pedis, or concomitant onychomycosis, systemic antifungals such as terbinafine, itraconazole, and fluconazole [21]. Preventative measures for athletes are particularly emphasized. Given that fungi thrive best in moist, warm environments, aquatic sports athletes must take precautions by maintaining proper personal hygiene of their feet and ensuring thorough drying of their feet after exposure to water [20, 21]. Moreover, wearing sandals in places such as swimming pools and locker room floors can also help to decrease infection rates as these are locations with high dermatophyte concentration rates [20].

2.2.8 Verruca

Verruca vulgaris colloquially referred to as "warts" are among the most common dermatoses of swimmers—a study found swimmers to be 1.81 times more likely to have warts compared to non-swimmers [20]. Caused by the HPV virus, warts are particularly prevalent in swimmers due to their transmission via contact with contaminated surfaces such as swimming pools and shared bathing areas [22]. Clinical presentation of warts is characteristic of well-defined, papillomatous or verrucous plaques with a rough surface, though the appearance may vary by location [4, 23]. Common sites affected in swimmers include the hands, feet, and other weight-bearing areas [23]. The decision to treat warts should balance the risk of persistence or spread against the inconvenience and potential complications of treatment [23, 24]. Initial treatment modalities consist of topical application of salicylic acid-containing compounds, which act by degrading the thickened stratum corneum and disrupting the viral life cycle within the wart [23, 25]. Other modalities include cryotherapy, which uses freezing temperatures to destroy the wart, laser ablation, which uses focused light energy to remove the wart, and immunotherapies that stimulate the body's immune system to clear the viral infection [23, 25]. Prevention strategies center around minimizing contact with contaminated pool surfaces and improving personal hygiene practices. Swimmers should be encouraged to wear proper foot protection such as water shoes when using shared pool facilities, and to thoroughly clean and disinfect their feet before and after swimming [26].

2.2.9 Pitted Keratolysis

Pitted keratolysis is a bacterial skin infection that manifests as distinctive small pits or depressions on the soles of the feet and toes [4]. Caused by *Corynebacterium sp.* or *Kytococcus sedentarius*, it is always preceded by water exposure or excessive sweating [4]. Athletes affected by pitted keratolysis present with malodorous, pitted lesions on the weight-bearing areas of the foot, which can be accompanied by discomfort or pain [4, 27]. Treatment options include topical antibacterial agents such as clindamycin and erythromycin for at least 10 days; oral antibiotics may be required depending on severity. Antimicrobial washes such as 4% chlorohexidine are also recommended [27]. Prevention strategies focus primarily on good foot hygiene, including thorough drying of feet after swimming or sweating, and wearing well-ventilated footwear to discourage the warm, moist conditions that enable bacteria to proliferate [27].

2.3 Pool Sport Associated Contact Dermatoses

Contact dermatitis is a common occurrence among aquatic sports athletes, particularly those that use equipment such as goggles, swim caps, nose clips, swim fins, and ear plugs (Fig. 2.1) [4]. The findings of contact dermatitis are often attributed to chemical irritants and allergens found in swimming equipment [28]. Clinical features include redness, itching, scaling, blisters, and occasionally vesicles on the areas that were in direct contact with the offending agent [29]. Cutaneous patch testing can aid in identifying the specific allergen responsible for contact dermatitis [16]. Management of aquatic sports-related dermatitis often involves the use of topical or systemic corticosteroids and antihistamines to control acute symptoms [4, 16]. Preventive measures involve avoidance of the causative agents and using hypoallergenic alternatives such as latex-free swim goggles or silicone-based equipment [4, 16]. Aquatic sports related contact dermatitis is further summarized in Table 2.2.

2.3.1 Pool & Pool-Water Dermatitis

Pool dermatitis is an irritant contact dermatitis to chemicals, like bromine and chlorine, used in pool water to increase its pH in order to prevent microbial growth and preserve water clarity. In contrast, pool water dermatitis is an allergic contact dermatitis to chlorinated or brominated compounds found in the water such as 1-bromo-3-chloro-5,5-dimethylhydantoin [4, 30].Clinical presentation of pool water dermatitis presents on exposed areas of the body with pruritic, erythematous, scaling plaques [4, 30]. General management primarily includes avoiding

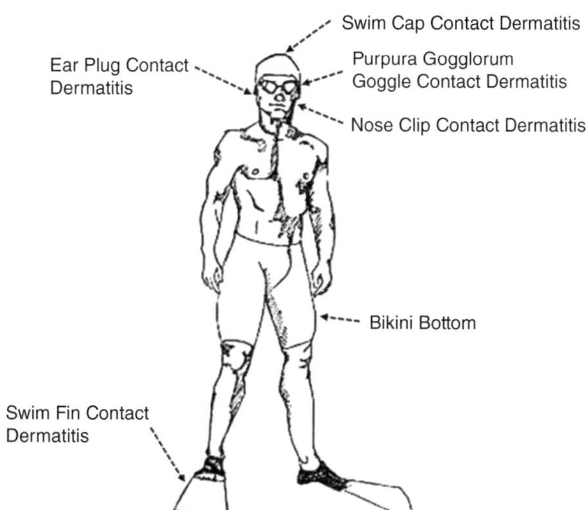

Fig. 2.1 Swimming Equipment-associated Dermatoses

Table 2.2 Aquatic sports contact dermatoses

Disease/condition	Symptoms and physical exam findings	treatment recommendations
Pool & Pool-water Dermatitis	Pruritic, erythematous, scaling plaques	Topical steroids and moisturizers
Bleached swimmer syndrome	Blonding or loss of hair, erythematous macular rashes, dry skin, and eczematous plaques	Rince body immediately after swimming
Swimmer's shoulder	Red erythematous plaque on the shoulder	More regular facial shaving

swimming in halogenated waters and treatment with topical steroids and moisturizers [4, 30–32]. Eruptions from pool dermatitis are also seen in exposed areas and present as urticarial or eczematous plaques [4].

2.3.2 Bleached Swimmer Syndrome

More common among high-intensity swimmers, such as collegiate athletes, bleached swimmer syndrome is caused by prolonged exposure to chemically treated pools. Common symptoms include blonding or loss of hair, erythematous macular rashes, and dry skin and eczematous plaques [4]. While chlorine is the most frequent cause of this dermatitis, bromine exposure is associated with more severe reactions; bromine pools are less common resulting in fewer but more consistent cases [4]. In rare instances, potassium peroxymonosulfate, a sanitation chemical used in hot tubs may result in similar bleaching symptoms with frequent exposure [29]. While bleaching of hair remains benign, it is important to monitor pool chemical levels in the case of more severe symptoms like eczema and rash. It is also suggested that athletes rinse their bodies immediately after swimming to reduce prolonged contact outside of necessary practice time.

2.3.3 Swimmer's Shoulder

Generally only seen in men, swimmer's shoulder is a mild contact dermatitis caused by repetitive friction of an unshaven beard against the skin [33]. A red erythematous plaque may be seen on the shoulder, particularly following lots of freestyle and is generally prevented with more regular facial shaving [33]. While mild on its own, recognition of the condition is important when determining the etiology of a shoulder rash, in order to rule out more serious dermatoses.

2.4 Miscellaneous Dermatoses Associated with Pool-Based Sports

2.4.1 *Purpura Gogglorum*

First described in 1997, purpura gogglorum is a pressure-induced dermatitis characterized by erythematous, purpuric rash around and over the eyelids [34]. While the redness and irritation of the rash is relatively harmless, appearance of the rash may indicate the potential for the development of ocular injuries like blindness and corneal erosion due to intense pressure applied over the eye [34]. This injury is entirely preventable and is generally attributed to poorly made or old goggles. An improper, leaky seal results in attempts to over-tighten goggles resulting in high levels of suction pressure applied directly over the eye [34]. Athletes and parents of young swimmers should retire goggles with a malfunctioning seal and be cautious of over-tightening. Miscellaneous dermatoses associated with pool-based sports are summarized in Table 2.3.

Table 2.3 Miscellaneous dermatoses associated with pool-based sports

Disease/Condition	Symptoms and Physical Exam Findings	Treatment Recommendations
Purpura Gogglorum	Erythematous, purpuric rash around and over the eyelids	Avoid use of malfunctioned goggles and overtightening
Platform "Diving" Purpura	Purpuric rash and erythema on regions affected by impact	OTC pain relivers
Chlorotrichosis	Slightly green discoloration of lighter hair tones	Optional penicillamine shampoo
Pool Palms	Benign, erythematous lesions with a smooth, shiny appearance on hands and toes	Spontaneous resolution with avoidance of irritant
Aquagenic Pruritis	Pruritic tingling/burning sensation without visible skin changes	Narrow-band UVB phototherapy, interferon-alpha, or SSRIs
Aquagenic Urticaria	Pruritic wheals	Second generation antihistamines
Cold Urticaria	Pruritic, erythematous, edematous papules	Second generation antihistamines
Swimmer's Xerosis	Dryness, scaling, and itching of the skin	Moisturizing before and after entering water and topical corticosteroids to alleviate symptoms

2.4.2 Platform "Diving" Purpura

Platform divers are at risk of platform purpura when unsuccessfully performing dives due to impact trauma. Platform purpura is characterized by a purpuric rash and erythema that develop on regions affected by impact trauma, often associated with local pain or numbness [35]. Unfortunately, as an entirely accidental injury, little can be done for athletes to prevent it. Treatment can include NSAIDs or similar over-the-counter pain relievers, but only time will heal the rash.

2.4.3 Chlorotrichosis (Green Hair)

Green hair, or chlorotrichosis, is another unique, but relatively benign dermatitis caused by pool water that results in slightly green discoloration of lighter hair tones (especially bleached blondes) [36]. Well documented, research beginning in 1977 with a case study by Lampe et al., indicates that most frequently green discoloration of hair is caused by a deposition of copper on the hair cuticle [37]. Historically, this is the result of copper-based green algicides or deteriorating copper pipes [37]. These days, green hair is more common in older, private pools which still have copper plumbing and for those with highly damaged hair cuticles [38]. Interestingly, one case study has revealed that even with normal copper concentrations of pool water and no significant copper deposition on the cuticle, one girl developed chlorotrichosis, thereafter referred to as pseudo green hair due to its unknown etiology [36]. As a benign condition, treatment is optional, but is best performed with penicillamine shampoo and clear water, which will remove copper deposits within a few days [39]. Otherwise, development can be presented by monitoring copper levels of pool water and limiting damage to the cuticle by reducing heat or chemical treatments. Green hair will eventually grow out and can be removed with a standard haircut if the athlete decides not to treat it.

2.4.4 Pool Palms

Numerous case reports have been made documenting the onset of benign, asymptomatic erythematous lesions with a smooth, shiny appearance on the fingers, palms, and toes after repeated contact with rough pool surfaces [4, 40]. Pool palms are more often seen in childhood resulting from a greater degree of skin fragility and the propensity for children to more regularly play in pools [40]. Spontaneous resolution can be achieved by avoidance of the irritating activity [4, 41].

2.4.5 Aquagenic Pruritis

A prickling, stinging, pruritic, tingling, or burning sensation, aquagenic pruritus presents without any visible skin changes on sites of contact with water, lasting between ten minutes to two hours [4, 42]. It can be either idiopathic or associated with Hodgkin's disease, myelodysplastic syndrome, essential thrombocytopenia, polycythemia vera, sarcoidosis, hypereosinophilic syndrome, iron deficiency, and juvenile xanthogranuloma [42]. Antihistamines show mixed-to-no efficacy in relieving symptoms; PUVA and narrow-band UVB phototherapy may relieve pruritus [4, 42]. Other effective forms of treatment include interferon-alpha, as it was shown to be effective in 81% of patients, and selective serotonin reuptake inhibitors, which were efficacious in 8 of 10 patients [42].

2.4.6 Aquagenic and Cold Urticaria

A rare form of urticaria, aquagenic urticaria manifests as pruritic wheals upon contact with water from any source regardless of the temperature [4, 43]. Some cases have shown aquagenic urticaria to be salt dependent with patients developing skin lesions only with exposure to tap water or sweat, but remaining asymptomatic in ocean water [42]. Cold urticaria presents with pruritic, erythematous, edematous papules along skin surfaces exposed to the cold [4]. These are mainly differentiated by placing an ice cube on the forearm and noting the development of a square urticarial plaque upon rewarming of the skin [4, 43]. First-line treatment for both forms of urticaria are second generation antihistamines [4, 43]. PUVA and UVB may prove effective as alternative treatments for aquagenic urticaria [4].

2.4.7 Swimmer's Xerosis

Pools lead to the dilution of the skin's sebum and draw out moisture out of the skin through osmosis [4, 44]. Therefore, those engaging in aquatic sports are prone to developing swimmer's xerosis, characterized dryness, scaling, and itching of the skin [4, 44]. Prolonged hot showers shortly after swimming can further exacerbate the dryness [4]. Moisturizing prior to and after entering the water is critical to treat and prevent swimmer's xerosis by minimizing water loss from the skin [45]. Topical corticosteroids may be used to alleviate eczematous changes and symptoms [4].

2.5 Open Water Marine Bacteria Infections

Marine bacterial infections may occur via direct inoculation injury or can be secondary to numerous other marine injuries. Implicated species include the more common skin pathogens of *Staphylococcus* or *Streptococcus*, among others. Vibrio (e.g. *V. vulnificus)* is a halophilic marine bacterial genus (Gram-negative halophilic) of bacteria that is a causal organism for cellulitis and necrotizing fasciitis that can be treated with tetracyclines or quinolones antibiotics (with wound debridement in necrotizing fasciitis) [46, 47]. The pathogenicity of *Vibrio* is linked to endotoxins that can cause cutaneous findings of bullae and ecchymoses [46]. *Aeromonas hydrophila* (Gram-negative fresh & saltwater marine pathogen) can cause wound infections that are treated with a combination of trimethoprim–sulfamethoxazole and fluroquinolones with incision and drainage *Myobacterium marinum* (acid-fast bacillus marine bacteria) wound infections (ulcerating lesions) are generally treated with clarithromycin [46]. Various other conditions including swimming pool granuloma, swimmer's ear, and bikini bottom, discussed above, can be encountered in both fresh and saltwater environments and should be considered.

2.6 Vertebrate-Induced Injuries

Aquatic vertebrates may cause cutaneous manifestations secondary to trauma or envenomation. There are nearly 250 fish and shark species that possess toxins capable of injury to humans [48]. Toxic mechanisms are also central to injury via chondrichthyans, known as the cartilaginous marine group. Stingrays, for example, use their tail spines to break the skin to deliver venom. The class Osteichthyes, also known as bony fishes, are capable of envenomation, bites, or puncture wounds. Fresh water catfish, a type of Osteichthye, are the culprits of common puncture wounds in the Southern United States regions [48]. Weaverfish, *Echiicthys vipera, E aranus, E radiatus,* and *E lineatus*, live often invisibly to swimmers yet are the most venomous fish in European and North American water (Fig. 2.2).

Finally, the Spopaenidae family, containing scorpionfish, lionfish, and stonefish, also possess dangerous venomous potential. In all cases of toxic injury, pain, pallor, erythema, edema, and even necrosis can occur. In more serious cases, seizures,

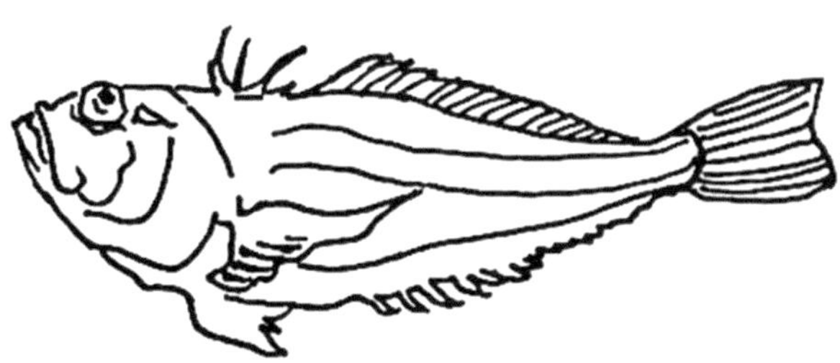

Fig. 2.2 Weaverfish

cardiac arrhythmias, and shock may occur. Wound debridement and removal of any remnants may be necessary following traumatic envenomation. Prophylactic antibiotics and antivenom may also be indicated. Aside from envenomation from vertebrates, bites, and lacerations also pose a danger to swimmers. The most common shark species known for attack are the white shark (*Carcharodhon carcharias*), the tiger shark (*Galeocerdo cuvier*), and the bull shark (*Carcharhinus leucas*) [49]. More recently, cookiecutter sharks have been identified in the Hawaiian channels [50]. Treatment for bites may include debridement and removal of any structures including spines and glandular tissue.

2.7 Invertebrate-Induced Dermatoses

Aquatic athletes taking part in sports in both fresh and especially saltwater environments are at risk of numerous invertebrate-induced dermatoses. While most commonly attributed to various forms of envenomation, this can also include the notable "swimmer's itch" rash caused by animals of the Platyhelminthes phylum [51]. Invertebrates–an artificial classification–define all animal species characterized by no central backbone. Marine life is notable for its wide array of invertebrates, many of which are responsible for both common and potentially life-threatening dermatoses in aquatic athletes. In this section, we will explore the six major phyla associated with aquatic invertebrate dermatoses: Cnidarians, Porifera, Echinoderms, Mollusca, Annelida, and Platyhelminths. We will also delve deeper into their most notable hazardous species and associated symptoms.

2.7.1 Cnidarians

As one of the most diverse phyla of aquatic invertebrates, the Cnidarians are characterized by perhaps the most notorious of stinging aquatic animals, the jellyfish, among others. Jellyfish are part of three distinct classes within this phylum: Scyphozoa, Hydrozoa, and Cubozoa [52]. The other three classes comprising the Cnidarians include Anthozoa (soft corals and sea anemones), Myxozoa (obligate parasites of fish), and Staurozoa (stalked jellyfish). Of these, only Anthozoa are recognized as a notable threat to aquatic athletes; Myxozoa is generally only harmful to humans when ingested via infected fish and Staurozoa stings appear to be poorly documented despite their theoretical capability [51, 53, 54].

The general anatomy of most Cnidarians consists of an active polyp stage possessing a central gastrovascular cavity with a mouth surrounded by stinging tentacles [55]. This gross anatomy is common to all of the colloquial jellyfish and the stalk jellyfish. For Hydrozoa and Anthozoa, functional units are composed of colonies while Scyphozoa, Cubozoa, and Staurozoa with each operating as individual organisms [55]. For all of these classes, the potential for envenomation is derived from nematocysts, which are small capsular organelles along the Cnidarian tentacles containing barbed, venomous threads. Upon stimulation, these nematocysts are mechanically discharged at very high speed [51]. In humans, barbed or thread-like microtubules from the ejected nematocyst embed themselves into fine dermal capillaries, by which injected venom can lead to local or systemic damage [51, 56]. While the nature of Cnidarian stings are diverse due to a wide range of species producing venoms with vastly different biochemical mechanisms, the general approach to initial treatment and diagnosis, especially in the absence of a confirmed culprit remains consistent [57]. Following a review of each class, their associated symptoms, and the most notable species responsible for human attack, we will go over relevant treatment, diagnosis and first aid strategies.

2.7.2 *Scyphozoa*

The Scyphozoa, or "true jellyfish", is responsible for the vast majority of Cnidarian envenomations worldwide, however most stings remain mild, with life-threatening complications being rare [57]. In general, Scyphozoa injury begins with an immediate linear vesicular urticarial reaction at the site of contact between the athlete's skin and the tentacle [51, 57]. These rashes are characterized by a rapid-onset burning sensation, generally accompanied by itching and erythema [51, 57]. For all stings, severity of the initial rash varies according to the species of jellyfish and the amount of time in contact with the tentacles and is generally a poor indicator of what species caused the injury. In more severe circumstances, stings can manifest with delayed systemic reactions including ocular injury, headache, abdominal pain and nausea [51]. For most stings, resolution of pain, itch and erythema generally occur within hours to days; however, evidence of the rash may remain far longer due to hyperpigmentation and scarring [57].

The species of Scyphozoa most frequently associated with stings in humans vary based on geographic location, but are often attributed to *Nemopilema nomurai, Rhopilema nomadica, Pelagia noctiluca, Rhizostoma pulmo, Aurelia aurita, Cyanea capillata, and Chrysaora quinquecirrha. N. nomurai* is an especially massive, edible species endemic to the East Asian marginal seas causing stings that range from moderately painful to potentially fatal, although evidence for the latter is poorly established in a clinical setting (Fig. 2.3) [52, 58]. *R. nomadica* is notable for its drastic population increases in the Mediterranean sea over the past four decades, and while generally mild is associated with less common delayed reactions prone to hyperpigmentation [52, 59]. Arguably the most dangerous Scyphozoa to humans, the mauve stinger (*P. noctiluca*), is responsible for some of the most severe "true jellyfish" stings across the Mediterranean and Northern Atlantic [52]. The mauve stinger is unusual due to being covered in nematocysts across its bell as well as the tentacles and is characterized by more intense pain and itching which can result in edema, papules, and scabs [60].

Fig. 2.3 True jellyfish envenomation

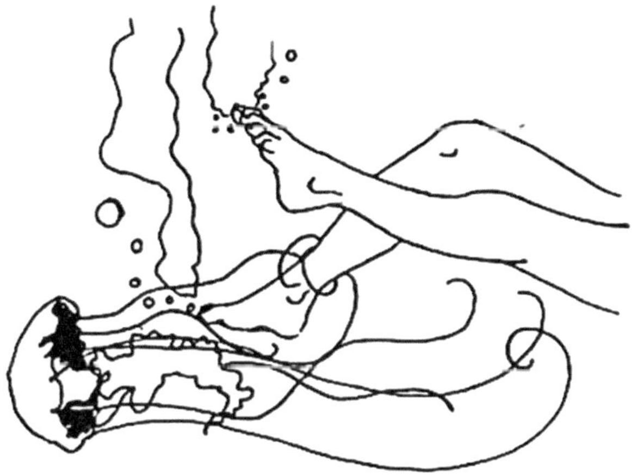

R. pulmo, colloquially the barrel jellyfish, which is common to the Mediterranean and Adriatic Seas has rather less recorded on the nature of its stings, but is believed to have the potential for recurrent cutaneous eruptions [52]. Another of the more harmful jellyfish, *A. auretia*, the moon jelly, has stings that tend to persist for days as vesicular rashes with the potential for necrosis [61]. The species has wide range, in vast regions of the Atlantic and Pacific oceans, and they may be increasing in size [52, 61]. The large *C. capillata*, commonly referred to as the lion's mane jellyfish, is the largest known species of jellyfish, typically only affecting open-ocean divers. Cutaneous manifestations of the lion's mane's sting are generally wheals, pain and swelling as with other species, but may rarely present with systemic symptoms reminiscent of decompression sickness such as extremity numbness and tingling [62]. Physicians by coastal waters should be aware of the potential for lion's mane-related injury in divers and evaluate the potential for both decompression sickness and stings when presented with neurological symptoms. The last of these common offenders, *C. quinquecirrha* (the sea nettle), are somewhat unique in that their endemic range remains very small–limited to the Chesapeake Bay and the surrounding Atlantic Coast [63].

2.7.3 Seabather's Eruption

Seabather's eruption is an ocean dermatosis characterized by a pruritic, urticarial, and papular rash that plagues swimmers [51]. In the last few decades, the cause of seabather's eruption has been elucidated as being uniquely from the larval stage of the Scyphozoa *Linuche unguiculata* and *Linuche aquila*, which can cause the rash with prolonged contact with skin [64]. This is unique from all other Scyphozoa, which tend to be venomous as polyps. A landmark symptom of seabather's eruption is a rash isolated to the bathing suit area due to trapped larva, with symptoms elsewhere on the body tending to be less severe or altogether absent [51]. Rashes are common to the Atlantic coast of the Americas, particularly in the warmer waters of Florida and the Caribbean [64]. Less frequently, the rash is associated with the larval stage of the sea anemone *Edwardsiella lineata* in the Northern Atlantic [51].

2.7.4 Hydrozoa

Hydrozoa stings are attributed to a few major organisms including the monotypic *Physalia physalis* (Portuguese man o' war), stinging hydroids, fire corals, and *Limnomedusae* [51]. These organisms are a very diverse class, with highly varying morphology and clinical manifestations. The Portuguese man o' war, a name referencing eighteenth century tall ships due to its appearance, is a species with broad geographic range, and is most commonly seen in warmer waters of the Mediterranean and Atlantic (Fig. 2.4)[52]. Unlike other 'jellies', the man o' war is not an individual organism, but rather a colony of zooids composing one symbiotic unit. This colony can be readily recognized by its floating gaseous bladder, which enables the man o' war to move based on directional winds; the species is often recognized after being washed ashore. *Physalia* stings are characterized by significant localized pain and a linear and beaded papulovesicular rash with significant swelling [51]. Prolonged or large stings are recognized for their musculoskeletal potential, and in rare cases, stings can be lethal [65]. Long-term effects of stings include scarring, hyperpigmentation, and keloids in those prone to them [52]. *Limnomedusae*, known as clinging jellyfish, are small, coldwater dwellers with stings similar in clinical presentation to the man o' war [51]. Divers and snorkelers are most at risk reporting with fairly severe pain and redness that can be potentially lethal, fortunately though, stings remain uncommon due to limited range [66].

Fig. 2.4 Portuguese Man O' War

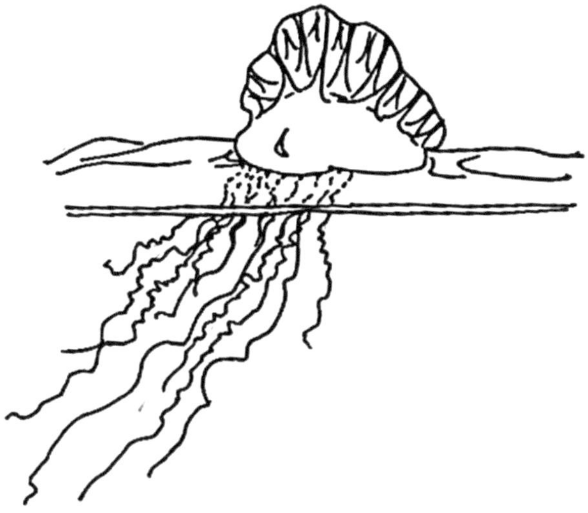

Unlike *Physalia* and *Limnomedusae*, the stinging hydroids and fire coral are sessile, decreasing the risk of sting for shallow water athletes. Fire coral stings, of the genus *Millepora* have less severe short term stings than their motile hydrozoan counterparts, although pain, redness, and swelling remains common [51]. However, the fire coral has been implicated in risk of type I hypersensitivity reactions and neuropathy, putting aquatic athletes at risk of more severe allergic reactions and prolonged sensitivity of the nervous system [67]. The stinging hydroids, or fireweed, of genus *Lytocarpus* present more severely and can result in zosteriform rashes and more significant pain [51].

2.7.5 Cubozoa

The class Cubozoa, colloquially box jellyfish, houses some of the most venomous species on the planet. Much like Syphozoa, Cubozoa are individual organisms composed of a bell (body) and multiple stinging tentacles, however unlike Scyphozoa, stings are nearly always severe and for many can be rapidly fatal if left untreated [51]. Common culprits include *Chironex fleckeri*, *Chironex yamaguchii*, *Alatina alata*, and *Carybdea rastonii* [52]. Easily the most notable of this class, *C. fleckeri* has been labeled the most venomous species on the planet to humans with at least 77 recorded fatalities occurring between 1920 and 2020 [51, 68]. While the range is limited to coastal waters of northern Australia and Southeast Asia, *C. fleckeri* is common in shallow waters posing a threat to most ocean athletes [52, 68]. Contact with tentacles inities an immediate and extremely painful dermatopathic rash with significant erythema in a linear, whip-like pattern that rapidly forms plaques [51, 52]. However, despite the severe pain, danger from *C. fleckeri* stems from is likelihood to induce severe systemic reactions such as pulmonary edema, vasospasms, cardiac arrhythmias and arrest, and hypotensive episodes [51, 68]. Venom toxicity is attributed to its highly necrotic effects via cell membrane pore formation and ion channel manipulation; immediate dermatological treatment following the sting can help reduce systemic symptoms, highlighting the need to uniform first aid protocols [68].

Both *C. yamaguchii*, endemic to Japanese coastal waters, and *A. alata*, endemic to Hawaiian waters, are significantly less dangerous than *C. fleckeri* [69]. Although both may generate severely painful stings and a similar linear, whip-like erythematous rash, systemic symptoms tend to be milder and thus fatalities more rare [52, 69]. *Carybdea spp.* are somewhat unique in that many species tend to present initially with relatively mild dermatopathology, characterized by mild pain, tingling, and erythema, however, severe delayed systemic symptoms may appear later [51]. This delayed response, called Irukandji Syndrome, will be covered in more detail below.

2.7.6 Anthozoa

Anthozoa include the true corals and sea anemones. Of these, sea anemones are responsible for envenomations via a similar mechanism to the previously discussed Cnidaria, while the true corals, although potentially venomous, tend to be more dangerous due to the risk of fine lacerations [51]. Both genera are sessile organisms in their mature state, much like the fire corals and stinging hydroids. Sea anemones are a soft tissue, solitary organism characterized by long floral-like tentacles while the corals tend to grow in colonial branch-like arrangements and produce a hard calcium carbonate-derived exoskeleton [51]. Notable sea anemones associated with stings include *Condylactis gigantea*, *Actinodendron plumosum*, *Phyllodiscus semoni*, and *Lebrunia danae*, with symptoms varying significantly between species [51, 70]. *C. gigantea*, one of the largest species of sea anemone, native to the tropical Atlantic, tends to generate relatively mild stings as compared with the extremely painful, vesicular rash caused by *A. plumosum* [51]. *L. danae* can induce more systemic reactions like abdominal pain and nausea [51]. However, perhaps the most interesting of these culprits, *P. semoni* in addition to is fulminant dermatopathic rash, which tends to cause pain, erythema, and notable dryness, is also nephrotoxic [70]. Victims experiencing nephrotoxicity typically present with acute renal failure similar to hemolytic uremia in the absence of other organ system toxicity [70, 71]. Cutaneous coral injuries can be caused by both envenomation and laceration, with envenomations presenting much like those of mild jellyfish stings. The rash might take on a more unique swirling pattern representative of the growth pattern of the coral species [72]. Lacerations on the other hand can be much more serious due to the risk of microbial inoculation at numerous contact points; skin ulceration and necrosis risk increase significantly if the wounds are left untreated [73, 74]. Ocean athletes of all kinds, but surfers in particular, are at risk of coral lacerations and stings when swept under by crashing waves.

2.7.7 Complications from Cnidarian Envenomation

In rare cases, Cnidarian stings may induce long-term, delayed, or recurrent reactions leading to widespread and chronic damage [75–77]. These more persistent symptoms are generally attributed to allergic dermatoses and are characterized histologically by high immunoglobulin levels and eosinophil infiltrates at sites of cutaneous damage and inflammation, which may manifest distally from the initial sting [75–77]. Other cases of systemic damage induced by severe envenomations are characterized by Irukandji Syndrome, which is usually attributed to numerous Cubozoans, but has constantly developing list of potential culprits. Irukandji Syndrome is notable for is apparent delayed, but potentially life threatening symptoms, with generally mild initial stings at the site of cnidarian contact, but eventual progression to potentially life-threatening systemic disorders [78]. Notable symptoms include hypertension, severe pain, nausea, and pulmonary edema. The disorder is still poorly understood, but may be induced by a sepsis-like "cytokine storm" or "catecholamine surge" [69]. Case studies of the most severe persistent syndromes reveal the need for species diagnosis and immediate treatment and monitoring by medical professionals even with seemingly minor initial reactions.

2.7.8 *Treatment & First Aid for Cnidarian Envenomation*

The treatment and first aid of cnidarian stings, while variable based on sting severity, should all follow the same general course. Immediate removal of remaining tentacles followed by washing of the wound site with vinegar is critical for the care of nearly every sting as acetic acid has been proven as an effective inactivator of nematocyst tubule discharge in box jellyfish and *Physalia* [52]. Baking soda slurries have been suggested as a superior alternative for many species of true jellyfish [79]. In the absence of vinegar or baking soda, sea water can be used as an emergency substitute for sting flushing, although evidence for its efficacy is unclear and thus should remain a last resort; freshwater is an inappropriate flushing agent [52]. Further first aid treatment includes the use of hot or cold compresses and local anesthetics like lidocaine for immediate pain management [52]. Beach lifeguards and patrols or aquatic athletes training in remote locations should keep vinegar, baking soda and emergency ice packs handy in the case of unexpected stings. It is important to note that acetic acid, while effective in preventing the progression of stings, is not capable of inactivating already released venom [78]. Thus, it is critical to monitor all victims of cnidarian envenomation for potentially life threatening system symptoms. Further treatment for severe stings, such as those by *C. fleckeri*, should always involve application of antivenom when available, wound site compression, and electrocardiographic monitoring by emergency personnel [80]. Proactive precautions can help reduce the risk of life-threatening side effects. Long-term care of wounds may include oral and topical antihistamines and topical corticosteroids, but only in the case of delayed hypersensitivity reactions; topical corticosteroids in particular have little efficacy in the short-term and have been shown to potentially delay healing and increase wound site infections [79, 81]. In general, athletes, clinicians and first responders should be aware of species endemic to their area, typical symptoms and the best course of immediate wound treatment to reduce the risk of lethal injury.

2.7.9 *Porifera*

Porifera, or the sea sponges, are less dangerous than many of their cnidarian counterparts, but are still a potential hazard for aquatic athletes. While usually understood to be a saltwater threat, cases of freshwater sponge dermatoses have arisen in recent years–attributed to *Drulia uruguayensis* and *D. ctenosclera* [51]. Initial clinical manifestations of sponge dermatoses can appear similar to those of corals due to the hard calcium carbonate or silicon dioxide exoskeletons which can produce many fine lacerations on contact [51]. Initial pruritic dermatitis is responsive for short term reactions and results in severe itching and burning accompanied by local edema, vesicular rashes and erythema [82]. However unlike most corals, irritant dermatitis results in prolonged symptoms due to spicule trauma or crinotoxin envenomation; these include desquamation, recurrent eczema and arthralgia of local joints [82]. Sponge spicules are microscopic needle-like protrusions that can penetrate the skin and remain for months to cause prolonged itching and irritation [51]. Effective removal of spinules can be achieved with adhesive tape, while crinotoxins respond to acetic acid (immediate deactivation) and topical corticosteroids (delayed hypersensitivity) via similar mechanisms as nematocyst toxins [51].

2.7.10 Echinoderms

Echinoderms are another highly diverse phylum, which includes the Echinoidea (sea urchins), Asteroidea (sea stars), and Holothuroidea (sea cucumbers). Each of these classes contain species with the potential to be hazardous to humans, with roughly 80 species capable of human envenomation [51, 83]. Mechanisms of injury range from penetrating venoms and sharp spines as often seen from sea urchins to environmentally released toxins from the sea cucumbers [51]. As bottom dwellers, Echinoderms pose the greatest threat to divers and snorkelers, but can less frequently impact other ocean athletes as well.

2.7.11 Echinoidea

The sea urchins possess numerous spines, which are typically long and brittle. When contact is made, these spines have a tendency to puncture the skin and break, leading to deep cutaneous embedding that has been observed to reach joints [84]. The penetration of these spines can cause notable injury of its own leading to intense itch, pain, edema and the potential for significant bleeding, however envenomation by some species can exacerbate these symptoms [51, 84]. If improperly treated, wound sites are at risk of secondary bacterial infections often caused by *Mycobacterium marinum*–a relative of *M. tuberculosis*–which can cause prolonged lesions and ulcers [84]. In rare cases, severe envenomation can result in systemic effects like hypotension, paralysis and respiratory distress, particularly when in contact with the neurotoxic Toxopneustes pileolus [51, 84]. Fortunately, long-term complications are primarily associated with residual spine tissue that was improperly removed from the wound site, highlighting the value of effective, immediate treatment. Proper first aid involves the careful removal of residual spine fragments with tissue forceps, or in the case of deeper penetration, surgical debridement of the wound [51, 84]. Delayed reactions associated with retained spines typically include synovitis or tenosynovitis, neuropathy, arthropathy, and even osteomyelitis [84]. Additional care should be taken to perform hot water soaks, even when toxicity is unknown, due to its efficacy in deactivating the heat-labile venoms of sea urchins [51, 84]. Additional long-term complications also include the formation of granulomas and granulomatous lesions, likely the result of the introduction of foreign matter at the site of tissue injury [84].

2.7.12 Asteroidea

Most sea star injuries are clinically insignificant, inducing few symptoms and requiring no medical intervention. The exception to this are injuries induced by *Acanthaster planci*, or the crown-of-thorns starfish, which is a large sea star covered in venomous spines endemic to waters of the Indo-Pacific [51]. Beyond the localized edema, itch, pain and erythema, which are similar to those of Echinoidea injuries, *A. planci* envenomation can induce neurotoxicity, nephrotoxicity, and hemolytic effects [85]. The primary toxins responsible for these effects effects include phospholipases, which degrades cellular membranes, and plancinin (an anticoagulant factor) [51]. Treatment protocols are relatively unchanged from those of sea urchins and must always involve effective removal of spines via tissue forceps or debridement, as well as hot water soaks to deactivate the heat-labile toxins [51, 85]. Presentation of nausea and vomiting indicate the need for oral antibiotics and when no puncture wounds have been made, topical corticosteroid treatment can be used to resolve symptoms of prolonged contact dermatitis [85].

2.7.13 Holothuroidea

Sea cucumbers have two primary mechanisms for inducing human dermatoses. Many species produce their own defensive holothurin toxins which are acutely damaging to epithelial tissue like skin and the mucous membranes of the eyes and mouth [86]. Symptoms include a painful, erythematous rash on the skin and significant irritation of the ocular conjunctiva that may result in permanent blindness [51, 86]. Unlike many of the other invertebrates covered, these animals utilize their venom by release into the surrounding environment; this means contact can occur over much wider areas and there is less likely to be a discernible central rash site [86]. To a lesser extent, they are also responsible for indirect Cnidarian stings due to their ability to ingest nematocysts and present them later as a secondary defense mechanism [51]. Appropriate treatment of irritant dermatitis includes a combination of hot water soaks and acetic acid flushing to deactivate the partially heat-stable holothurin toxins [86]. Unfortunately, the sensitive nature of the conjunctiva lends itself to a more cautious approach consisting only of water flushing and local anesthetics with prolonged monitoring for more severe complications [86].

2.7.14 Mollusca

Gastropoda (sea slugs and snails) and Cephalopoda (octopi, squid and cuttlefish) are major branches of the phylum Mollusca known to induce significant dermatoses in humans. To a lesser extent Pelecypods (bivalves) may result in lacerations or puncture wounds, but these generally require only typical wound first aid and confirmation of tetanus vaccination [87]. Within Gastropoda, sea snails are significantly more dangerous than their sea slug counterparts, but both have the potential to induce injury. Sea slugs, in a nearly identical mechanism to the aforementioned sea cucumbers, are capable of utilizing the toxins of ingested Cnidarian nematocysts, but are not known to be directly venomous on their own [88]. Appropriate treatment should occur in the same manner as if caused by a direct Cnidarian sting, and include vinegar flushing and monitoring for more dangerous systemic complications.

By contrast, sea snails, particularly the cone snails of the genus *Conus* are highly venomous animals that have caused known fatalities [89]. *Conus* snails initiate injury by the discharge of venomous harpoon-like teeth, called radula, that are typically used for feeding, but are also deployed for self defense; puncture by radula releases potent neurotoxic conotoxins [51]. Localized pain at the site of injury manifests first, followed by radiating inhibition of neuromuscular junctions via calcium channel blockade which induces flaccid paralysis and respiratory distress [51, 89]. The most dangerous of these are *C. geographus*, which is found in large swathes of the Indo-Pacific and is responsible for the vast majority of human fatalities [89]. Unfortunately, research on these species is limited meaning there is no known antivenom; treatment is supportive for pain and respiratory paralysis [51, 89].

Technically, all Cephalopoda are venomous, which use their venom to immobilize prey via bites with their chitinous beaks, but many are not clinically significant to humans [51]. For the vast majority of these bites, the only damage involves lacerations or puncture wounds of the skin, which require treatment for bleeding and potential secondary bacterial infection [87]. However, a few species of octopus of the genus *Haplochlaena* are significantly toxic to humans, possessing neuroinhibitory tetrodotoxin venoms significantly more dangerous than species in other genera; it is believed that these toxins are derived from a symbiotic relationship with bacteria in the *Haplchlaena* salivary glands [87, 51]. Interestingly, localized reactions to the bites are usually characterized by mild pain and free bleeding [87]. Supportive treatment is currently the only option and is focused on alleviating respiratory paralysis [87]. It is very important to recognize that the blue-ringed octopi are not naturally aggressive to humans and bites have only been recorded in cases of aggravation, making injuries entirely preventable [87]. Divers and snorkelers should be careful to leave octopi alone to mitigate the risks of potentially lethal envenomations.

2.7.15 *Annelida*

The phylum Annelida, segmented worms, includes many aquatic and terrestrial species including the common earthworms. The most clinically relevant classes in terms of aquatic dermatopathology are the Hirudinea (leeches), Polychaeta (bristleworms and fireworms) and Aphroditidae (sea mice) [51, 90]. Lethal reactions to all groups are limited and generally result from untreated secondary infections.The bristleworms and fireworms of Polychaeta and sea mice of Aphroditidae all possess fine, chitinous spines along their bodies that appear like fur; when threatened, these worms contract their bodies to cause their spines to stand on end [90]. There is little evidence of clinical toxicity, but localized reactions to the skin tend to include intense itching, pain, erythema, and edema [90]. Appropriate treatment involves careful removal of the chitinous spines and hot water or vinegar soaking, with one case study following sea mouse injury suggesting that ineffective treatment may rarely result in permanent granulomatous damage due to persistent irritation by foreign bodies [90].

2.7.16 *Hirudinea*

Hirudinea (leeches) are well known for their bloodsucking nature; in reality, most species feed by predation or scavenging, but those that are obligate warm-blooded parasites are both clinically significant and notorious [51]. Parasitic leeches have broad geographic ranges: freshwater, terrestrial and marine environments across every major ocean and continent. Feeding of these organisms is initiated when they bite human skin with chitinous jaws and then inject hirudin (an anticoagulant) into the wound site [51]. Leeches may then be removed by sliding a fingernail or thin card beneath their terminal sucker or flushing with vinegar [51]. Unfortunately vinegar rinses increase the risk of regurgitation which can lead to bacterial infections of the open wound, particularly infections with the bacteria *Aeromonas* [51]. Interestingly, leeches are frequently therapeutic in addition to pathologic, having been used for centuries to treat a wide range of conditions. *Hirudo medicinalis*, the primary species used for treatment, can help remove stagnant blood following surgery or even mitigate infectious abscesses [91]. Appropriate removal of a biting leech is critical though, as prolonged contact or residual jaw chitin is implicated in basal cell malignancy due to chronic nickel dermatitis [92].

2.7.17 Platyhelminthes (Swimmer's Itch)

The last of our major dermatopathic aquatic invertebrates, Platyhelminthes (flatworms) are obligately parasitic worms responsible for a wide range of diseases. However, only a small collection of species of the genus *Schistosoma* are notable for aquatic dermatoses. *Schistosoma* are the primary cause of the cercarial dermatitis nicknamed swimmer's itch. It is characterized by a maculopapular rash typically distinct from seabather's eruption as a result of its indiscriminate manifestations (seabather's eruption is usually worst in covered areas) [51]. Symptoms usually begin with stinging and are later followed by an intensely pruritic, vesicular rash that lasts between 1 and 2 weeks [51, 93]. Any marine athlete is at risk of swimmer's itch, with prevention effectively impossible. Treatment is generally supportive and typically involves pain and itch relief through topical creams or ointments [93].

Invertebrates can pose a significant risk to all aquatic athletes, with sessile bottom dweller being more dangerous to divers and snorkelers. Beach safety and patrols and coastal clinicians should be readily familiar with species endemic to their region and maintain appropriate first aid kits or medication respectively. Athletes can take precautions to avoid unnecessary injury by observing local risk announcements for relevant species (Cnidarians in particular). Appropriate bathing attire like wetsuits, large goggles, and water shoes and gloves are exceptional first-line defenses that work by blocking initial contact to begin with and should be used whenever possible.

2.8 Open Water Environmental Injuries

In the setting of compression and decompression, divers may experience various cutaneous insults including decompression sickness, nitrogen rashes, and diver's hand. Decompression sickness occurs due to nucleation of nitrogen or inert gas bubbles in the vasculature during ascent of divers, flight after diving, violating decompression limits, through experiencing decreased pressure, or other physiological means during or post-dive. This serious condition may initially appear on the skin with pallor and mottling. Patients with these signs require prompt decompression chamber therapy [94]. Following extensive periods of saturation diving, divers may experience what is known as divers hand, characterized by extensive scaling of the palms and soles. No effective protection or treatment exists, although the condition typically resolves spontaneously [95]. Finally, nitrogen exposure may cause nitrogen rashes, presenting as tender, erythematous purpura of the elbows and flanks. Avoidance of diving until spontaneous resolution is recommended.

Frostbite and hypothermia are additional environmental injuries posing a threat to those exposed to extremes of temperature. Frostbite can occur in conditions at subfreezing temperatures (skin <-4 °C), and presents with the physical exam findings of anesthesia, paresis, grey-yellow discoloration, bullae, and potential eschar formation if not promptly treated [96]. Those in contact with saltwater conditions may be vulnerable to impaired wound healing. Studies conducted in rats immersed in salt water have revealed slower healing times and rates of wound epithelialization [97, 98].

2.9 Paddlesport-Specific Dermatoses

Paddlesports, including kayaking, rowing, and paddle boarding pose risks of injuries from falls on deck and from capsizing. Those involved in rowing fleet may be subject to rowing blisters. These are typically painful erythematous lesions around the ventral hands [99]. Sculler's knuckles, occurring when crossing the arms, are due to chronic knuckle friction. The dorsum of the hands, particularly at the proximal interphalangeal or metacarpophalangeal joints, may experience contact abrasions [99]. For all these conditions, protective hand gear and lubricating jellies should be worn. Spontaneous resolution often occurs.

Rowers may also experience what is known as rower's rump, or lesions on the buttocks that resemble lichen simplex chronicus. These often are secondary to improperly fitted rower seats and may cause uncomfortable pruritus. Acne mechanica is a similar condition of the buttocks following long periods of mechanical friction. Papules, pustules, and tender nodules may develop and management includes a combination of steroids, isotretinoin, and antibiotics. Immersion (trench) foot may occur following long trips as well, due to moisture exposure to the feet [100]. Finally, particular susceptibility to staphylococcal skin infections is seen in those participating in common United States water rafting locations [100].

2.10 Board Sport-specific Dermatoses

Board sports include surfing, windsurfing, kitesurfing, wakeboarding and more casually bodyboarding (alternatively boogie boarding). Paddle boarding is also in this category, posing potential risks from both the paddles and the board. For all board sports, but surfing in particular, dermatoses from the board itself are common due to repetitive friction or trauma [73, 101]. Board sport lacerations are a risk that should be treated as any other open wound and may be the result of cuts from sharp areas of the board or underwater contact with hard corals and sponges [73]. These cuts are particularly at risk of secondary bacterial infections making it important to monitor for signs of unusual swelling, oozing or pain to begin antibiotic therapy [73]. Surfer's nodules, which present as fibrotic nodules of increased collagen deposition, are typically seen on the bony prominences of surfers' bodies [101]. These injuries are the result of repetitive trauma typically to the bony regions of the leg and foot, although can manifest anywhere [101]. Manifestation of these lesions can result in their characterization as nodules, knots, cysts, or ulcers, with further subcategories assigned according to body location [101]. Treatment involves chemical exfoliants like salicylic or lactic acid and they can be prevented by using protective padding on sensitive areas [101]. Repetitive friction of skin in contact with the board may induce an irritant contact dermatitis called surf rider's dermatitis; this may be exacerbated by allergic hypersensitivities to the waxes and polymers present on these boards [101]. Treatment is supportive for pain and itch, but further development of irritation is best prevented by use of protective clothing such as wetsuits and rash guards. A few dermatoses unique to windsurfers may also be encountered. Windsurfers use a distinct black rubber handle nicknamed the "wishbone" that may cause erythematous and pruritic plaques on the hands believed to be the result of allergic contact dermatitis; prevention involves using aluminum handles instead of the black rubber that are more common [101].

References

1. Owens DW, Knox JM. Influence of heat, wind, and humidity on ultraviolet radiation injury. Natl Cancer Inst Monogr. 1978;50:161–7.
2. De Castro-Maqueda G, Gutierrez-Manzanedo JV, Lagares-Franco C, de Troya-Martin M. Sun exposure during water sports: do elite athletes adequately protect their skin against skin cancer? Int J Environ Res Public Health. 2021;18(2):800.
3. Freiman A, Barankin B, Elpern DJ. Sports dermatology part 1: common dermatoses. CMAJ. 2004;171(8):851–3.
4. Tlougan BE, Podjasek JO, Adams BB. Aquatic sports dermatoses: part 1. In the water: freshwater dermatoses. Int J Dermatol. 2010;49(8):874–85.
5. Lipska J, Hamerska J, Hamerska L, Bocianiak B, Antczak J, Kajka A, et al. Swimmer's ear: prevention, diagnosis, treatment, and management strategies for athletes. Quality Sport. 2024;18:53330.
6. Strauss MB, Dierker RL. Otitis externa associated with aquatic activities (swimmer's ear). Clin Dermatol. 1987;5(3):103–11.
7. Rosenfeld RM, Schwartz SR, Cannon CR, Roland PS, Simon GR, Kumar KA, et al. Clinical practice guideline: acute otitis externa. Otolaryngol Head Neck Surg. 2014;150(1 Suppl):S1–s24.
8. Sjövall A, Pätäri-Sampo A, Silvola J, Aarnisalo A, Laulajainen-Hongisto A. Acute otitis externa and auricular erysipelas; causative pathogens, antimicrobial susceptibility and treatment strategies of tertiary referral centre patients. Eur J Clin Microbiol Infect Dis. 2023;42(8):1025–9.
9. van Balen FA, Smit WM, Zuithoff NP, Verheij TJ. Clinical efficacy of three common treatments in acute otitis externa in primary care: randomised controlled trial. BMJ. 2003;327(7425):1201–5.
10. Wipperman J. Otitis externa. Prim Care. 2014;41(1):1–9.
11. Jacob JS, Tschen J. Hot tub-associated pseudomonas folliculitis: a case report and review of host risk factors. Cureus. 2020;12(9):e10623.
12. Yu Y, Cheng AS, Wang L, Dunne WM, Bayliss SJ. Hot tub folliculitis or hot hand-foot syndrome caused by Pseudomonas aeruginosa. J Am Acad Dermatol. 2007;57(4):596–600.
13. Schiavano GF, Carloni E, Andreoni F, Magi S, Chironna M, Brandi G, Amagliani G. Prevalence and antibiotic resistance of Pseudomonas aeruginosa in water samples in central Italy and molecular characterization of oprD in imipenem resistant isolates. PLoS One. 2017;12(12):e0189172.

14. Silvestre JF, Betlloch MI. Review Cutaneous manifestations due to infection. Int J Dermatol. 1999;38(6):419–31.
15. Segna KG, Koch LH, Williams JV. "Hot tub" folliculitis from a nonchlorinated children's pool. Pediatr Dermatol. 2011;28(5):590–1.
16. Freiman A, Barankin B, Elpern DJ. Sports dermatology part 2: swimming and other aquatic sports. CMAJ. 2004;171(11):1339–41.
17. Fiorillo L, Zucker M, Sawyer D, Lin AN. The pseudomonas hot-foot syndrome. N Engl J Med. 2001;345(5):335–8.
18. Meza-Romero R, Navarrete-Dechent C, Downey C. Molluscum contagiosum: an update and review of new perspectives in etiology, diagnosis, and treatment. Clin Cosmet Investig Dermatol. 2019;12:373–81.
19. Davies HD, Jackson MA, Rice SG. Infectious diseases associated with organized sports and outbreak control. Pediatrics. 2017;140(4):e20172477.
20. Field LA, Adams BB. Tinea pedis in athletes. Int J Dermatol. 2008;47(5):485–92.
21. Leung AK, Barankin B, Lam JM, Leong KF, Hon KL. Tinea pedis: an updated review. Drugs Context. 2023:12.
22. Al-Mutairi N, AlKhalaf M. Mucocutaneous warts in children: clinical presentations, risk factors, and response to treatment. Acta Dermatovenerol Alp Pannonica Adriat. 2012;21(4):69–72.
23. Herman BE, Corneli HM. A practical approach to warts in the emergency department. Pediatr Emerg Care. 2008;24(4):246–51; quiz 52–4.
24. Berman B, Weinstein A. Treatment of warts. Dermatol Ther. 2000;13(3):290–304.
25. Esterowitz D, Greer KE, Cooper PH, Edlich RF. Plantar warts in the athlete. Am J Emerg Med. 1995;13(4):441–3.
26. Metelitsa A, Barankin B, Lin AN. Diagnosis of sports-related dermatoses. Int J Dermatol. 2004;43(2):113–9.
27. Palaniappan V, Murthy AB, Karthikeyan K. Pitted keratolysis. Clin Exp Dermatol. 2023;48(9):978–83.
28. Lazarov A, Nevo K, Pardo A, Froom P. Self-reported skin disease in hydrotherapists working in swimming pools. Contact Derm. 2005;53(6):327–31.
29. Sridhar SC, Deo SC. Marine and other aquatic dermatoses. Indian J Dermatol. 2017;62(1):66–78.
30. Cohen PR. Pool Toes: case report and review of pool-associated pedal dermatoses. Cureus. 2020;12(11):e11756.
31. Loughney E, Harrison J. Irritant contact dermatitis due to 1-bromo-3-chloro-5,5-dimethylhydantoin in a hydrotherapy pool. Risk assessments: the need for continuous evidence-based assessments. Occup Med (Lond). 1998;48(7):461–3.
32. Khodaee M, Grothe HL, Seyfert JH, VanBaak K. Athletes at high altitude. Sports Health. 2016;8(2):126–32.
33. Kockentiet B, Adams BB. Contact dermatitis in athletes. J Am Acad Dermatol. 2007;56(6):1048–55.
34. Jowett NI, Jowett SG. Ocular purpura in a swimmer. Postgrad Med J. 1997;73(866):819–20.
35. Dokic Y, Engeln K, McCann SE. Purpura and erythema associated with cutaneous numbness and hyperesthesia. JAAD Case Rep. 2020;6(10):970–2.
36. Tomas X, Nogueras M, Bartolome A, Ferrando J. Pseudo green hair. Int J Trichology. 2022;14(2):65–7.
37. Lampe RM, Henderson AL, Hansen GH. Green hair. JAMA. 1977;237(19):2092.
38. Connor CJ, Vidal NY, Liu V. Persistent chlorotrichosis with chronic sun exposure. Cutis. 2020;105(2):E25–e7.
39. Person JR. Green hair: treatment with a penicillamine shampoo. Arch Dermatol. 1985;121(6):717–8.
40. Novoa A, Klear S. Pool palms. Arch Dis Child. 2016;101(1):41.

41. Morgado-Carrasco D, Feola H, Vargas-Mora P. Pool Palms. Dermatol Pract Concept. 2020;10(1):e2020009.
42. Hamie L, Abou-Rahal J. Water-related dermatoses. Int J Dermatol. 2019;58(5):515–29.
43. Rujitharanawong C, Kulthanan K, Tuchinda P, Chularojanamontri L, Metz M, Maurer M. A systematic review of aquagenic urticaria-subgroups and treatment options. J Allergy Clin Immunol Pract. 2022;10(8):2154–62.
44. De Luca JF, Adams BB, Yosipovitch G. Skin manifestations of athletes competing in the summer olympics: what a sports medicine physician should know. Sports Med. 2012;42(5):399–413.
45. Basler RSW, Basler GC, Palmer AH, Garcia MA. Special skin symptoms seen in swimmers. J Am Acad Dermatol. 2000;43(2):299–305.
46. Oliver JD. Wound infections caused by Vibrio vulnificus and other marine bacteria. Epidemiol Infect. 2005;133(3):383–91.
47. Wong KC, Brown AM, Luscombe GM, Wong SJ, Mendis K. Antibiotic use for Vibrio infections: important insights from surveillance data. BMC Infect Dis. 2015;15:226.
48. Haddad JV. Aquatic animals of medical importance in Brazil. Rev Soc Bras Med Trop. 2003;36(5):591–7.
49. Scala VA, Hayashi MS, Kaneshige J, Haut ER, Ng K, Furuta S. Shark-related injuries in Hawai'i treated at a level 1 trauma center. Trauma Surg Acute Care Open. 2020;5(1):e000567.
50. Scala VA, Ng K, Kaneshige J, Furuta S, Hayashi MS. Cookiecutter shark-related injuries: a new threat to swimming across the Ka'iwi channel. Hawaii J Health Soc Welf. 2021;80(11 Suppl 3):31–7.
51. Ottuso P. Aquatic dermatology: encounters with the denizens of the deep (and not so deep) a review. Part I: the invertebrates. Int J Dermatol. 2013;52(2):136–52.
52. Peng X, Liu KT, Chen JB, Yan ZH, Danso B, Wang MK, et al. Jellyfish stings: a review of skin symptoms, pathophysiology, and management. Med Sci Monit. 2024;30:e944265.
53. Molnár K, Eszterbauer E. Specificity of infection sites in vertebrate hosts. In: Myxozoan evolution, ecology and development. Springer; 2015. p. 295–313.
54. Miranda LS, Mills CE, Hirano YM, Collins AG, Marques AC. A review of the global diversity and natural history of stalked jellyfishes (Cnidaria, Staurozoa). Mar Biodivers. 2018;48(4):1695–714.
55. D'Ambra I, Lauritano C. A review of toxins from cnidaria. Mar Drugs. 2020;18(10):507.
56. Beckmann A, Özbek S. The nematocyst: a molecular map of the cnidarian stinging organelle. Int J Dev Biol. 2012;56(6–8):577–82.
57. Remigante A, Costa R, Morabito R, La Spada G, Marino A, Dossena S. Impact of scyphozoan venoms on human health and current first aid options for stings. Toxins (Basel). 2018;10(4):133.
58. Kawahara M, Uye S, Burnett J, Mianzan H. Stings of edible jellyfish (Rhopilema hispidum, Rhopilema esculentum and Nemopilema nomurai) in Japanese waters. Toxicon. 2006;48(6):713–6.
59. Silfen R, Vilan A, Wohl I, Leviav A. Mediterranean jellyfish (Rhopilema nomadica) sting. Burns. 2003;29(8):868–70.
60. Mariottini GL, Giacco E, Pane L. The mauve stinger Pelagia noctiluca (Forsskål, 1775). Distribution, ecology, toxicity and epidemiology of stings. A review. Mar Drugs. 2008;6(3):496–513.
61. Simmons BJ, Griffith RD, Falto-Aizpurua LA, Nouri K. Moon jellyfish stings. JAMA Dermatol. 2015;151(4):454–6.
62. Trevett A, Sheehan C, Wilkinson A, Moss I. Lion's mane jellyfish (Cyanea capillata) envenoming presenting as suspected decompression sickness. Diving Hyperb Med. 2019;49(1):57–60.
63. Burnett JW, Pierce LH Jr, Stone JH. Studies on sea nettle stings. Arch Dermatol. 1968;98(6):587–9.
64. Tomchik RS, Russell MT, Szmant AM, Black NA. Clinical perspectives on seabather's eruption, also known as 'sea lice'. JAMA. 1993;269(13):1669–72.

65. Alam JM, Qasim R. Toxicology of Physalia's (Portuguese man-o' war) venom. Pak J Pharm Sci. 1991;4(2):159–68.
66. Govindarajan AF, Källström B, Selander E, Östman C, Dahlgren TG. The highly toxic and cryptogenic clinging jellyfish Gonionemus sp. (Hydrozoa, Limnomedusae) on the Swedish west coast. PeerJ. 2019;7:e6883.
67. Moats WE. Fire coral envenomation. J Wilderness Med. 1992;3(3):284–7.
68. Piontek M, Seymour JE, Wong Y, Gilstrom T, Potriquet J, Jennings E, et al. The pathology of Chironex fleckeri venom and known biological mechanisms. Toxicon X. 2020;6:100026.
69. Reinicke J, Kitatani R, Masoud SS, Galbraith KK, Yoshida W, Igarashi A, et al. Isolation, structure determination, and synthesis of cyclic tetraglutamic acids from box jellyfish species Alatina alata and Chironex yamaguchii. Molecules. 2020;25(4):883.
70. Mizuno M, Nozaki M, Morine N, Suzuki N, Nishikawa K, Morgan BP, Matsuo S. A protein toxin from the sea anemone phyllodiscus semoni targets the kidney and causes a severe renal injury with predominant glomerular endothelial damage. Am J Pathol. 2007;171(2):402–14.
71. Kim AY, Cho KH, Kang SH, Park JW, Do JY, Kim MK. Hemolytic uremic syndrome caused by sea anemone sting: a case report. BMC Nephrol. 2021;22(1):14.
72. Lause M, McIntyre M 2nd, Trinidad J. Coral dermatitis. JAMA Dermatol. 2019;155(1):107.
73. Zoltan TB, Taylor KS, Achar SA. Health issues for surfers. Am Fam Physician. 2005;71(12):2313–7.
74. Byun JY, Choi YW, Choi HY, Myung KB. A case of dedifferentiated Liposarcoma that developed in the dermis. Ann Dermatol. 2008;20(4):204–8.
75. Burnett JW, Calton GJ. Jellyfish envenomation syndromes updated. Ann Emerg Med. 1987;16(9):1000–5.
76. Loredana Asztalos M, Rubin AI, Elenitsas R, Groft MacFarlane C, Castelo-Soccio L. Recurrent dermatitis and dermal hypersensitivity following a jellyfish sting: a case report and review of literature. Pediatr Dermatol. 2014;31(2):217–9.
77. Naumann D, Hejmadi RK, Evriviades D. Ocean enemy's lasting sting: chronic cutaneous reaction after Cnidarian attack. J R Nav Med Serv. 2013;99(3):169–70.
78. Carrette TJ, Underwood AH, Seymour JE. Irukandji syndrome: a widely misunderstood and poorly researched tropical marine envenoming. Diving Hyperb Med. 2012;42(4):214–23.
79. Burnett JW. Treatment of Atlantic cnidarian envenomations. Toxicon. 2009;54(8):1201–5.
80. Beadnell CE, Rider TA, Williamson JA, Fenner PJ. Management of a major box jellyfish (Chironex fleckeri) sting. Lessons from the first minutes and hours. Med J Aust. 1992;156(9):655–8.
81. Thaikruea L, Siriariyaporn P. Severe dermatonecrotic toxin and wound complications associated with box jellyfish stings 2008-2013. J Wound Ostomy Continence Nurs. 2015;42(6):599–604.
82. Cahn BA, Elston DM. Aquatic antagonists: sponge dermatitis. Cutis. 2021;107(1):34–6. e5
83. Bonamonte D, Verni P, Filoni A, Angelini G. Dermatitis caused by echinoderms; 2016. p. 89–104.
84. James M, Bakkour W, Checkley A, Calonje E, Walker SL. Long-term management options for sea urchin injury: a case series. Clin Exp Dermatol. 2022;47(12):2251–4.
85. Sato H, Tsuruta Y, Yamamoto Y, Asato Y, Taira K, Hagiwara K, et al. Case of skin injuries due to stings by crown-of-thorns starfish (Acanthaster planci). J Dermatol. 2008;35(3):162–7.
86. Ellis CR, Elston DM, Joustra JPL, Haddad V Jr. Aquatic antagonists: sea cucumbers (Holothuroidea). Cutis. 2021;108(2):68–70.
87. Whatley RE. Marine mollusks and the skin. Dermatol Ther. 2002;15(1):38–42.
88. Ottuso PT. Aquatic antagonists: indirect nematocyst envenomation and acute allergic contact dermatitis due to nudibranchs. Cutis. 2009;83(5):237–9.
89. Haddad V 2nd, de Paula Neto JB, Cobo VJ. Venomous mollusks: the risks of human accidents by conus snails (gastropoda: conidae) in Brazil. Rev Soc Bras Med Trop. 2006;39(5):498–500.
90. Smith ML. Cutaneous problems related to coastal and marine worms. Dermatol Ther. 2002;15(1):34–7.

91. Singh AP. Medicinal leech therapy (hirudotherapy): a brief overview. Complement Ther Clin Pract. 2010;16(4):213–5.
92. Shamsaddini S, Dabiri S. Basal cell carcinoma on nickel dermatitis after leech applying. East Mediterr Health J. 2000;6(1):197–9.
93. Hoeffler DF. "Swimmers' itch" (cercarial dermatitis). Cutis. 1977;19(4):461–5. 7
94. Davis JC. Hyperbaric oxygen therapy. J Intensive Care Med. 1989;4(2):55–7.
95. Ahlén C, Iversen OJ, Risberg J, Volden G, Aarset H. Diver's hand: a skin disorder common in occupational saturation diving. Occup Environ Med. 1998;55(2):141–3.
96. Knapik JJ, Reynolds KL, Castellani JW. Frostbite: pathophysiology, epidemiology, diagnosis, treatment, and prevention. J Spec Oper Med. 2020;20(4):123–35.
97. Fan ZF, Wang JH, Li ZQ, Yi CH. Influence of sea water immersion on inflammation and healing of the wounds in scalded rats. Zhonghua Shao Shang Za Zhi. 2006;22(3):215–7.
98. Yang YX, Wang JH, Liu L, Zou Q, Zhang Y, Bai Z. Effects of seawater immersion on the inflammatory response and oxygen free radical injury of rats with superficial partial-thickness scald at early stage. Zhonghua Shao Shang Za Zhi. 2017;33(6):361–7.
99. Rumball JS, Lebrun CM, Di Ciacca SR, Orlando K. Rowing INJURIES. Sports Med. 2005;35(6):537–55.
100. Spittler J, Gillum R, DeSanto K. Common Injuries in whitewater Rafting, Kayaking, Canoeing, and stand-up paddle boarding. Curr Sports Med Rep. 2020;19(10):422–9.
101. Tlougan BE, Podjasek JO, Adams BB. Aquatic sports dermatoses: part 3. On the water. Int J Dermatol. 2010;49(10):1111–20.

Chapter 3
Running Sports

Hannah Metheny, Isabel Rodriguez, Rachel Cohen, Ryan Scheinkman, and Keyvan Nouri

3.1 Introduction

Track and field, cross-country, and marathon/ultramarathon running are among the world's oldest sports. Track and field originated in ancient Greece, where the first recorded Olympic Games had been held in 776 BCE. The earliest events included foot races, with other athletic disciplines introduced later in the games. During the nineteenth century, the modern version of track and field began to take shape, culminating in its inclusion in the first modern Olympic Games in 1896. Today, track and field forms a central part of the Summer Olympic Games, encompassing sprint, endurance, and field events [1, 2]. Cross-country running evolved from organized running races in rural Britain during the early nineteenth century. The first documented cross-country competition—a 'hare and hounds' race—occurred in 1837 at Rugby School. By the late nineteenth century, cross country became formalized with the establishment of local and national championships. Cross country was included in the Olympic Games from 1912 to 1924, and it remains relevant at collegiate, national, and international levels [3].

Marathon running traces its roots to the Greek legend of Pheidippides, who is said to have run from Marathon to Athens in 490 BCE to deliver news of a Greek military victory. This myth inspired the introduction of the modern marathon in the 1896 Olympics, with a standard distance of 42.195 kilometers established at the 1908 London Olympics. Throughout the twentieth century, marathon running became increasingly popular, bolstered by events like the Boston Marathon and a recreational running boom in the 1970s [4]. Ultramarathon running—races exceeding the

H. Metheny · I. Rodriguez · R. Cohen · R. Scheinkman (✉) · K. Nouri
Dr. Phillip Frost Department of Dermatology and Cutaneous Surgery, University of Miami, Miami, FL, USA
e-mail: hannah.metheny@med.miami.edu; ixr294@miami.edu; rachelcohen@med.miami.edu; scheinkman@med.miami.edu; knouri@med.miami.edu

K. Nouri (ed.), *Sport-Related Skin Conditions*,
https://doi.org/10.1007/978-3-031-90444-8_3

traditional marathon distance—emerged more recently, with organized events gaining momentum in the mid-twentieth century. Ultramarathons now occur worldwide, often featuring extreme conditions such as mountainous terrain or deserts [5, 6].

The physiologic demands of running predispose athletes to distinct dermatological manifestations. Prolonged physical exertion, environmental exposure, and repetitive friction contribute to these conditions. Dermatological complaints represent a significant portion of medical consultations among athletes, comprising up to 10% of all medical visits in endurance sports like running [7]. Common manifestations include friction blisters, calluses, and talon noir in long-distance runners, while sprinters more frequently present with acne mechanica and equipment-related dermatoses [8].

The temporal progression of cutaneous conditions in runners varies between acute presentations during specific training periods or competitions and chronic manifestations developing over extended training intervals. For example, research demonstrates that long-distance runners frequently develop tinea pedis due to sustained moisture exposure and occlusive footwear [9]. Moreover, UV exposure during outdoor events significantly increases the risk of acute sunburn and chronic photodamage, particularly in ultramarathon participants [10].

Dermatological conditions significantly impact athletic performance, causing discomfort, disruption of training schedules, and potentially necessitating competition withdrawal. Friction injuries and fungal infections represent the predominant causes of dermatoses among all athletes [11]. Addressing dermatological conditions afflicting running athletes is paramount to maintaining athletic performance and health. This chapter examines dermatoses encountered among running athletes and explores evidence-based approaches for prevention, treatment, and optimization of skin health.

3.2 Special Considerations by Event

3.2.1 Sprinting Events

Sprinters demonstrate increased susceptibility to acute skin trauma due to the explosive movement-generated forces involved in their sport. During the acceleration phases, ground reaction forces often exceed 4–5 times the athlete's body weight, creating conditions that place significant stress on the skin, making it more prone to injuries such as abrasions and friction burns [12, 13]. Block starts, deceleration phases, and curve running generate mechanical shear forces, which commonly result in localized friction injuries [14]. These forces create ideal conditions for skin trauma, especially in vulnerable areas. Additionally, synthetic track surfaces, commonly used for sprint events, frequently cause friction burns, particularly when athletes fall [15]. The severity of these injuries can vary depending on factors such as track temperature, humidity, and surface composition [15, 16]. Hurdle events add another layer of risk, with athletes susceptible to trauma from direct contact with barriers [13].

Sprinters are also at risk for sweat-induced skin irritation, particularly in high friction areas like the groin and axillae. These areas may develop conditions such as miliaria or intertrigo due to the combination of sweat and friction [13, 14]. Friction and moisture significantly contribute to the development of such conditions in athletes [13]. Additionally, prolonged exposure to sweat and friction can exacerbate irritation, leading to more severe skin conditions like contact dermatitis, often caused by exposure to materials in starting blocks or the components of spike shoes [13, 16]. The friction and pressure from starting block contact, combined with the lateral motion generated during the run, can further aggravate skin irritation [13, 14].

The specialized footwear required for sprinting contributes to distinct skin manifestations. Spike shoes, designed to support forefoot loading and lateral pressure during curved running, can create characteristic callus patterns and focal trauma on the feet [14]. Repeated contact with starting blocks during practice sessions can worsen these skin irritations, creating the need for careful management [13, 14]. Friction-induced calluses and abrasions are commonly observed in athletes due to the combined impact of specialized footwear and repetitive contact with surfaces like starting blocks and track turf [14].

3.2.2 *Middle-Distance Track*

Middle-distance runners experience moderate environmental exposure when compared to sprinters or long-distance runners, but still face significant challenges. Events lasting between 4 and 15 minutes place a considerable thermoregulatory burden on the body, and the resulting heat stress can compromise skin barrier function, increasing susceptibility to irritation [17]. Training in cooler months, particularly during early spring or late autumn, subjects athletes to cold-weather conditions that can lead to frostnip or windburn, which may impair the skin's ability to recover effectively after exercise [18]. Despite the relatively shorter duration of middle-distance events, UV exposure remains significant, and runners are at an increased risk of sunburn and other sun-related skin conditions. Sun protection during outdoor competitions is essential for preventing long-term skin damage [19]. Post-competition blister formation is also a common occurrence in middle-distance running. Repetitive motion during races can cause friction between the skin and footwear, emphasizing the importance of preventive strategies such as the use of lubricants and properly fitted shoes [20].

3.2.3 Long-Distance Track, Cross-Country, Marathon/ Ultramarathon

Long-distance runners are predisposed to a variety of skin conditions due to prolonged training and racing paired with the repetitive movements of running. They are at an increased risk of chafing, particularly in high-friction areas such as the groin, inner thighs, axillae, and under-breast regions. Movement combined with sweat accumulation can exacerbate friction, leading to intertrigo or maceration in these areas. Prolonged exposure to moisture also predisposes runners to pitted keratolysis, a bacterial infection that thrives in humid environments, particularly on the soles of the feet [21, 22]. Similarly, tinea pedis, athlete's foot is common among runners, especially when damp footwear is worn for extended periods without adequate drying. Blisters are frequently observed, especially in areas of high pressure or friction such as the heels and toes. Ill-fitting or worn-out footwear can further increase the risk of blisters, as well as calluses, corns, and subungual hematomas ("runner's toe") [23]. Long-term repetitive trauma can lead to onychodystrophy and chronic paronychia, which may require medical intervention for resolution [24].

Sunburn is a significant concern during daytime training or races, especially when sunscreen is not applied or re-applied appropriately. Chronic ultraviolet (UV) exposure increases the risk of actinic keratosis and skin cancer, including melanoma [25]. Research indicates that endurance athletes may have an elevated risk of skin cancers due to cumulative UV exposure [26]. In cooler climates, runners may develop windburn, characterized by erythema and irritation on exposed areas such as the face and hands [27]. Additionally, rain or humid weather increases the risk of moisture-associated dermatoses, while cold weather predisposes runners to chilblains or frostbite, especially in poorly protected extremities [28].

The combination of sweat and prolonged skin contact with synthetic or tight-fitting clothing can lead to contact dermatitis, either irritant or allergic, depending on the material and exposure. For example, adhesives, dyes, or seams in technical running gear may cause localized irritation or an allergic response [29]. Compression wear and hydration packs, frequently used by long-distance runners, can also exacerbate friction and sweat retention, contributing to conditions such as miliaria (heat rash) or worsening of intertrigo [30].

3.2.4 Field Events, Steeple Chase

Field event athletes participate in any of the following events, including shot put, discus, javelin, hammer throw, long jump, high jump, pole vault, and triple jump. The steeplechase event combines distance running with water jumps and barriers. Athletes in each of these specialties encounter dermatoses related to friction, pressure, and environmental exposures.

The repetitive motions and forceful grips required in throwing events often lead to frictional skin injuries. Athletes may develop calluses and blisters on their palms and fingers from handling equipment like shot puts, discuses, and javelins [22, 31]. Repetitive mechanical stress can compromise the skin's integrity, increasing susceptibility to infections such as cellulitis or fungal colonization [32].

Similarly, common dermatologic conditions found among steeplechase athletes are friction-induced injuries, including blisters and calluses. These occur primarily on the feet, particularly when the athlete's footwear becomes saturated during water jumps, leading to increased friction and maceration [22, 31]. The moisture from water jumps can exacerbate the risk of fungal infections such as tinea pedis [32].

Field events and steeplechase are typically outdoor events, subjecting these athletes to prolonged sun exposure. This can lead to sunburn and increase the risk of long-term photodamage, including actinic keratoses and melanoma [25, 26]. These athletes also frequently encounter allergens or irritants in equipment materials, chalk, or athletic tape. These exposures can cause contact dermatitis [29, 33]. Exposure to varying weather conditions, such as wind and rain, can exacerbate contact dermatitis [34].

3.3 Equipment-Related Dermatoses

3.3.1 Contact Dermatitis

Contact dermatitis is an inflammatory skin condition triggered by exposure to external agents, resulting in erythema, swelling, and itching. It can be classified into two main types: irritant contact dermatitis (ICD) and allergic contact dermatitis (ACD). The former involves direct damage to the skin's stratum corneum, leading to the release of pro-inflammatory cytokines that cause inflammation and disruption of the skin barrier. In contrast, ACD is a type IV hypersensitivity reaction, where T lymphocytes recognize a sensitizing agent as an allergen and initiate an inflammatory cascade upon subsequent exposure [35].

Running athletes experience both ICD and ACD. Contact dermatitis results from gear (e.g., shirts and shoes) they wear as well as topical medications these athletes use [36]. Irritant dermatitis of the nipples resulting from contact with running shirts is called Jogger's nipples (discussed later in this chapter). Rubbers, leathers, glues, and dyes used to manufacture running shoes can induce ACD, as the increased moisture within shoes leaches out specific chemicals that cause it [36]. Indeed, previous studies have shown ethyl butyl thiourea in neoprene innersoles of Nike shoes and rubber insoles from tennis shoes containing mercaptobenzothiazole and dibenzothiazyl disulfide all can cause dermatitis eruptions on the feet [37–39]. Lastly, anti-inflammatory creams and gels, topical salicylates, and analgesic sprays have been shown to cause ACD in athletes [40–43]. Picolinamine salicylate, indomethacin and diclofenac gels, as well as eucalyptus oil were among the allergens cited in these cases. Furthermore, a case series studying the incidence of ACD in student athletes identified benzocaine and lanolin as the most prevalent allergens triggering contact dermatitis in runners [44].

The distribution of dermatitis relates to the location where the skin encounters the causative agent. ICD lesions present with dry and fissured skin with less distinct borders and symptoms of burning, pruritis, and pain. The predominant symptom of ACD lesions is pruritis, presenting as vesicles and bullae with distinct angles, lines, and borders. Contact dermatitis lesions can have characteristics of both ICD and ACD [45]. Both ACD and ICD are primarily clinical diagnoses. ACD is confirmed through patch testing, and ICD is diagnosed based on clinical presentation and the exclusion of other causes, as it results from direct damage to the skin barrier rather than an immune-mediated response [22, 35].

Management focuses on identifying and eliminating the causative agents. Topical corticosteroids are commonly used to reduce inflammation, while emollients aid in restoring the skin barrier and reducing transepidermal water loss. In severe cases of dermatitis, systemic corticosteroids may be required to control widespread inflammation [22, 46]. Preventive measures include wearing appropriate protective clothing to minimize friction and reduce exposure to potential irritants. Barrier creams can help shield the skin, and proper hygiene practices, such as washing off sweat and irritants promptly, are essential. Athletes should consider hypoallergenic products to lower the risk of allergic reactions, especially in individuals with a history of ACD [3, 47].

3.3.2 Acne Mechanica

Acne mechanica is a localized form of acne caused by mechanical friction, pressure, occlusion, and heat acting on the skin, often exacerbated by sweat [48, 49]. Repetitive mechanical trauma to hair follicles leads to follicular occlusion, microtrauma, and subsequent inflammation [33, 50]. Acne mechanica is commonly seen in athletes wearing tight and/or protective gear, and athletes engaging in repetitive physical activity. While not common among running athletes, the use of synthetic fabrics traps heat and sweat, developing a favorable microenvironment for the development of acne mechanica. Furthermore, the constant cradling of the shot put against the neck may produce acne mechanica among shot putters [31, 51].

This condition presents as erythematous papules or pustules in areas of repetitive friction or occlusion, such as the back, chest, shoulders, and areas under straps or seams [52]. Diagnosis is primarily clinical, and treatments include benzoyl peroxide or salicylic acid to reduce inflammation and prevent follicular occlusion. For moderate or severe cases, topical or oral antibiotics may be prescribed [50, 53]. Severe or refractory cases may require retinoids to normalize follicular turnover [53]. Preventive strategies include wearing loose, moisture-wicking fabrics to reduce heat and friction, showering promptly after exercise to remove sweat and bacteria, and using barrier creams on high-friction areas [49, 50]. Ensuring proper fit and padding for gear such as hydration packs or compression wear can also minimize mechanical stress [31].

3.4 Environmental-Related Dermatoses

3.4.1 *Miliaria Rubra (Heat Rash)*

Miliaria rubra (heat rash, or "prickly heat") is considered a mild heat-related illness generally caused by exercising in a hot environment [53]. Excessive sweating saturates the skin and occludes the sweat ducts, leading to leakage of eccrine sweat into the epidermis [54]. This causes vasodilation of skin vessels and obstructed sweat ducts/pores from macerated stratum corneum [55]. Secondary infection, especially with staphylococcus, is possible and may produce prolonged symptoms [54, 55]. The risk of miliaria rubra among running athletes increases with increased heat and humidity of the training and/or racing environment, increased duration and/or intensity of training/racing in such an environment, and increased occlusion of the skin by excessive clothing or equipment [54]. Miliaria rubra was observed on the forearms, inner thighs, and calves of ultramarathon runners in the 29th Sultan Marathon des Sables run in Morroco in 2014 after they removed their compression garments [56].

Miliaria rubra presents with erythematous, pruritic papules (often appearing papulovesicular) and can evolve to miliaria pustulosa when miliaria rubra papules become pustules [53, 54]. Skin occluded by clothing and areas of friction are most often affected and commonly include the neck, upper extremities, trunk, and groin [54, 55]. Classically, malaria rubra will have rapid onset in sweaty areas in the setting of a history of excessive heat exposure and sweating. A stinging or "prickling" sensation associated with the rash is a common finding [57]. Entering a cooler environment, reducing clothing coverage, and cooling the area with cold compresses help resolve the rash [53, 54]. While a benign skin lesion, the rash typically takes a week or more to resolve completely [58]. The use of a mild anti-inflammatory lotion like desonide may be useful to relieve symptoms and shorten the duration of the rash [56]. Prevention strategies include wearing loose-fitting, light-colored clothing, avoidance of activities during extreme temperatures, and scheduled rest periods and adequate hydration when avoidance of extreme temperatures is not possible [59].

3.4.2 *Frostnip and Frostbite*

Frostnip is a milder version of frostbite, consisting of superficial freezing of the skin and subcutaneous tissue [60]. It is the most common superficial skin injury caused by cold weather [60–64]. The presence of a windchill factor combined with below-freezing temperatures may induce frostnip, which most often affects the skin covering the cheeks, chin, nose, and ears [61, 63–65].

However, a case of penile frostnip in a long-distance runner after running in subfreezing temperatures and severe winds while wearing polyester trousers and cotton underwear with an anterior opening has been previously reported [66]. Frostnip initially presents with gray-white skin. The skin becomes mottled bluish-purple and swells, stings, and burns as sensation is lost as freezing progresses. Within 24–36 hours, blisters may form (indicative of frostbite) and resolve with crusting over 2 weeks; a burning or throbbing sensation may linger for weeks, and the affected skin may remain sensitive to cold for months after [60, 62, 64].

Frostbite involves the freezing of the skin, subcutaneous tissue, muscle, and/or bone [67]. Running athletes are at an increased risk of developing frostbite when competing and training in subzero conditions associated with rain and wind for extended periods of time [53]. Athletes competing at higher altitudes are also at an increased risk for frostbite due to decreased ambient oxygen tension, which, along with cutaneous vasoconstriction that occurs to maintain core body temperature in a cold environment, exacerbates hypoxia of cutaneous tissues [68]. Additionally, metal can cause frostbite instantaneously through direct contact with exposed [and especially moist] skin because it is a heat conductor [69]. This may have implications for field event athletes, particularly shot putters and javelin, hammer, and discus throwers, as the objects they throw are made of metal. Exposed and unexposed areas are at risk for frostbite, but the anterior of the neck is the most affected [64].

The pathophysiology of frostbite has four phases: cooling, thawing and rewarming, extension of injury, and resolution. During the cooling phase, there is cyclic vasoconstriction and vasodilation as extracellular ice and intracellular ice crystals form. Intravascular ice formation leads to erythrocyte sludging and vessel occlusion. Ice melts during the thawing and rewarming phase, and dehydrated cells start to swell. This paired with loss of vessel wall integrity and compromise of vascular tone contributes to edema and vasodilation. Inflammatory mediators are released, leading to platelet and leukocyte aggregation, causing thrombosis. During extension of injury and resolution, thromboxane A2 levels increase and platelet and leukocyte aggregation extends into bordering tissue, creating vascular compromise. Tissue re-epithelializes or dessicates and mummifies. It is possible that vasomotor instability persists indefinitely [70, 71].

Likewise, there are four categories of frostbite based on severity. The first is frostnip, described above. Second-degree frostbite consists of hyperemia, edema, blistering, and clear fluid in the bullae. Third-degree is characterized by full-thickness dermal loss with hemorrhagic bulla and/or the development of waxy, dry, mummified skin. Lastly, fourth-degree frostbite demonstrates full-thickness necrosis leading to skin, tendon, muscle, and bone damage as well as tissue loss. As with frostnip, healing does occur with second-degree frostbite, with patients having long-term sensory neuropathy. Waxy, dry, mummified skin is a poor prognostic indicator for tissue loss, and injuries form fourth-degree frostbite often require amputation [70, 71].

Treatment of frostnip and frostbite involves rapid rewarming in a 38–44 °C water bath for 20-minute intervals [22, 72, 73]. Prevention is crucial with frostnip and frostbite. Exercise, wind, cold, and water from immersion or perspiration in combination can reduce the insulation effect of clothing to 10% of its normal value [74]. Therefore, wet clothes should be removed as soon as possible; wearing multiple layers of thin clothing is also imperative as it allows for the trapping of heat between the layers and reabsorption of excess perspiration [67, 74]. The application of petroleum jelly or zinc oxide to exposed areas serves as a barrier and seals in moisture and heat. Waiting to shower and shave until after cold exposure takes advantage of the natural insulating effects of sebum and helps prevent skin damage induced by cold training/racing conditions as well [61]. Since the neck is an especially vulnerable region to frostbite, wearing either an absorbent terry-cloth towel or a synthetic breathable neck garment around the neck when training in extremely cold temperatures is advisable [64, 73, 75].

3.4.3 Cholinergic Urticaria and Exercise-Induced Anaphylaxis (EIA)

Athletes have an increased likelihood of developing physical urticarias, with physical urticarias representing 15% of urticarial types among athletes as compared to 2.5% of urticarial types among the general population [76]. Physical urticarias are most common among running sports, especially cholinergic urticaria [22]. Cholinergic urticaria results from an elevated core body temperature, usually after the start of sweating, that occurs during exercise, passive warming, and emotional stress. It presents within 2–30 minutes of overheating of the body as 2–5 mm punctate wheals surrounded by erythematous large flares that may coalesce [77, 78]. The lesions usually occur on the upper thorax and neck and spread distally [79]. Development of urticaria after asking an athlete to exercise is diagnostic [80]. Treatment for athletes begins with non-sedating antihistamines, like cetirizine and xyzal. Taking beta-blockers or Danazol may also be helpful. Prevention involves prophylactic antihistamines, avoidance of heat, exercise, and other triggers [77].

The development of vibratory angioedema, which presents with transient erythema and wheals at the sight of vibration, occurs with increased frequency among those who develop cholinergic urticaria. In one case, a 28-year-old female developed vibratory angioedema on the posterior aspect of her thighs because of repetitive pounding related to running. She was treated with prophylactic terfenadine [81, 82].

While cholinergic urticaria may cause bronchospasm, it rarely progresses to exercise-induced anaphylaxis (EIA) [77]. EIA is a distinct physical allergy and the most life-threatening dermatological manifestation among runners [78]. Pruritis and wheals (10–15 mm) present after the initiation of exercise and can relate to cofactors such as specific food ingestion, personal history of atopy, aspirin or NSAID use, insect stings, exposure to high pollen levels, humidity, extremes of weather, and menses [82–86]. In addition to wheals, an individual with EIA may develop laryngealoedema, angioedema, bronchospasm, gastrointestinal symptoms, hypotension, and/or syncope [79, 87]. A few mechanisms have been proposed to describe the pathophysiology of EIA. One involves the activation of the alternative complement pathway, while the other is lactate-, creatine phosphokinase,- or IgE-mediated mast cell degranulation, increasing serum levels of histamine [22, 88].

The diagnosis of EIA is not completely straightforward. Diagnosis requires a history of symptoms suggesting anaphylaxis with involvement of cutaneous, respiratory, gastrointestinal, and cardiovascular systems within two hours [often within 30 minutes] from exposure to the causative agent [89, 90]. For EIA, the causative agent is physical exertion, but often, a cofactor is needed to elicit the reaction; therefore, the clinical history taken must be very accurate to identify the cofactor. A challenge is used for diagnosis, with physical exercise alone proving sufficient. The use of food followed by physical exercise is used for challenges in cases in which food is the cofactor [91]. Furthermore, athletes that show a relation with food should be evaluated with prick tests and radioallergosorbent blood tests (RAST) [92]. Acute treatment includes airway and cardiovascular support and epinephrine if necessary. Antihistamines are not effective for the prevention of EIA. Avoidance of exposure to triggers is useful for preventing EIV, and monitoring, which may consist of training with a medically-trained companion or wearing a medical alert device, is key [93].

3.5 Sun and Ultraviolet Radiation-Related Dermatoses

3.5.1 Cheilitis Simplex (Chapped Lips)

Cheilitis simplex, also known as chapped lips, is one of the most common forms of cheilitis (inflammation of the lips). It may be caused by acute and chronic sun exposure, atopic dermatitis, seborrheic dermatitis, and allergic and irritant contact dermatitis [94]. In a cross-sectional study of road runners in Brazil, 14.5% of runners reported getting cheilitis simplex, and it was more prevalent among athletes running more than 64 kilometers per week [95]. Repetitive biting, licking, and rubbing of the lips can further cause and exacerbate cheilitis simplex by promoting dryness and irritation, causing the mucosa of the lips to separate. It presents with cracking, fissuring, and scaling of both lips, but it is most common on the lower lip. The lesions can progress to crusting, hemorrhage, and blister formation in chronic cases [94]. Cheilitis simplex is a clinical diagnosis. Both treatment and prevention strategies involve the aggressive use of barrier lubricants, like petroleum jelly, on a regular basis [94].

3.5.2 Acute Solar Erythema (Sunburn)

Acute solar erythema, or sunburn, is caused by skin exposure to ultraviolet (UV) rays and is the most common skin disorder [53]. Running athletes are at risk due to long training hours in the sun. Sunburn is a biological marker indicating exposure to high-dose UV radiation (UVR). Exposure to UVA rays with wavelengths between 320 and 400 nm and UVB rays with wavelengths between 295 and 320 nm can cause sunburn and DNA damage. UVA rays cause oxidative DNA damage and UVB rays induce the formation of thymine-thymine cyclobutane dimers, as they are directly absorbed by DNA [95–97]. The dimers trigger the DNA repair response, inducing cell apoptosis and release of inflammatory markers [e.g., prostaglandins, reactive oxygen species, and bradykinin] [98]. This leads to vasodilation, edema, and pain. UVB ray exposure specifically can elevate levels of chemokines, such as C-X-C-motif chemokine 5 (CXCL5), and activate peripheral nociceptors, leading to overactivation of the skin's pain receptors [99, 100].

In a 2014 cross-sectional study of road runners in Brazil, 19.7% of runners experienced sunburn, and it was a common, recurrent dermatosis regardless of the distance ran [101]. Importantly, the prevalence of sunburn among running athletes may vary, especially in the context of sun protection practices. In the same 2014 Brazil study, 57% of the athletes trained before 10 a.m., 86% wore clothing and accessories for sun protection, and 62% wore sunscreen [101]. A 2014 study examining skin manifestations among ultramarathon runners observed during the Marathon des Sables noted sunburn was infrequent because most runners used sunscreen [56]. Athletes who take photosensitizing drugs and athletes with fair skin (Fitzpatrick skin type I-III, these skin types exhibit less melanin pigment that acts to shield the skin cells against UVR) are at a higher risk of developing sunburn [53, 102].

Sunburn usually occurs between 10 am and 3 pm on exposed skin. It presents with erythema and pain in the most superficial layers of the skin. Deep burns damage deeper skin layers, including nerves, causing blisters and bullae [53]. Affected sunburned skin may be warm and painful to the touch, and severe cases of sunburn can induce systemic symptoms like nausea, chills, and fever. Within 3–7 days, erythema will usually subside, while blisters take 7–10 days to heal. Furthermore, skin peeling may continue for 7–10 days after sun exposure; individuals may develop solar lentigines [age spots], which are pale, brown macules that remain after the sunburn has resolved [102].

When treating sunburns, it is important for running athletes to remove themselves from the sun and stay hydrated. Treatment options for symptomatic minor burns include cold compresses, possibly low-dose topical steroids, anesthetics, or antihistamines [53]. More severe burns may benefit from warm soaks, petroleum jelly, sarna lotion, gauze, topical corticosteroids in a cream or spray, and NSAIDs (aspirin, indomethacin) [22, 63, 64, 103–105] Oral fluids and other forms of supportive treatment may be needed in athletes with severe burns [53]. Preventing sunburn requires athletes to avoid training during peak sun exposure (between 10 am and 3 pm), wear protective clothing/headgear, and wear sunscreen. Sunscreen protecting against UVA and UVB rays should be applied 30 minutes before exercise and reapplied after sweating and/or water exposure. Sunscreen formulas that are waterproof provide increased protection [53].

3.5.3 Melanoma and Non-Melanoma Skin Cancers (NMSCs)

Experiencing high levels of UVR is considered the most important environmental risk factor for melanoma and non-melanoma skin cancers (NMSCs) [106]. The intensity of UVR varies with latitude, altitude, atmospheric conditions, seasons, time of day, and photo-protection practices of an individual [107–109]. While no previous relative risk studies have assessed the risk of developing skin cancer among runners, a study has evaluated the risk factors of malignant melanoma among marathon runners as compared to a matched control group. This study found that, compared to the control group, marathon runners presented with more atypical meanlocytic nevi, solar lentigines, and lesions suggestive of NMSC, which correlated with increasing training intensity [110]. Given that the number of atypical melanocytic nevi and solar lentigines has been shown to be the strongest independent indicator of an increased risk of the development of malignant melanoma, this study concluded marathon runners presented with an increased risk for malignant melanoma and NMSCs [110, 111].

The main NMSCs include basal cell carcinoma (BCC) and squamous cell carcinoma (SCC). In addition to UVR exposure, major risk factors for BCC include ionizing radiation and immunosuppression (e.g., organ transplantation). While BCC can occur on any skin surface, it most commonly occurs on sun-exposed areas, especially the head and neck. It presents as a pearly, telangiectatic papule or as a small, crusted area that bleeds and becomes a nonhealing sore. Aggressive forms of BCC include morpheaform, sclerosing, micronodular, and infiltrative subtypes. BCCs are characterized by slow growth and a rare rate of metastasis, approximately 0.0028% to 0.55%. Although they rarely metastasize, BCCs can be locally destructive, invading neighboring skin, muscle, cartilage, and bone. Treatments include malignant destruction with electrodes- iccation and curettage, curettage and cryotherapy, and excision with 4 mm margins around the tumor. Mohs micrograph surgery is another procedure to treat BCC [112].

While UVR exposure is also a major risk factor for SCC, darkly pigmented athletes are more likely to develop SCC, and it is usually related to an underlying chronic scarring condition or ulcer. It occurs in less pigmented skin of digits and has been connected to immunosuppression (organ transplantation and chronic lymphocytic leukemia), HIV infection, and HPV infection (strains 16 and 18). Additional risk factors include a history of exposure to arsenic, x-rays, and inherited skin disorders like xeroderma pigmentosum and DOCK-8 deficiency. Generally, SCC starts as a scaly papule that can become indurated with mounds of scale on the surface on. It can occur on sun-exposed and non-sun-exposed areas of the skin, and often arises from premalignant lesions known as actinic keratoses, which present as red, scaly patches or papules on sun-exposed skin. Lesions of SCC can also present as volcano-like lesions with a central crater and sharply demarcated edges and SCC *in situ* presents as a flat, pink-to-red scaling plaque. On the genitalia, SCC presents as an erosion, ulceration, or sessile papule. Additionally, SCC sometimes occurs in area of chronic scarring, such as burns, and is called a Marjolin ulcer. Overall, SCCs do not bleed as readily as BCC. Treatment of SCC is similar to that of BCC, but SCC has a higher risk of metastasis and treatment depends on staging. Curettage and topical treatments, such as 5-fluorouracil and imiquimod, are used to treat SCC *in situ*. For SCC, excisional biopsies or MMS is the standard of treatment. Radiation therapy works, but it is costly and labor intensive [112].

There are four main types of melanomas: superficial spreading, nodular, lentigo maligna, and acral lentiginous. The risk of developing melanoma increases with UVR exposure, number of atypical nevi, number of benign nevi, large and giant congenital melanocytic nevi, pale skin and/or blonde or red hair and blue or green eyes, immunosuppression, family history of melanoma, and genetic predisposition (defects in the CD-KN2A and/or CDK4 gene, xeroderma pigmentosum) [112]. Visual identification of melanoma is based on the ABCDE mnemonic: A for asymmetry, B for irregular borders, C for uneven color, D for a diameter greater than 6 mm and E for evolving in that it changes size, shape, and color. Any tumor suspicious of melanoma should be biopsied or removed. Once diagnosis is confirmed [biopsy], complete excision of the tumor treats melanoma, with excisional margins based on Breslow tumor thickness. Lymphatic mapping and sentinel lymph node biopsies can be performed as a staging tool for melanoma. Advanced disease may require medical management, surgery, and/or radiation therapy [112]. Prevention of NMSCs and melanoma among running athletes requires reducing exposure to UVR, as detailed in the acute solar erythema section.

3.6 Friction and Pressure-Related Dermatoses

3.6.1 Runner's Rump

Runner's rump is the hyperpigmentation of the skin, specifically on the superior aspect of the gluteal cleft, in long-distance runners. It is caused by friction resulting from continual contact/rubbing of each buttock during every stride, producing small, asymptomatic ecchymoses. Variations in running form may contribute to the appearance of runner's rump, as only certain runners are prone to developing the condition [73, 113]. A physical exam and history of long-distance running are adequate for diagnosis [80]. Runner's rump tends to spontaneously resolve during periods of decreased training [73, 113]. Prevention may include choosing softer clothing material to run in and application of topical lubricants to the area before, during, and after a run [80].

3.6.2 Athlete's Nodules ("Nike Nodules")

Athlete's nodules are cutaneous nodules caused by chronic pressure trauma or friction trauma [53]. Basler and Jacobs described a nodular lesion they termed "pseudobursae" on the dorsum of the foot that were transient in nature. These were observed in a woman who wore tight-fitting athletic shoes; they therefore referred to the condition as "Nike nodules" [114]. These nodules are soft, flesh-colored keratinized nodules ranging in size from 0.5 cm to 4.0 cm and occur on the malleolus or foot dorsum. A biopsy confirms the diagnosis [77]. While dermatofibromas appear similar, on histology, athlete's nodule will have tumorous proliferation of fibroblasts in the dermis and reactive hypertrophy of the epidermis [115]. Surgical excision is the preferred treatment if the athlete is symptomatic; otherwise, watchful waiting is recommended [53].

3.6.3 Nipple Fissure (Jogger's Nipple)

Nipple Fissure, commonly known as "jogger's nipple," is a form of exercise-induced chafing that occurs due to repetitive friction between the nipple and clothing. In severe cases, the keratin separates from the granular sublayer in the epidermis, eventually resulting in a crusted and cracked lesion [116]. The condition is worsened with longer runs in coarse material. In a study measuring the injuries in a variety of marathons in the United States, researchers found that up to 16.3% of runners experienced jogger's nipple [78]. This cutaneous condition typically presents with painful, erythematous erosions of the nipple with occasional bleeding [22]. Although quite uncomfortable, it is fortunately preventable to a certain degree. Prophylactic measures include bandages or tape over the nipples, petroleum jelly lubricants, and soft, moisture-wicking shirts (or no shirts if applicable). Treatment may include applying a topical hydrocortisone cream [116].

3.6.4 Physical Intertrigo

Intertrigo is a dermatosis that occurs due to repetitive skin-on-skin rubbing in large and small body folds [117]. This can become worrisome as it can lead to secondary bacterial and fungal infections [118]. In the stride of a runner, almost all body folds of the body rub against each other, notably the axilla, inguinal, and inframammary regions. Physical intertrigo may present as mild to severe erythema with possible abrasion and fissuration [119]. Patients should aim to keep the areas cool and dry with absorptive powders, barrier creams, and light, absorbing clothing [118]. Any secondary infection, bacterial or fungal, should be addressed and treated accordingly.

3.6.5 Blisters (Friction Blisters/Bullae)

Blisters are the most frequent dermatological condition that runners face [120]. Even though they are extremely common, they are not as easily prevented or treated. In a survey on marathon runners, up to 39% of runners presented to the medical tent due to blisters [78]. During an ultra endurance run study, 76% of participants experienced blisters by day 4 of running, with the majority located on the toes, ball of the foot, heel, and sole [120]. The sheer force of running on feet causes epidermal splits that fill with blood or tissue transudate [78]. There is a lack of evidence to determine the best preventative measures, although paper tape may prove effective as well as moisture-wicking socks and antiperspirants for the feet [78, 121]. Research of prevention and treatment of blisters varies, and a consensus is yet to be reached. However, treatment may include incision and drainage while maintaining the blister roof within 24 hours of blister development. Moleskin may reduce the likelihood of additional trauma to a blister, and hydrocolloid dressings and silvadene or antibacterial ointments may decrease discomfort and prevent secondary infection [77].

3.6.6 Calluses

The skin naturally adapts to an increased thickness as a defense mechanism to protect the soft underlying tissues from repeated pressure or friction [122]. Common risk factors for runners include improper or ill-fitting running shoes, irregularities within the sock or shoe, repetitive force on a specific location, and abrupt increases in the intensity or duration of the run [122]. Prevalence of calluses may also be determined by the footedness (preferred or dominant lower limb) of the runner [123]. Calluses present as diffuse hyperkeratotic lesions at sites of pressure and/or friction that may vary in color and degree of pain [122]. Treatments for runners include padding and modification of activity and footwear, although surgery or sharp debridement may be necessary in severe cases [124].

3.6.7 Longitudinal Melanonychia

Longitudinal Melanonychia presents as a tan, brown, or black single or multi-band streak within the nail plate that can occur due to a variety of factors. The most important differential diagnosis is subungual melanoma, although it can also be caused by chronic or acute trauma such as that from running [125]. Improper footwear should be discussed with patients as ill-fitting running shoes may have an association with the darkened streaks in toenails [126]. In the case of running induced longitudinal melanonychia, treatment includes removal of the trauma, such as finding better fitting shoes or trying different forms of running exercises [127].

3.6.8 *Nail Dystrophy*

With every step a runner takes, pressure is exerted from the knee to the ankle, and eventually, to the toes. This continuous exposure to repeated pressure can cause minor trauma to the toenail. Nail dystrophy is a condition in which the nail bed gradually thickens, develops ridges, and becomes discolored due to the thrusting of the toes on the toe box of the sneaker [22]. The extreme force on the nail may cause subungual hematomas resulting in darkened discolorations that may need to be drained in severe, painful cases [128]. Treatment of trauma-induced nail dystrophies that runners experienced mainly involves prevention of further injury such as wearing properly fitted sneakers with trimmed toenails. There is sparse research on various clinical treatments that are available for this type of trauma-induced injury.

3.7 Trauma-Induced Dermatoses

3.7.1 *Contusions*

Contusions are the second leading cause of morbidity from sports-related injuries [129]. Although running is an extremely low-contact sport, various injuries causing contusions (more commonly called "bruises") are not uncommon. Runners may trip and fall or bump into one another on crowded tracks or paths leading to injury. When a runner falls or bumps his/her knee on the ground, the integrity of the underlying vessel is compromised, leading to leakage of blood into the surrounding areas. A contusion is a form of trauma-induced bruise in which larger quantities of blood extravasate the tissue without exiting the skin [130]. There is very little evidence on how to best treat contusion injuries, especially since research heavily relies on animal models rather than humans, although researchers in New Zealand aim to provide change [131].

3.7.2 *Lacerations and Abrasions*

Runners vary greatly based on the environment in which they perform their sport. The course in which a runner exercises can range from a paved or turf track, to a dirt-filled or rocky terrain, to a sidewalk through a grassy park. Running is possible in almost every environment; this readily widens the realms of possible scrapes and tears athletes may experience. Abrasions are more minor, superficial wounds affecting more commonly the epidermis, only rarely leaving a scar [132]. These forms of scrapes can occur after falling on pavement or brushing against a rough object while running. Treatment involves inspecting the injury for any foreign body and irrigating the wound with water or saline. Abrasions usually heal by primary intention, but may need further treatment for those susceptible to keloid hyperplasia [132].

Lacerations, unlike abrasions, occur from more traumatic injuries. If a runner were to trip and land on a sharp tree branch or rock, they could tear through much deeper than the epidermis or dermis. Deep cuts from blunt trauma need emergent medical attention as deeper structures and tissues are at risk of injury and infection. Initially, direct pressure should be used to stop the bleeding. Then, the medical professional should evaluate the wound to determine which structures are affected. Various factors such as location and severity of the injury determine which kind of medical professional can treat the patient, as well as further prognosis [133]. Follow up care is important for removal of sutures and prevention of infection.

3.7.3 Piezogenic Pedal Papules

Runners may experience piezogenic papules, or small, sometimes painful, herniations of footpad's subcutaneous fat, in their feet upon weight bearing due to continuous pressure on the heels [134]. It is hypothesized that the pressure may cause small tears in the plantar fascia for the fat to seep through [135]. Through a case review of athletes with piezogenic pedal papules, it was found that 52.2% of the cohort had the painful variety of piezogenic pedal papules [136]. Patients present with skin-colored papules bilaterally around the heels which become accentuated with weight-bearing [77]. Biopsy is typically unnecessary for diagnosis [135]. Painless cases are often ignored and can be treated conservatively, however the painful variety requires much more attention. Firstly, the feet should be treated with restrictive therapy including heel cups, compression socks, and taping [137]. If these interventions do not help, steroid therapy or electro-acupuncture may be attempted [137]. In 2018, Turkmani reported the first case report of deoxycholic acid injections for painful piezogenic pedal papules which showed efficacy on a small scale [134]. Surgery is only appropriate in severe, recurrent cases [77]. If the piezogenic pedal papules are symptomatic, runners may consider reduction of weight-bearing exercises as there are no other preventative measures.

3.7.4 Talon Noir (Calcaneal Petechiae)

Talon Noir, or "black heel syndrome", is a relatively common running-related dermatological condition characterized by its asymptomatic dark brown and/or black macules of irregular pattern surrounding the heels and soles of athletes' feet [138]. It primarily affects young athletes, likely caused by the shear stress of abrupt contact of the heel of the foot with a hard surface [139]. Talon noir can be differentiated from melanoma by scarification of paring, which should show black pigment of extravasated red cells [140]. This condition resolves without intervention within one month [78]. No treatment is necessary [141]. Prevention may include additional or thicker socks, heel lubricant, heel cups, and reduction in running [78].

3.7.5 Subungual Hematoma (Runner's/Jogger's Toe)

Subungual hematomas are collections of blood under the toenail typically due to trauma such as the force of the toe against a sneaker while running. If enough blood pools under the nail bed, the pressure may cause a throbbing sensation [142]. Subungual hematomas typically resolve spontaneously with cessation of running, however, a heated sterile needle through the nail plate may be used to quickly relieve pressure in such painful cases [31]. In recent years, the FDA has approved nail trephination devices that can puncture through the nail plate with more precision to better protect the underlying vasculature [143]. Runners should be encouraged to wear proper fitting shoes, especially in the toe box region.

3.7.6 Onychomadesis (Complete Nail Shedding)

Onychomadesis is a condition in which the proximal nail plate separates and then painlessly sheds from the nail matrix. It is commonly associated with diseases and infections but can also be due to local trauma such as that faced by runners [144]. In a cross-sectional study reporting on sport-related dermatoses in southern Brazil, onychomadesis was reported in 31.5% of the road runners [101]. Ultrasound imaging may be a useful diagnostic tool to visualize the proximal and distal nail plate separation, as well as the timeframe of the injury [145]. Cases of onychomadesis frequently self-resolve; there is no universal treatment noted [146]. In a 2021 analysis of microtrauma associated with footwear and running, researchers found that a urea 40% cream aided in nail improvement [147]. Runners should be especially cautious in caring for their feet. Physicians may recommend proper fitting shoes and maintaining well-trimmed toenails.

3.7.7 Onychocryptosis (Ingrown Toenails)

Onychocryptosis, or ingrown toenail, is a common, often painful, nail condition in which the edge of the nail penetrates into the periungual dermis [148]. The great toes are the most commonly affected, with primary causes being ill-fitting footwear and half-circle cut toenails [149]. In a 2017 analysis of nail conditions in runners, it was found that young male runners had the highest rates of onychocryptosis at a staggering 71.4% of participants [150]. Participation in sports may cause production of nail spicules that pierce skin lateral of the nail. If left untreated, ingrown toenails can progress to infection and difficulty walking [151]. First line treatments include taping, cotton packing, and gutter application, while more severe cases may include surgical procedures ranging in a variety of techniques [148].

3.8 Infection-Related Dermatoses

3.8.1 Bacterial Infections

Impetigo contagiosum is a bacterial infection that often results from the breakdown of skin due to abrasions and is commonly caused by *Staphylococci* and *Streptococci* species. Although Impetigo is more frequently seen in contact sports, it is highly contagious, and running athletes may be at risk through direct contact with infected lesions or through shared equipment [22, 152]. Clinically, Impetigo presents as well-demarcated erythematous plaques with yellow-colored crusts typically seen on the face, neck, or extremities [152].

Diagnosis can be made upon history and physical with differentials that may include atopic dermatitis, tinea corporis gladiatorum, and acne. First-line treatments are topical and oral antibiotics, such as cefalexin or dicloxacillin. Management and prevention strategies may include removing yellow-colored crust to allow for better antibiotic penetration, improvement in more thorough hygiene practices, and avoiding sharing sporting equipment or towels. Additionally, as the infection is often contacted through open lesions or abrasions, extra care should be taken to make sure any open wounds are covered and well-dressed [22].

Folliculitis is characterized by inflammation of a hair follicle that is more superficial often accompanied by small pustules around the follicle. Furunculosis is a deeper infection of the hair follicle, and painful boils may be seen. These diseases can appear around where clothes fit, especially with the tighter-fitting uniforms of running athletes (3). The pustules characteristic of folliculitis can be found anywhere on the body, sparing the palms and soles and can be infected by various organisms such as *Staphylococcus* or *Pseudomonas* [152].

Diagnosis and treatment of Folliculitis and Furunculosis are relatively straightforward, with the diagnosis being based on clinical presentation, and the treatment including topical and oral antibiotics. It may also be helpful to recommend athletes to limit intensity of their activity and avoid contact with other team members for at least 3 days after initiating treatment [153]. Prevention strategies involve not sharing personal items such as towels and limiting frequent shaving of areas impacted by high friction [152].

Pitted keratolysis is a bacterial infection that causes multifocal, crater-like lesions on the toes and soles of the feet. It is usually accompanied by a foul odor and may appear brown in color. Although it is most often asymptomatic, patients may experience symptoms such as pain, burning sensations, hyperhidrosis, or irritation [154].

Pitted keratolysis is common among athletes, especially those who frequently wear occlusive footwear such as runners [155]. Other risk factors include humid environments, poor foot hygiene, and excessive sweating [154].

Diagnosis can be made clinically based on its characteristic presentation of crater lesions and malodor. A Wood's lamp examination is often negative or may demonstrate coral-red fluorescence if *Corynebacterium* is the causative organism. Treatment involves topical antibiotics, such as clindamycin or erythromycin, as first-line management. This regimen is usually effective, with resolution in about three weeks. Oral antibiotics are reserved for cases that did not resolve with topical medications. Preventative measures can include good foot hygiene, rotating footwear often in addition to frequent sanitation, and the use of synthetic socks along with regular changes [155].

3.8.2 Viral Infections

Molluscum Contagiosum is a highly infectious poxvirus infection that is most frequently seen among contact sports athletes. It may be spread through direct contact with an infected lesion or through moist surfaces including shower floors, exercise mats, or the benches of saunas. Running athletes may encounter this infection in such locations, such as locker room showers, or other shared facilities and equipment, like towels [153]. On physical examination, Molluscum Contagiosum appears as small, flesh-colored papules that are raised and round with a central dimple. Several dozen papules may be present at the time of diagnosis [156].

Diagnosis is made based on clinical characteristics, but curettage may be performed with histological verification that is both diagnostic and therapeutic [152]. While Molluscum Contagiosum is self-limiting and does not require treatment in most cases, it is highly recommended that any cases in athletes are actively dealt with as soon as possible to help prevent any further spread of infection. In terms of treatment, curettage allows for complete removal of the lesions and is more effective than the use of topical medications, or a hyfrecator can be used to lightly burn the bases of the papules. It is of the most importance to make sure that the affected areas are covered during the healing period [156]. Prevention of Molluscum Contagiosum includes good hygiene practices, using only disinfected mats and other sporting equipment, and the use of protective footwear in open moist areas like showers [153].

Verruca Plantaris, also known as Plantar Warts, are benign bumps found on the soles of the foot that are caused by human papillomavirus. They are acquired either from direct contact with someone who is infected or by surfaces such as shower floors or other warm, moist areas. The running athlete may encounter plantar warts if exposed to such environments, and they are at an increased risk of infection if their skin is wet or broken [152]. Plantar warts appear as thick, hyperkeratotic plaques that may be misdiagnosed as calluses. They can be skin colored with small black dots on the surface. They may also be especially debilitating to running athletes due to being painful with applied pressure [157].

Plantar warts are diagnosed by their clinical characteristics, with careful inspection and exclusion of other differential diagnoses. Treatment includes removal options, such as liquid nitrogen, laser, or curettage, or topical and oral medications like imiquimod or cimetidine [152]. Thorough hygiene practices are the mainstay of management and prevention, including only using one's personal, clean towel, avoiding walking around barefoot, and good sanitation and upkeep of shoes. Any lesions should be covered in order to limit the spread to other teammates [157].

3.8.3 *Fungal Infections*

Athletes, especially runners, contract tinea pedis in increased proportions. Two studies reported prevalences of 22% and 31% in runners, almost twice the prevalence of that in the general population [158, 159]. Tinea pedis, also known as athlete's foot, is a fungal infection affecting the foot. It can vary in its clinical presentation, either presenting with scale and may be erythematous or non-erythematous, or it can have inflammatory vesicles. It may also manifest in between the toe, with scaly plaques. Symptoms include itchiness, burning, or stinging [160]. Tinea pedis is more frequently encountered in locations such as communal showers or locker room floors. Additionally, runners are at an increased risk due to their feet being more commonly exposed to athletic footwear, repeated trauma, and moist environments [161].

Clinical presentation can aid in the diagnosis of Tinea pedis along with a positive potassium hydroxide examination for confirmation. Treatment can involve topical antifungal medications like azoles, and in more severe cases, oral antifungals may be necessary. Preventative measures can include the use of protective footwear, such as sandals, in showers or other moist areas. In addition, runners can use synthetic socks that keep their feet cool and dry to try avoiding the creation of an environment where such organisms may grow. Lastly, some athletes may choose to participate in the routine use of antifungal agents in order to prevent infection [162].

Tinea corporis, also known as Ringworm, presents as erythematous, well-demarcated plaques with a central clearing. It is often spread from person to person but may also be contracted from animals or surfaces that have been contaminated. Tinea corporis is used to describe fungal infections on parts of the body not otherwise specified by a given name, like Tinea pedis or Tinea capitis. Runners may be at risk of infection through humid environments, like showers, that increase the survival of fungal organisms as well as mechanical trauma that cause microinjuries on the feet and may create a pathway for infection [152, 153]. Diagnosis is based on the clinical picture and is confirmed with a positive potassium hydroxide examination. Similar to tinea pedis, topical antifungals are the first-line treatment, with oral antifungals reserved for more severe presentations. Hygiene practices are important in the prevention of infection with tinea corporis, and certain habits like decontaminating communal surfaces and showering as soon as possible after events may help limit the spread [22, 153].

Onychomycosis, also known as tinea unguium, is a fungal infection of the nails. The nails may present as brittle, thickened, and discolored, such as yellow, brown or white. Toenail infections are more common than those presenting in the fingernails, about seven more times prevalent. Athletes are 2.5 times more likely to be infected when compared to the general population. Runners are at a particular risk for fungal toenail infections due to their use of occlusive footwear, interactions with warm, moist environments, and repeated trauma to their feet and toenails [163]. Separation from the nail bed can occur which may predispose the athlete to secondary infection by bacteria or mold [153].

Diagnosis can be made clinically, based on the patient's history and physical examination, along with a confirmatory potassium hydroxide preparation. Treatment can include oral antifungals, nail polishes or creams, and other measures such as nail removal or laser treatments. However, onychomycosis treatment may be accompanied by significant side effects and recurrence of infection. Thus, preventive measures are crucial in the management of onychomycosis. Synthetic socks and proper foot hygiene, such as regular toenail trimmings, can play important roles in the prevention of fungal infection [163].

3.9 Inflammatory and Immune-Related Dermatoses

Exercise-induced vasculitis (EIV) is a small-vessel vasculitis that can occur after strenuous activity such as running. It is also known as exercise-induced purpura, which refers to the appearance of the rash. It most frequently presents on the lower extremities, resulting in a urticarial or petecheial rash with surrounding erythema. There may be associated pain, edema, or itchiness, but any skin compressed by socks is usually spared [164]. Long distances and hot weather are two major risk factors for acquiring this condition and can impact the severity of the disease presentation. EIV presents more often in females and is more severe in patients with pre-existing edema [165].

Diagnosis is made clinically based on physical characteristics and patient history, but EIV is often misdiagnosed and underrecognized despite its prevalence among runners. Any autoimmune diseases or coagulopathies should be investigated and excluded in order to make a diagnosis of exercise-induced vasculitis. It is self-limiting and usually resolves within a few days. Non-steroidal antiinflammatory drugs or steroids may be helpful in symptom management. Elevation of the legs may also be beneficial for patients [164]. Prevention strategies can include well-fitted compression socks, prophylactic use of steroids, or other methods effective for edema prevention [165].

3.10 Prevention on a Macroscopic Level

Dermatoses prevention among running athletes begins at the individual level, where adequate precautions help the athletes reduce their risk of acquiring a skin disease. Such precautions can include wearing properly fitted shoes and socks to prevent friction blisters, or heel cups to help relieve some of the discomfort from piezogenic pedal papules [166, 167]. However, prevention should not be limited to the personal care of the running athletes. All other personnel involved in the sport must be aware and do their part to help prevent the acquisition of skin disease and the potential spread of infection.

Track and field, and most other running sports, is considered an individual sport, with limited to no contact with other teammates or opponents. Still, there must be care and attention in personal care and hygiene to limit the prevalence of skin infections. Shared equipment and facilities increase the risk of spreading infection, and skin disease in one individual may put others at risk. Runners are at a notably higher risk of certain infections, like Tinea pedis, which thrives in warm and moist environments. It is thought that Tinea pedis may originate in places like pools, showers, and locker rooms [168]. The National Athletic Trainers' Association 2010 Position Statement stresses the importance of hygiene practices, such as providing appropriate hygienic materials to athletes, like antimicrobial soap, and maintaining contact with a team dermatologist that aids in diagnosing, treating, and preventing skin diseases. The statement also recommends the cooperation of all sports staff members in infectious control, including coaches, administrators, custodians, and athletes. Most importantly, education about skin diseases must be emphasized among all members to help increase awareness and participation in prevention strategies [169]. If a skin disease is contracted, treatment and management depend on the etiology, and return-to-play guidelines also vary. The guidelines for noncontact sports or sports that do not frequently share equipment, like track and field or cross country, are managed on a case-by-case basis [170].

Illnesses and injuries can burden medical personnel involved in athletic events, such as marathon and ultramarathon races. These races pose unique challenges due to race distance and environmental conditions. Having medical services on-site can help reduce the rate of medical complications and encourage race participant safety. Skin trauma is a frequent complaint to event medical teams and makes up most encounters, around 74.3% in multi-day ultramarathons. Foot trauma, such as blisters, is a prevalent complication of running sports. Thus, implementing initiatives like mandatory foot care kits for participants and educating them on self-care may reduce the burden of care placed on medical professionals [171]. Previous intervention studies have focused on participant risk identification before race events and implementing a thorough, high-quality medical operations protocol. One study featured the Two Oceans Marathon in Cape Town, South Africa, where runners participated in online prerace medical screening. There was also an educational program and a risk stratification based on a mandatory questionnaire for race participants. By identifying high-risk runners and providing them with appropriate educational materials, all medical encounters were reduced by 29% at both the 56 km and half-marathon races [172]. Such intervention strategies can drastically reduce medical burden, improve athlete safety, and reduce community resource costs.

Running athletes face a wide range of potential dermatological complications, specific to their respective sport and conditions they compete in. In order to best address this, prevention must not be restricted solely to the level of the athlete's efforts but rather be best implemented and carried out as a whole team approach.

References

1. Miller SL. Ancient Greek athletics. Yale University Press; 2004.
2. Young DS. A brief history of track and field. J Olympic Hist. 2003;11(3):20–3.
3. Collins T. The origins of modern sports: cross-country running in Britain. Routledge; 2013.
4. Noakes TD. Lore of running. 4th ed. Human Kinetics; 2002.
5. Hoffman MD, Wegelin JA. The Western States 100-mile endurance run: participation and performance trends. Med Sci Sports Exerc. 2009;41(12):2191–8.
6. Knechtle B, Nikolaidis PT. Ultramarathon running: pacing, performance, and physiology. Front Physiol. 2018;9:634.
7. Adams BB. Sports dermatology: skin conditions in athletics. Am J Clin Dermatol. 2002;3(7):473–8.
8. Mailler-Savage EA, Adams BB. Skin infections in athletes. Sports Med. 2006;36(10):851–8.
9. Curtis CF, Lewis CJ. Athletes' foot and other tinea pedis infections. Clin Dermatol. 2006;24(3):195–201.
10. Moehrle M. Ultraviolet exposure in the Ironman triathlon. Med Sci Sports Exerc. 2001;33(8):1385–6.
11. Goh CL, Lau PC. Common dermatological conditions in sports. Sports Med Arthrosc Rehabil Ther Technol. 2010;2:33.
12. Weyand PG, Sternlight DB, Bellizzi MJ, Wright S. Faster top running speeds are achieved with greater ground forces not more rapid leg movements. J Appl Physiol. 2000;89(5):1991–9.
13. Adams BB. Dermatologic disorders of the athlete. Am J Sports Med. 2002;30(3):411–20.
14. Bolognia JL, Jorizzo JL, Schaffer JV. Dermatology. 4th ed. Elsevier; 2017.
15. Nigg BM, Yeadon MR. Biomechanical aspects of playing surfaces. J Sports Sci. 1987;5(2):117–45.
16. McMahon TA, Greene PR. Synthetic surfaces for athletic tracks and field events: a biomechanical evaluation. J Biomech. 1979;12(4):301–12.
17. Maughan RJ, Shirreffs SM, Leiper JB. Heat stress and the physiological response to exercise in the heat. Int J Sports Med. 2004;25(Suppl 1):S71–3.
18. McGinnis R. Cold injuries in sport: frostbite and hypothermia. In: Wenzel H, editor. Textbook of sports medicine. Wiley-Blackwell; 2015. p. 295–305.
19. Soter NA, Dinehart SM. Dermatologic considerations in the athlete. In: Greco AJ, editor. Clinical sports medicine. 3rd ed. Elsevier; 2019. p. 142–59.
20. Martens M, Anderson S, Desjardins A, et al. Preventing sports-related skin injuries: friction and blister management. J Sports Med Phys Fitness. 2016;56(1–2):41–7.
21. Smith EW, Maibach HI. Percutaneous penetration enhancers. 2nd ed. Boca Raton: CRC Press; 2005. p. 305–8.
22. Adams BB. Dermatologic disorders of the athlete. Sports Med. 2002;32(5):309–21.
23. Knapik JJ, Reynolds KL, Duplantis KL, Jones BH. Friction blisters: pathophysiology, prevention, and treatment. Sports Med. 1995;20(3):136–47.

24. Hillstrom HJ, Song J, Kraszewski AP, Hafer JF. Footwear and orthotic devices: implications for running injuries. Clin Sports Med. 2020;39(1):93–110.
25. Gilchrest BA, Eller MS, Geller AC, Yaar M. The pathogenesis of melanoma induced by ultraviolet radiation. N Engl J Med. 1999;340(17):1341–8.
26. Wright TI, Spencer JM, Flowers FP. Prevention and treatment of excessive sun exposure in athletes. Sports Med. 2002;32(7):389–94.
27. Papageorgiou PP, Chu AC. Chloracne and acneiform eruptions. In: Burns T, Breathnach S, Cox N, Griffiths C, editors. Rook's textbook of dermatology. 8th ed. Hoboken: Wiley-Blackwell; 2010. p. 73.1–10.
28. Blauvelt A, Ellis CN. Cutaneous frostbite injuries in athletes. Am J Sports Med. 1994;22(1):74–7.
29. Zug KA, Warshaw EM, Fowler JF Jr, Maibach HI, Belsito DV, Pratt MD, et al. Patch-testing North American contact dermatitis group data, 2005–2006. Dermatitis. 2009;20(3):149–60.
30. Pandya AG, Guevara IL. Disorders of hyperpigmentation. Facial Plast Surg Clin North Am. 2004;12(4):407–20.
31. Adams BB. Sports dermatology. New York: Springer; 2006.
32. Likness LP. Common dermatologic infections in athletes and return-to-play guidelines. J Am Osteopath Assoc. 2011;111(6):373–9.
33. Adams BB, Adatto M. Sports dermatology. In: Bolognia JL, Schaffer JV, Cerroni L, editors. Dermatology. 4th ed. Philadelphia: Elsevier; 2018. p. 2052–63.
34. Kuehl KS, Perrier ET. Skin conditions in endurance athletes. Curr Sports Med Rep. 2014;13(5):320–4.
35. Rietschel RL, Fowler JF. Fisher's contact dermatitis. 5th ed. Philadelphia: LippincottWilliams & Wilkins; 2001. p. 1–25.
36. Kockentiet B, Adams BB. Contact dermatitis in athletes. J Am Acad Dermatol. 2007;56(6):1048–55.
37. Fisher AA. Allergic contact dermatitis: practical solutions for sports-related rashes. Phys Sportsmed. 1993;21:65–72.
38. Roberts JL, Hanifin JM. Athletic shoe dermatitis. Contact allergy to ethyl butyl thiourea. JAMA. 1979;241:275–6.
39. Jung JH, McLaughlin JL, Stannard J, Guin JD. Isolation, via activity-directed fractionation, of mercaptobenzothiazole and dibenzothiazyl disulfide as 2 allergensresponsible for tennis shoe dermatitis. Contact Derm. 1988;19:254–9.
40. Camarasa JG. Analgesic spray contact dermatitis. Dermatol Clin. 1990;8:137–8.
41. Vilaplana J, Romaguera C. Allergic contact dermatitis due to eucalyptol in an anti-inflammatory cream. Contact Derm. 2000;43:118.
42. Gamboa P, Jauregui I, Fernandez JC, Antepara I, Urrutia I. Contact sensitization to topical salicylate. Contact Derm. 1995;33:52.
43. Gomez A, Florido JF, Quiralte J, Martin AE, de San S, Pedro B. Allergic contact attdermatitis due to indomethacin and diclofenac. Contact Derm. 2000;43:59.
44. Usatine RP. Contact dermatitis. In: Usatine RP, Smith M, Mayeaux Jr EJ, et al., editors. Color atlas of family medicine. New York: McGraw-Hill; 2009.
45. Ventura MT, Dagnello M, Matino MG, Di Corato R, Giuliano G, Tursi A. Contact dermatitis in students practicing sports: incidence of rubber sensitisation. Br J SportsMed. 2001;35:100–2.
46. Usatine RP, Smith M, Mayeaux EJ Jr, et al. Contact dermatitis. In: Color atlas of family medicine. New York, NY: McGraw-Hill; 2009.
47. Roberts JL, Hanifin JM. Athletic shoe dermatitis: contact allergy to ethyl Butylthiourea. JAMA. 1979;241:275–6.
48. Basler RS. Acne mechanica in athletes. Cutis. 1992;50(2):119–20.
49. Mills OH Jr, Kligman AM. Acne mechanica. Arch Dermatol. 1975;111(4):481–3.
50. Wojtachnio D, Nowakowska I, Bartoszewicz J. Mechanical acne—a review of contributing factors and diagnostic-therapeutic approach. J Educ Health Sport. 2022;12(8):474–81.

51. Hannam S, Smith ML. Environmental and sports-related skin diseases. In: Bolognia JL, Schaffer JV, Cerroni L, editors. Dermatology. 5th ed. Philadelphia: Elsevier; 2025. p. 1585–610.
52. Dreno B, Bettoli V, Perez M, Bouloc A, Ochsendorf F. Cutaneous lesions caused by mechanical injury. Eur J Dermatol. 2015;25(2):114–21.
53. Franks RR. Skin problems in the athlete. In: Madden CC, Putukian M, Young CC, McCarty EC, editors. Netter's sports medicine. 3rd ed. Philadelphia: Elsevier; 2023. p. 305–17.
54. Howe AS, Boden BP. Heat-related illness in athletes. Am J Sports Med. 2007;35(8):1384–95.
55. Lipman GS, Eifling KP, Ellis MA, Gaudio FG, Otten EM, Grissom CK. Wilderness medical society practice guidelines for the prevention and treatment of heat-related illness. Wilderness Environ Med. 2013;24(4):351–61.
56. Descamps V, Claessens YE, Doumenc B, Trotters D. Skin manifestations in ultramarathon runners: experience in the Marathon des Sables 2014. Br J Dermatol. 2017;177(2):562–3.
57. Habif TP. Clinical dermatology: a color guide to diagnosis and therapy. 4th ed. St. Louis, MO: Mosby; 2004. p. 162–94.
58. Seto CK. Environmental illness in athletes. Clin Sports Med. 2005;24:695–718.
59. Gauer R, Meyers BK. Heat-related illnesses. Am Fam Physician. 2019;99(8):482–9.
60. Pharis DB, Teller C, Wolf JE. Cutaneous manifestations of sports participation. J Am Acad Dermatol. 1997;36:448–59.
61. Basler RSW. Skin lesions related to sports activity. Prim Care. 1983;10:479–94.
62. Levine N. Dermatologic aspects of sports medicine. J Am Acad Dermatol. 1980;3:415–24.
63. Atton AV, Tunnessen WW. The athlete and his skin. Clin Rev Allergy. 1988;6:403–29.
64. Basler RSW. Sports-related skin injuries. In: Callen JP, Dahl MV, Golitz LE, et al., editors. Advances in dermatology, vol. 4. Chicago: Year Book Medical Publishers; 1989. p. 29–50.
65. Kantor GR, Bergfeld WF. Common and uncommon dermatologic diseases related to sports activities. Exerc Sport Sci Rev. 1988;16:215–53.
66. Hershkowitz M. Penile frostbite, an unforeseen hazard of jogging. N Engl J Med. 1977;292:178.
67. Washburn B. Frostbite: what it is, how to prevent it, emergency treatment. N Engl J Med. 1962;266:974–89.
68. Pugh LG. Cold stress and muscular exercise, with special reference to accidental hypothermia. Br Med J. 1967;1:333–7.
69. Dover JS. Sports dermatology. In: Fitzpatrick TB, Eisen AZ, Wolff K, et al., editors. Dermatology in general medicine. New York: McGraw-Hill; 1991. p. 1617–23.
70. Hallam MJ, Cubison T, Dheansa B, et al. Managing frostbite. BMJ. 2010;341:c5864.
71. Meffert JJ. Environmental skin diseases and the impact of common dermatoses on medical readiness. Dermatol Clin. 1999;17:1–17.
72. Adams BB. Sports dermatology. Dermatol Nurs. 2001;13:347–63.
73. Basler RSW. Skin injuries in sports medicine. J Am Acad Dermatol. 1989;21:1257–62.
74. Pugh LG. Clothing insulation and accidental hypothermia in youth. Nature. 1966;209:1281–6.
75. Fisher AA. Sports-related cutaneous reactions, part I: dermatoses due to physicalagents. Cutis. 1999;63:134–6.
76. Mikhailov P, Berova N, Andreev VC. Physical urticaria and sport. Cutis. 1977;20(381–4):389–90.
77. De Luca JF, Adams BB, Yosipovitch G. Skin manifestations of athletes competing in the summer Olympics: what a sports medicine physician should know. Sports Med. 2012;42(5):399–413.
78. Mailler-Savage EA, Adams BB. Skin manifestations of running. J Am Acad Dermatol. 2006;55(2):290–301.
79. Nichols AW. Exercise-induced anaphylaxis and urticaria. Clin Sports Med. 1992;11:303–12.
80. Carr PC, Cropley TG. Sports dermatology: skin disease in athletes. Clin Sports Med. 2019;38(4):597–618.

81. Lawlor F, Black AK, Breathnach AS, Greaves MW. Vibratory angioedema: lesion induction, clinical features, laboratory and ultrastructural findings, and response to therapy. Br J Dermatol. 1989;120:93–9.
82. Patterson R, Mellies CJ, Blankenship ML, Pruzansky JJ. Vibratory angioedema: a hereditary type of physical hypersensitivity. J Allergy Clin Immunol. 1972;50:174–86.
83. Gerth van Wijk R, Roovers MH, Dieges PH. Exercise-dependent anaphylaxis. Ned Tijdschr Geneeskd. 1991;135:2293–5.
84. Shadick NA, Liang MH, Partridge AJ, et al. The natural history of exercise-induced anaphylaxis: survey results from a 10-year follow-up study. J Allergy Clin Immunol. 1999;104:123–7.
85. Wade JP, Liang MH, Sheffer AL. Exercise-induced anaphylaxis: epidemiologic observations. Prog Clin Biol Res. 1989;297:175–82.
86. Volcheck GW, Li JT. Exercise-induced urticaria and anaphylaxis. Mayo Clin Proc. 1997;72(2):140–7.
87. Lee HB, Ahn IS, Choi JH, et al. A case of wheat-dependent exercise-induced anaphylaxis. Ann Dermatol. 2009;21:447–9.
88. Adams BB. Exercise-induced anaphylaxis in a marathon runner. Int J Dermatol. 2002;41(5):394–6.
89. Simons FE, Ebisawa M, Sanchez-Borges M, et al. 2015 Update of the evidence base: World allergy organization anaphylaxis guidelines. World Allergy Organ J. 2015;8:32.
90. Muraro A, Roberts G, Worm M, et al. Anaphylaxis: guidelines from the European academy of allergy and clinical immunology. Allergy. 2014;69:1026–45.
91. Pravettoni V, Incorvaia C. Diagnosis of exercise-induced anaphylaxis: current insights. J Asthma Allergy. 2016;9:191–8.
92. Romano A, Di Fonso M, Giuffreda F, et al. Diagnostic work-up for food-dependent, exercise-induced anaphylaxis. Allergy. 1995;50:817–24.
93. Schwartz LB, Delgado L, Craig T, et al. Exercise-induced hypersensitivity syndromes in recreational and competitive athletes: a PRACTALL consensus report (what the general practitioner should know about sports and allergy). Allergy. 2008;63:953–61.
94. Shyam N, Cohen BA. Oral cavity. In: Cohen BA, editor. Pediatric dermatology. 5th ed. Philadelphia: W.B. Saunders; 2022. p. 260–85.
95. Shih BB, Farrar MD, Cooke MS, Osman J, Langton AK, Kift R, Webb AR, Berry JL, Watson REB, Vail A, de Gruijl FR, Rhodes LE. Fractional sunburn threshold UVR doses generate equivalent vitamin D and DNA damage in skin types I-VI but with epidermal DNA damage gradient correlated to skin darkness. J Invest Dermatol. 2018;138(10):2244–52. https://doi.org/10.1016/j.jid.2018.04.003.
96. Mancuso JB, Maruthi R, Wang SQ, Lim HW. Sunscreens: an update. Am J Clin Dermatol. 2017;18(5):643–50. https://doi.org/10.1007/s40257-017-0317-1.
97. Seité S, Fourtanier A, Moyal D, Young AR. Photodamage to human skin by suberythemal exposure to solar ultraviolet radiation can be attenuated by sunscreens: a review. Br J Dermatol. 2010;163(5):903–14. https://doi.org/10.1111/j.1365-2133.2010.09894.x.
98. Lopes DM, McMahon SB. Ultraviolet radiation on the skin: a painful experience? CNS Neurosci Ther. 2016;22(2):118–26. https://doi.org/10.1111/cns.12451.
99. Dawes JM, Calvo M, Perkins JR, Paterson KJ, Kiesewetter H, Hobbs C, Kaan TK, Orengo C, Bennett DL, McMahon SB. CXCL5 mediates UVB irradiation-induced pain. Sci Transl Med. 2011;3(90):90ra60. https://doi.org/10.1126/scitranslmed.3002147.
100. Bishop T, Marchand F, Young AR, Lewin GR, McMahon SB. Ultraviolet-B-induced mechanical hyperalgesia: a role for peripheral sensitisation. Pain. 2010;150(1):141–52. https://doi.org/10.1016/j.pain.2010.03.018.
101. Purim KS, Leite N. Sports-related dermatoses among road runners in Southern Brazil. An Bras Dermatol. 2014;89(4):587–92.
102. Guerra KC, Crane JS. Sunburn. In: StatPearls [Internet]. Treasure Island (FL): StatPearls Publishing; 2023 [cited 2024 Dec 29]. Available from: https://www.statpearls.com.
103. Conklin RJ. Common cutaneous disorders in athletes. Sports Med. 1990;9(2):100–19.

104. Adams BB. Skin and sports: common skin conditions in athletes and tips on treatments. Skin Aging. 2003;11(2):65–70.
105. Houston SD, Knox JM. Skin problems related to sports and recreational activities. Cutis. 1977;19(5):487–91.
106. Gloster HM Jr, Brodland DG. The epidemiology of skin cancer. Dermatologic Surg. 1996;22(3):217–26.
107. D'Acri AM, Bakos RM, Purim KSM. Dermatoses no esporte. In: Lupi O, Cunha PR, editors. Rotinas de diagnóstico e tratamento da Sociedade Brasileira de Dermatologia. 2nd ed. Itapevi (SP): AC Farmacêutica; 2012. p. 165–9.
108. Bakos RM, Wagner MB, Bakos L, Derose EH, Grangeiro Neto JA. Queimaduras e hábitos solares em um grupo de atletas brasileiros. Rev Bras Med Esporte. 2006;12(5):275–8.
109. Purim KSM, Leite N. Fotoproteção e exercício físico. Rev Bras Med Esporte. 2010;16:224–9.
110. Ambros-Rudolph CM, Hofmann-Wellenhof R, Richtig E, Müller-Fürstner M, Soyer HP, Kerl H. Malignant melanoma in marathon runners. Arch Dermatol. 2006;142(11):1471–4. https://doi.org/10.1001/archderm.142.11.1471.
111. Garbe C, Buttner P, Weiss J, et al. Risk factors for developing cutaneous melanoma and criteria for identifying persons at risk: multicenter case-control study of the Central Malignant Melanoma Registry of the German Dermatological Society. J Invest Dermatol. 1994;102(5):695–9.
112. Hall JC, editor. Sauer's manual of skin diseases. 11th ed. Philadelphia: Wolters Kluwer; 2016.
113. Fisher AA. Sports-related cutaneous reactions, part III: sports identification marks. Cutis. 1999;63:256–8.
114. Basler RSW, Jacobs SI. Athlete's nodules [letter reply]. J Am Acad Dermatol. 1991;24:318.
115. Uchiyama M, Tsuboi R, Mitsuhashi Y. Athlete's nodule. J Dermatol. 2009;36:608–11.
116. Eiland G, Ridley D. Dermatological problems in the athlete. J Orthop Sports Phys Ther. 1996;23(6):388–402.
117. Mistiaen P, van Halm-Walters M. Prevention and treatment of intertrigo in large skin folds of adults: a systematic review. BMC Nursing [Internet]. 2010;9(1):1–9.
118. Janniger CK, Schwartz RA, Szepietowski JC, Reich A. Intertrigo and common secondary skin infections. Am Family Physician [Internet]. 2005;72(5):833–8.
119. Verzì AE, Nasca MR, Dall'Oglio F, Cosentino C, Micali G. A novel treatment of intertrigo in athletes and overweight subjects. J Cosmet Dermatol. 2021;20(S1):23–7.
120. Scheer BV, Reljic D, Murray A, Costa RJS. The enemy of the feet: blisters in ultraendurance runners. J Amer Podiatric Med Assoc. 2014;104(5):473–8.
121. Worthing RM, Percy RL, Joslin JD. Prevention of friction blisters in outdoor pursuits: a systematic review. Wilderness Environ Med. 2017;28(2):139–49.
122. Grouios G. Corns and calluses in athletes' feet: a cause for concern. Foot. 2004;14(4):175–84.
123. Grouios G. Footedness as a potential factor that contributes to the causation of corn and callus formation in lower extremities of physically active individuals. Foot. 2005;15(3):154–62.
124. Freeman DB. Corns and calluses resulting from mechanical hyperkeratosis. Am Family Physician. 2002;65(11):2277–80.
125. Baran R, Kechijian P. Longitudinal melanonychia (melanonychia striata): diagnosis and management. J Am Acad Dermatol. 1989;21(6):1165–75.
126. Baran R. Frictional longitudinal Melanonychia: a new entity. Dermatology. 1987;174(6):280–4.
127. Singal A, Bisherwal K. Melanonychia: etiology, diagnosis, and treatment. Indian Dermatol Online J [Internet]. 2020;11(1):1–11.
128. Paller AS, Mancini AJ. Disorders of hair and nails. Elsevier eBooks; 2011. p. 130–66.
129. Beiner JM, Jokl P. Muscle contusion injuries: current treatment options. J Am Acad Orthop Surg [Internet]. 2001;9(4):227–37.
130. Child Abuse and Neglect E-Book [Internet]. Google Books. 2024 [cited 2024 Dec 31].
131. Barnes MJ, Lomiwes DD, David MS. An experimental model of contusion injury in humans. PLoS One. 2022;17(11):e0277765.

132. Shrestha R, Krishan K, Ishaq H, Kanchan T. Abrasion [Internet]. Nih.gov. StatPearls Publishing; 2023 [cited 2024 Dec 31].
133. Forsch RT. Essentials of skin laceration repair. Am Fam Physician [Internet]. 2008;78(8):945–51.
134. Turkmani MG. Piezogenic pedal papules treated successfully with Deoxycholic acid injection. JAAD Case Rep. 2018;4(6):582–3.
135. Brown F, Cook C. Piezogenic Pedal Papule [Internet]. PubMed. Treasure Island (FL): StatPearls Publishing; 2022.
136. Redbord KP, Adams BB. Piezogenic pedal papules in a marathon runner. Clinical J Sport Med. 2006;16(1):81–3.
137. Doukas DJ, Holmes J, Leonard JA. A nonsurgical approach to painful Piezogenic pedal papules. Cutis. 2004;73(5):339–46.
138. King MJ. Dermatologic problems in podiatric sports medicine. Clin Podiatr Med Surg. 1997;14(3):511–24.
139. Wilkinson DS. Black heel a minor hazard of sport. Cutis [Internet]. 1977;20(3):393–6.
140. Karthikeyan K, Keerthi S, Madhavi S. Talon noir: a mirage of melanoma. Pigment Int. 2015;2(1):54.
141. Martin SB, Lucas JK, Posa M, Howell DM, Kelly MN. Talon Noir in a young baseball player: a case report. J Pediatr Health Care. 2021;35(2):235–8.
142. Akella A, Daniel AR, Gould MB, Mangal R, Ganti L. Subungual hematoma. Cureus. 2023;15(11):e48952.
143. Salter SA, Ciocon DH, Gowrishankar TR, Kimball AB. Controlled nail trephination for subungual hematoma. Am J Emerg Med. 2006;24(7):875–7.
144. León-Muiños E, Monteagudo-Sánchez B, Dutta A, Ghosh SK, Das A, Mishra V, et al. Images. Indian Pediatr. 2014;51(8):677–80.
145. Lee DK, Lipner SR. Optimal diagnosis and management of common nail disorders. Ann Med. 2022;54(1):694–712.
146. Salgado F, Handler MZ, Schwartz RA. Shedding light on Onychomadesis. Cutis [Internet]. 2017;99(1):33–6.
147. Sous D, Starace MVR, Chen L, Nieman EL, Anadkat MJ, Piraccini BM, et al. Recurrent Onychomadesis of the Toenails in children and adults: a case series. Skin Appendage Disord. 2021;8(1):31–3.
148. Geizhals S, Lipner SR. Review of onychocryptosis: epidemiology, pathogenesis, risk factors, diagnosis and treatment. Dermatol Online J. 2019;25(9):13030/qt9985w2n0.
149. Rook's Textbook of Dermatology [Internet]. Google Books. 2014 [cited 2024 Dec 31].
150. Pico AMP, Verjano E, Mayordomo R. Relation between nail consistency and incidence of ingrown toenails in young male runners. J Am Podiatr Med Assoc. 2017;107(2):137–43.
151. Khunger N, Kandhari R. Ingrown toenails. Indian J Dermatol Venereol Leprol. 2012;78(3):279.
152. Pujalte GGA, Costa LMC, Clapp AD, Presutti RJ, Sluzevich JC. More than skin deep: dermatologic conditions in athletes. Sports Health. 2023;15(1):74–85.
153. Nowicka D, Bagłaj-Oleszczuk M, Maj J. Infectious diseases of the skin in contact sports. Adv Clin Exp Med. 2020;29(12):1491–5.
154. Palaniappan V, Murthy AB, Karthikeyan K. Pitted keratolysis. Clin Exp Dermatol. 2023;48(9):978–83.
155. Fernández-Crehuet P, Ruiz-Villaverde R. Pitted keratolysis: an infective cause of foot odour. CMAJ. 2015;187(7):519.
156. Peterson AR, Nash E, Anderson BJ. Infectious disease in contact sports. Sports Health. 2019;11(1):47–58.
157. Esterowitz D, Greer KE, Cooper PH, Edlich RF. Plantar warts in the athlete. Am J Emerg Med. 1995;13(4):441–3.
158. Auger P, Marquis G, Joly J, Attye A. Epidemiology of tinea pedis in marathon runners: prevalence of occult athlete's foot. Mycoses. 1993;36(1–2):35–41.

159. Lacroix C, Baspeyras M, de La Salmonière P, Benderdouche M, Couprie B, Accoceberry I, Weill FX, Derouin F, Feuilhade de Chauvin M. Tinea Pedis in European marathon runners. J Eur Acad Dermatol Venereol. 2002;16(2):139–42.
160. Powell FC. Sports dermatology. J Eur Acad Dermatol Venereol. 1994;3:1–15.
161. Field LA, Adams BB. Tinea Pedis in athletes. Int J Dermatol. 2008;47(5):485–92.
162. Adams BB. Skin infections in athletes. Dermatol Nurs. 2008;20(1):39–44. PMID: 18380294
163. Daggett C, Brodell RT, Daniel CR, Jackson J. Onychomycosis in athletes. Am J Clin Dermatol. 2019;20(5):691–8.
164. Jud P, Hafner F. Exercise-induced vasculitis. CMAJ. 2018;190(7):E195.
165. Ramelet AA. Exercise-induced vasculitis. J Eur Acad Dermatol Venereol. 2006;20(4):423–7.
166. Adams BB. Sports dermatology. Adolesc Med. 2001;12(2):vii:305–22.
167. Freiman A, Barankin B, Elpern DJ. Sports dermatology part 1: common dermatoses. CMAJ. 2004;171(8):851–3.
168. Bassiri-Jahromi S, Sadeghi G, Paskiaee FA. Evaluation of the association of superficial dermatophytosis and athletic activities with special reference to its prevention and control. Int J Dermatol. 2010;49(10):1159–64.
169. Zinder SM, Basler RSW, Foley J, Scarlata C, Vasily DB. National athletic trainers' association position statement: skin diseases. J Athl Train. 2010;45(4):411–28.
170. Sedgwick PE, Dexter WW, Smith CT. Bacterial dermatoses in sports. Clin Sports Med. 2007;26(3):383–96.
171. Krabak BJ, Waite B, Lipman G. Injury and illnesses prevention for ultramarathoners. Curr Sports Med Rep. 2013;12(3):183–9.
172. Breslow RG, Giberson-Chen CC, Roberts WO. Burden of injury and illness in the road race medical tent: a narrative review. Clin J Sport Med. 2021;31(6):e499–505.

Chapter 4
Winter Sports

Daniel Green, Kristen Dean, Lea Tordjman, Ryan Scheinkman, Alexia Vignau, Rachel Summers, Rachel Cohen, Samuel San Antonio, and Keyvan Nouri

4.1 Introduction

Winter sports encompass a variety of sports, including skiing, snowboarding, sledding, snowshoeing, skating, hockey, and other sports performed in alpine and winter conditions. Winter sports expose athletes to a unique set of dermatological challenges. These activities combine harsh environmental factors, such as intense ultraviolet (UV) radiation at high altitudes and cold, dry air, with the physical demands of wearing insulated, moisture-retentive gear. Such conditions increase the risk of skin damage, ranging from sunburn and eczema flares to infections and inflammatory exacerbations. It is an especially prescient topic as winter sports continue to grow in popularity. One report discloses that participation in winter sports has increased in recent years. In the 2022–23 winter season, nearly 10% of the U.S. population aged six and older, engaged in winter sports activities [1]. Understanding these risks is essential for athletes to adopt effective preventive measures to ensure their skin health while enjoying their outdoor pursuits. Athletes can mitigate dermatological risks through preventive strategies, such as using broad-spectrum sunscreen, wearing properly fitted moisture-wicking gear, and maintaining proper hygiene. As winter sports continue to grow in popularity, spreading awareness and emphasizing the importance of skin protection will be vital in safeguarding athletes'

Daniel Green, Kristen Dean and Lea Tordjman contributed equally with all other contributors.

D. Green · K. Dean · L. Tordjman · R. Scheinkman (✉) · A. Vignau · R. Summers · R. Cohen
S. S. Antonio · K. Nouri
Dr. Phillip Frost Department of Dermatology and Cutaneous Surgery, University of Miami, Miami, FL, USA
e-mail: dag258@med.miami.edu; kkd45@med.miami.edu; lat91@med.miami.edu; scheinkman@med.miami.edu; axv200@med.miami.edu; rachelcohen@med.miami.edu; sxs3273@miami.edu; knouri@med.miami.edu

K. Nouri (ed.), *Sport-Related Skin Conditions*,
https://doi.org/10.1007/978-3-031-90444-8_4

dermatological health and enhancing their overall performance and enjoyment in these activities.

4.2 Environmental Exposures

4.2.1 UV Exposure and Skin Cancer Risk in Winter Sports

The practice of winter sports, including skiing and snowboarding, greatly increases ultraviolet (UV) exposure and the associated risk of skin cancer [2]. UV levels rise by approximately 10% for every 1000 meters of altitude [2]. This risk is intensified by the snows high reflectance (up to 80% of UV radiation), compared to 15% from dry beach sand and 25% from sea foam [2]. Consequently, individuals participating in winter sports face elevated UV radiation, both from direct sunlight and from intense reflections off snow and ice. Research indicates that skiers can experience severe sunburn in as little as six minutes of unprotected UV exposure at altitudes of 11,000 feet [3]. Despite a general awareness of these risks, compliance with sun protection practices remains significantly low [4]. A survey of 4837 adult skiers and snowboarders across 28 high-altitude ski areas revealed that only 4.4% adhered to comprehensive sunscreen guidelines [4]. While nearly half of the participants reported using sunscreen with an SPF of 15 or higher, only 20.4% re-applied it as recommended every two hours [4]. Compliance dropped during inclement weather and on low-UV days, highlighting significant gaps in protective behaviors, especially among male athletes and those who underestimate the seriousness of skin cancer [4]. To address these challenges, effective outreach and education on sun protection for winter sports participants are essential. Implementing preventive measures—such as regular application of broad-spectrum sunscreen with an SPF of 30 or higher, reapplication every two hours, and wearing protective clothing—can significantly enhance skin safety for winter sports enthusiasts [4]. As winter sports and high-altitude skiing become increasingly popular, educating athletes about sun protective strategies is essential to mitigate the risks of UV exposure and safeguard skin health, ultimately reducing the incidence of skin cancer in this vulnerable population.

4.2.2 Chilblains (Pernio) & Frostbite

Hypothermia can cause redness and numbness as skin temperature drops, potentially leading to cell death. Gradual rewarming and systemic monitoring are necessary to prevent deeper tissue damage [5]. However, if left untreated Chilblains may develop. Chilblains are a consequence of an abnormal vascular response, resulting after the initial vasoconstriction due to cold. Upon the rewarming of the skin the blood vessels dilate unevenly; causing endothelial damage and vascular leakage [6]. Symptoms manifest as itchy, red or purple swellings on the extremities after cold exposure and may persist for days to weeks; blistering may also develop. Management includes gradual warming, protective moisturizers, and topical corticosteroids or oral nifedipine for severe cases [7]. Frostbite is a severe condition marked by numbness, tingling, and a waxy, hard texture on affected areas. It occurs as a result of tissues being exposed to temperatures at or below freezing point, ~0 °C, for a sustained period of time [8]. Tissue necrosis can result due to ischemia, due to the constriction of blood vessels, usually in the extremities, to preserve core body temperature (Fig. 4.1).

Additional damage is caused by the formation of ice crystals with exposure to freezing temperature; further damaging cells. Common body parts that are affected include toes, fingers, feet, and the nose. Symptoms usually manifest as tingling and/or a numbness sensation; as well as red or pale skin, waxy or hard texture in affected areas, and, in severe cases, skin blistering. In recent times, the presentation of frostbite has increased, mainly among those who partake in winter sports such as skiing,

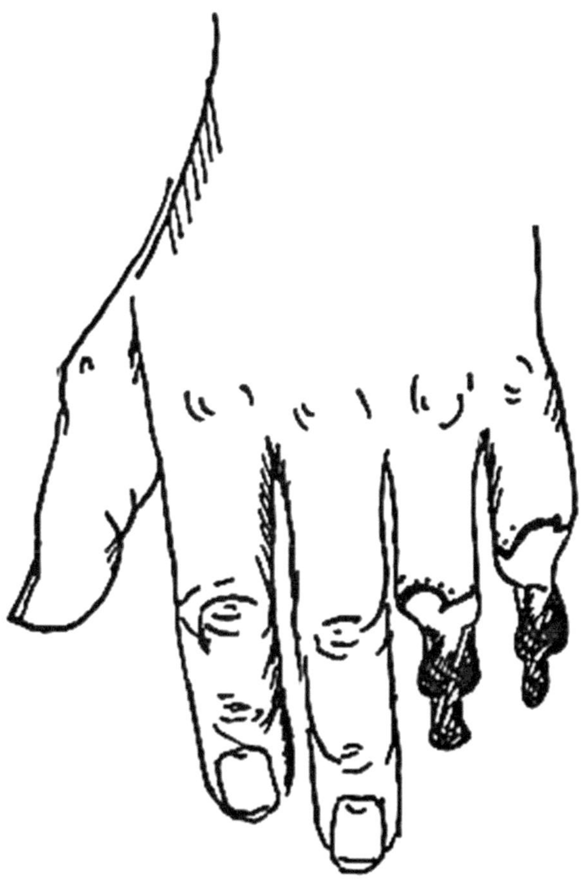

Fig. 4.1 Frostbite physical exam Findings

hiking, mountain and ice climbing; and especially among young adults [9]. Treatment involves rapid rewarming of frostbitten areas with warm water, pain management, wound care, and in severe cases, surgical intervention to remove necrotic tissue. As such, recovery from frostbite can range from complete resolution without significant sequelae to major limb amputation and its functional consequences [8].

4.3 Allergies/Irritation

While subzero temperatures are a prerequisite to participating in winter sports such as skiing, snowboarding, snowshoeing and sledding, such temperatures increase the risk for dermatologic allergies and irritations. Winter sports equipment such as helmets, goggles, boots, and multiple layers of clothing play a contributory role in symptom manifestations or flares in dermatologic risks (summarized in Table 4.1).

4.3.1 Eczema Flares

Winter sports exacerbate eczema flares due to the harsh environmental conditions athletes endure. Cold air, low humidity, and prolonged exposure to wind can lead to significant transepidermal water loss (TEWL), disrupting the skin barrier and triggering inflammatory processes [10, 11]. Additionally, the friction and occlusion of the skin barrier by heavy, insulated gear, can exacerbate irritation, especially in individuals with preexisting atopic dermatitis. Eczema in winter athletes often presents as erythematous, pruritic plaques with scaling or lichenification, commonly

Table 4.1 Allergies/Irritation associated with winter sports

Disease/ Condition	Symptoms and physical exam findings	Treatment recommendations
Eczema Flares	Erythematous, pruritic plaques with scaling or lichenification	Regular use of emollients, topical corticosteroids, moisture-wicking fabric
Contact Dermatitis	Erythematous, edematous plaques with vesiculation or scaling	Avoidance of irritant and topical corticosteroids or emmolients
Cold Urticaria	Erythematous, raised, and pruritic lesions	Antihistamines. Corticosteroids in severe presentations
Acne Mechanica	Comedones, papules, and pustules in areas of repetitive friction	Reduce friction. Benzoyl peroxide, salicylic acid, or retinoids. Oral antibiotics in severe presentations
Hyperkeratosis	Rough, thickened, scaly patches often on heels or sides of toes	Reduce friction. Mechanical debridement of the thickened area or use of topical keratolytic agents in severe presentations.

presenting on exposed skin areas, such as the face, hands, and neck [10]. Diagnosis is typically clinical, which typically includes a patient history of recurrent flares during colder months. Treatment includes regular use of emollients to restore the skin barrier, topical corticosteroids to reduce inflammation, and protective measures such as layering moisture-wicking fabrics under sports gear to decrease the amount of direct skin irritation. Preventive strategies are vital to managing eczema flares, which can include avoiding prolonged exposure to cold temperatures and applying hypoallergenic moisturizers immediately after activity [11].

4.3.2 *Contact Dermatitis*

Contact dermatitis is an inflammatory dermatologic condition that is caused by irritants or allergens present on surfaces or in the environment. In the context of winter sports, athletes may experience contact dermatitis from various equipment, clothing or environmental exposures. Materials such as rubber in ski goggles, adhesives in helmet padding, or nickel in gear buckles may act as common triggers in skiers, snowboarders, or snowshoers that use such equipment [12]. While contact dermatitis can occur in any temperature, it is particularly exacerbated by below-freezing temperatures that coincide with winter sports. Irritant contact dermatitis (ICD) is more common and arises from friction, occlusion, or direct exposure to chemicals. Allergic contact dermatitis (ACD) occurs when sensitized individuals encounter specific allergens. Athletes may develop erythematous, edematous plaques with vesiculation or scaling localized to areas in contact with the irritant or allergen [10]. Diagnosis is based on clinical history and patch testing to identify allergens. Treatment focuses on avoidance of the offending substance and use of topical corticosteroids or emollients to soothe affected areas. Athletes should ensure their gear is well-fitted and made from hypoallergenic materials. Antiperspirants or moisture-wicking liners can help reduce sweating, which often exacerbates ICD [12].

4.3.3 *Cold Urticaria*

Cold urticaria, also known as cold-induced hives, is a skin reaction characterized by the development of wheals or hives after exposure to cold temperatures, such as those encountered in winter sports [12]. This condition is triggered by rapid cooling of the skin, which results in the release of histamine and other inflammatory mediators from mast cells, which can lead to erythematous, raised, and pruritic lesions. Skiing, snowboarding, or snowshoeing athletes are particularly susceptible as they are frequently exposed to cold, windy, and wet conditions, all of which can provoke or exacerbate skin reactions [12, 13]. Cold urticaria can vary in severity, ranging from mild localized itching to more widespread rashes affecting large areas of the body. Diagnosis of cold urticaria is typically based on clinical symptomatology, including a history of cold exposure leading to the appearance of hives [13]. In some cases, a cold stimulation test is employed to confirm this diagnosis. If hives are present after exposing the skin to ice or cold water for a few minutes, the diagnosis is confirmed [12]. Management of cold urticaria includes the use of antihistamines for itching and swelling symptoms [13]. Severe presentations of cold urticaria may require corticosteroids or other immunomodulatory therapies. Athletes with known cold urticaria should be educated on this condition. For example, patients should be advised to avoid prolonged exposure to cold environments, wear insulated and moisture-wicking clothing, and carry antihistamines to either prevent or reduce symptom severity. Management of cold urticaria is particularly necessary when participating in winter sports to minimize symptoms and any discomfort while exposed to low temperature conditions required for winter sports.

4.3.4 Acne Mechanica

Acne mechanica is a form of acne vulgaris as a result of repetitive friction, pressure, and occlusion of the skin, that is common in athletes who wear tight, protective gear during physical activity [13]. Winter sports such as skiing and snowboarding, which involve the use of helmets, goggles, thermal attire and other equipment, serve as surrogates for such friction against the skin, and thus constitute frequent triggers of acne mechanica. The combination of physical contact with equipment with heat and moisture from perspiration, can lead to occluded pores and inflammation of the pilosebaceous units, resulting in the formation of comedones, papules, and pustules. Such skin reactions typically appear in areas where gear contacts the skin (e.g., forehead, chin, and jawline) due to the mechanism of friction and contact with equipment [13, 14].

Acne mechanica is primarily diagnosed based on a detailed history of gear use and the distribution of lesions. Patterns of lesions consistent with acne mechanica are often confined to areas of repetitive friction [13]. Treatment of this condition involves addressing the primary cause by reducing friction and moisture. Additional approaches for topical acne therapy such as benzoyl peroxide, salicylic acid, or retinoids may also help alleviate symptoms [13]. In more severe cases, oral antibiotics like doxycycline may be prescribed. In addition to these measures, athletes should be encouraged to cleanse their skin immediately after activity, ensure proper-fitting gear, and to use breathable materials while participating in high-risk activities, such as winter sports, to reduce friction and moisture buildup. Limiting prolonged use of occlusive equipment can also prevent flare-ups of acne mechanica; however, for athletes this may not always be possible and medications may be more feasible for managing symptoms while allowing patients to participate in their respective sports.

4.3.5 *Hyperkeratosis*

Hyperkeratosis can be described as a thicker outer layer of the skin (stratum corneum) that is a protective response to repeated friction, pressure, or environmental irritation. In winter athletes, hyperkeratosis commonly develops on the feet due to constant pressure from ski/snowboard/snowshoe boots [13, 14]. Hyperkeratotic lesions manifest as rough, thickened patches of skin, often appearing on the heels, or sides of the toes. While generally benign, hyperkeratosis can cause discomfort and may predispose athletes to other complications, such as blisters or calluses, if not managed properly. The diagnosis of hyperkeratosis is clinical, based on the macroscopic appearance of thickened, scaly skin, typically without any signs of infection [13]. For winter sports athletes, prevention involves wearing well-fitted gear that does not create excessive pressure on the skin. The use of moisture-wicking and cushioning materials in high-friction areas, and regular exfoliation or moisturizing these areas can help to maintain skin flexibility and reduce the formation of hyperkeratotic lesions. If hyperkeratosis becomes severe or symptomatic, treatment may include mechanical debridement of the thickened area or the use of topical keratolytic agents, such as salicylic acid. For athletes, minimizing friction through proper gear and keeping up with skincare regimens, as described, is key to preventing and managing hyperkeratosis.

4.4 Infections

Winter sports like skiing, snowboarding, snowshoeing, and sledding have increased infection risks due to extended periods in damp, insulated clothing and increased use of shared indoor spaces such as ski lodges [14, 15]. The cold weather also compromises the skin barrier, making athletes more susceptible to bacterial, fungal, viral, and yeast infections. Equipment and locker rooms in these sports, similar to warm-weather settings, serve as transmission points for infectious pathogens [13, 14].

4.4.1 *Bacterial Infections*

Bacterial infections in winter athletes are often influenced by a combination of heavy clothing that traps moisture and prolonged use of shared facilities. Cuts and abrasions from falls or equipment use can facilitate bacterial entry [15]. Staphylococcal infections are especially prevalent due to crowded ski resorts and close-contact training facilities. Impetigo is a highly contagious bacterial infection commonly caused by Staphylococcus aureus or Streptococcus pyogenes [16]. It can also be caused by methicillin-resistant Staphylococcus aureus (MRSA) infection which is much more serious. One study showed that 70% of team members with MRSA required hospitalization and intravenous antibiotics [17]. In winter sports, impetigo transmission is facilitated by shared helmets, goggles, and other equipment. The damp, insulated clothing can lead to skin maceration, increasing the risk of bacterial invasion. Impetigo presents as erythematous macules that evolve into vesicles or pustules [13]. These eventually rupture and form honey-colored crusts. They are often formed around the nose and mouth due to frequent facial exposure to equipment [16]. In cold-weather athletes, lesions may spread rapidly in areas under gear. A thorough history and clinical examination for impetigo is usually enough for the clinician to make a diagnosis, but a bacterial culture can confirm S. aureus or S. pyogenes involvement [13]. First-line treatment for impetigo is topical mupirocin thrice daily for 10 days [13]. To prevent spread, athletes should avoid sharing personal items, and surfaces should be disinfected. They can return to sports 72 hours after starting treatment if there are no moist exudative or draining oozing lesions [13].

Folliculitis is an inflammation of hair follicles often caused by Stapholococcus aureus infection [14]. It is common in winter sports where insulated gear creates warm, moist conditions [18]. This setting fosters bacterial proliferation, particularly in areas where friction from tight clothing or equipment traps sweat. Folliculitis appears as erythematous papules or pustules at the follicular openings [18]. In cold-weather athletes, it frequently affects the thighs, buttocks, and back, where skin contacts moisture-retentive gear. It can also turn into non-healing crusted sores anywhere on the skin except the palms and soles [13]. Clinical assessment for folliculitis is usually sufficient; however, bacterial culture may help rule out resistant organisms if the condition does not improve with treatment [13]. Treatment for folliculitits is typically Cephalexin 500 mg per oral four times daily for 7–10 days [15]. It is recommended for athletes to not shave over the infectious area during treatment and healing. Small lesions can also be treated with warm compresses four times daily, and large lesions can be treated with incision, drainage, and a wound culture obtained [13]. Athletes may return to play after 48 hours of no new lesions and at least 72 hours of antibiotic therapy [14].

An infected hair follicle that forms a perifollicular abscess is called a furuncle, and a carbuncle then forms from a collection of furuncles [14]. The deeper infections of furunculosis and carbuncles are also linked to S. aureus infection [16]. They can develop in winter athletes due to the constant pressure and friction from heavy, damp equipment. The shared facilities promote further bacterial spread, especially during prolonged indoor recovery times. Furuncles are painful, firm nodules with erythema, often evolving into pustules with a central necrotic core [15]. They typically form as an abscess within the hair follicle [13]. Carbuncles are larger clusters of furuncles involving multiple hair follicles and surrounding tissue. They are typically seen in areas subject to friction, such as the back, neck, and thighs [13]. Diagnosis of these conditions typically relies on clinical appearance, with cultures as needed for resistant strains or recurrent infections [15]. Treatment for furunculosis and carbuncles includes warm compresses four times daily [16]. For larger lesions, incision and drainage with systemic antibiotics is recommended. Antibiotics include mupirocin twice daily and dicloxacillin 500 mg thrice daily [16]. Athletes should avoid equipment that exacerbates friction until lesions heal. Athletes can return to competition after 72 hours of antibiotic therapy [13].

4.4.2 *Fungal and Dermatophyte Infections*

The fungal infections faced by winter athletes are often due to damp environments and the use of moisture-retentive, insulated clothing [14]. Fungal infections like Tinea pedis, Tinea cruris, and Onychomycosis thrive in these conditions, particularly within locker rooms or boot linings [13]. Tinea pedis is a dermatophyte infection caused by Trichophyton species that is common in athletes due to moist environments [14]. In winter sports, the prolonged use of insulated, moisture-trapping footwear promotes this fungal growth. Tinea pedis often presents as pruritic, fairly erythematous scaling plaques, particularly in the interdigital spaces [18]. In more severe cases, vesiculobullous lesions can appear on the plantar surface. In cold-weather athletes, symptoms can worsen due to prolonged moisture exposure in their gloves and boots. Clinical examination is generally sufficient, but a direct examination with a 10% or 20% KOH preparation or fungal culture can confirm dermatophyte infection [13]. Treatment for Tinea pedis is typically topical imidazole antifungals (clotrimazole, ketoconazole, miconazole) or allylamines (terbinafine, naftifine) applied thrice daily for seven days [13]. Ensuring dry footwear and changing socks frequently can help prevent recurrence. Athletes should return to sport after 72 hours of antibiotic therapy, but daily hygiene remains crucial [18].

Tinea cruris affects the groin region, and in winter sports, this area is especially vulnerable due to thick, insulating gear that promotes sweating [13]. Sharing of training attire or towels in the locker room further increases infection risk. Tinea cruris presents as pruritic, erythematous plaques with well-defined borders and scaling [14]. The lesions may spread in a bilateral, symmetrical pattern over the inner thighs [13]. Cold-weather athletes may experience more frequent exacerbations due to moist environments. Clinical examination is generally sufficient, but a direct examination with a 10% or 20% KOH preparation or fungal culture can confirm dermatophyte infection [13]. Treatment for Tinea cruris is either fluconazole 150 mg once per week for 3 weeks, itraconazole 200 mg per day for 2 weeks, or terbinafine 250 mg per day for 2 weeks [14]. Ensuring dry footwear and changing socks frequently can help prevent recurrence [15]. Athletes should return to sport after 72 hours of antibiotic therapy, but daily hygiene remains crucial [13].

Tinea corporis is primarily caused by Trichophyton rubrum, Trichophyton tonsurans, and Microsporum canis species [14]. It affects exposed skin and may arise from close contact with other infected athletes or contaminated gear. Damp, warm clothing also increases susceptibility to this infection. Tinea corporis appears as erythematous, annular plaques with central clearing and overlying scaling [14]. Lesions are often pruritic and may spread to various body areas [15]. In winter athletes, lesions may develop on covered or sweat-prone areas. Clinical examination is generally sufficient, but a direct examination with a 10% or 20% KOH preparation or fungal culture can confirm dermatophyte infection [13]. Treatment for Tinea corporis is either fluconazole 150 mg once per week for 3 weeks, itraconazole 200 mg per day for 2 weeks, or terbinafine 250 mg per day for 2 weeks [14]. Ensuring dry footwear and changing socks frequently can help prevent recurrence. Athletes should return to sport after 72 hours of antibiotic therapy, but daily hygiene remains crucial [13].

4.5 Inflammatory

Winter sports such as skiing, snowboarding, snowshoeing, sledding, skating, and hockey expose athletes to a range of environmental conditions that can exacerbate or trigger inflammatory skin conditions [19]. The cold, dry air, combined with high altitudes and prolonged snow and wind exposure frequently lead to dehydration of the skin barrier which can trigger inflammation [12]. In these winter sports, the combination of moisture from perspiration and sudden temperature changes can disrupt skin homeostasis, thus increasing the likelihood of skin inflammation and irritant reactions.

4.5.1 Acne Vulgaris

Acne vulgaris is a common inflammatory condition of the pilosebaceous unit of the skin that is characterized by comedones, papules, pustules, and in more severe cases, painful nodules and cysts [13]. Winter sports equipment such as helmets, masks, and goggles can contribute to acne mechanica, an acne subtype triggered by repetitive friction, occlusion, and heat under protective gear. This occlusive environment allows for the accumulation of sweat, sebum, and environmental debris which enhances the potential for follicular occlusion and inflammation. However, when compared with summer and fall, a study found that skin moisture was significantly lower in the winter ($P \leq 0.016$ for both seasons) [20]. Acne lesions are typically localized to areas where winter gear applies pressure, such as the forehead, cheeks, and chin. Inflammatory papules, pustules, and closed comedones are common, with erythematous macules persisting after active lesions resolve. Athletes who have preexisting microcomedones are more susceptible to progressing to acne mechanica [14]. Severe presentations may include painful nodulocystic lesions, which can lead to scarring if untreated. The diagnosis of acne vulgaris is primarily clinical and based on lesion morphology and distribution [13]. The history of consistent winter gear use in affected areas often distinguishes acne mechanica from other acne forms [14]. Treatment of acne vulgaris includes topical retinoids, benzoyl peroxide, or salicylic acid to reduce follicular occlusion and inflammation [13]. For more persistent cases in athletes, oral antibiotics like doxycycline or minocycline may be considered [13]. For winter athletes, minimizing time spent in occlusive gear and cleansing the skin immediately after sports activities is recommended to reduce acne load.

4.5.2 *Xerosis & Eczema Dermatitis*

Xerosis is a dermatologic condition that is marked by excessive dryness due to disrupted skin barrier function [11]. It can be exacerbated by the low humidity and cold winds experienced in winter sports environments. Xerosis can lead to eczema dermatitis by intensifying transepidermal water loss [10]. The repetitive exposure to these harsh environmental conditions to the skin predisposes winter athletes to the erythema, scaling, and pruritus seen in xerosis and eczema dermatitis. Xerosis presents as rough, flaky patches with scaling and is often seen on the shins, arms, and hands [10]. Eczema may present as pruritic, erythematous plaques with fine scale or as more severe, lichenified plaques with excoriations [10]. Winter athletes commonly experience exacerbated symptoms on exposed or semi-exposed skin areas due to the harsh winter environment. A clinical evaluation focused on lesion morphology and history of environmental exposure aids diagnosis for these conditions [10]. A positive history of atopic dermatitis or previous winter-related flare-ups supports the diagnosis of eczema. Management of these conditions includes liberal use of emollients and barrier creams to keep the skin moist and reduce water loss [10]. Topical corticosteroids or calcineurin inhibitors may also be indicated for inflammatory control during active flares [10]. Winter-specific athletes are advised to use skin moisturizers and wear moisture-wicking underlayers to prevent skin irritation while competing.

4.5.3 *Dermatitis Herpetiformis*

Dermatitis herpetiformis is a chronic, autoimmune blistering skin disorder. It is associated with celiac disease, a gluten-sensitive enteropathy [21]. It is predominantly seen affecting extensor surfaces. The friction of tight winter clothing may exacerbate dermatitis herpetiformis in affected athletes, leading to pruritus, papulovesicular eruptions, and skin trauma due to scratching. Dermatitis herpetiformis in athletes can interfere with comfort and performance, especially in high-friction sports like snowboarding. Dermatitis herpetiformis typically presents as pruritic clusters of vesicles, papules, and excoriations, primarily on the elbows, knees, and buttocks [22]. Vesicles may rupture, leading to erosions or crusts. Chronic lesions can appear as hyperpigmented or hypopigmented macules [22]. Diagnosis of dermatitis herpetiformis is confirmed through skin biopsy which shows granular IgA deposits at the dermal papillae on direct immunofluorescence [21]. Serological testing for anti-tissue transglutaminase (tTG) or anti-endomysial antibodies may support the diagnosis, particularly in athletes with underlying gluten-sensitive enteropathy. The primary treatment is a strict gluten-free diet, which can lead to significant improvement of dermatitis herpetiformis over time [21]. Symptomatic relief may include oral dapsone to reduce itching and lesion formation [22]. Athletes with dermatitis herpetiformis are encouraged to choose loose-fitting, breathable clothing to minimize friction with winter gear. Education on dietary management is also key to reducing dermatitis herpetiformis flares.

4.6 Mechanical Conditions

Mechanical skin conditions occur in winter sports due to the repetitive friction, pressure, and shear forces [19]. These occur frequently in skiing, snowboarding, snowshoeing, and sledding due to prolonged contact with equipment, such as boots and bindings (Fig. 4.2). The resulting blisters can compromise the athlete's performance by causing discomfort and increasing the risk of secondary infections if the skin barrier is breached.

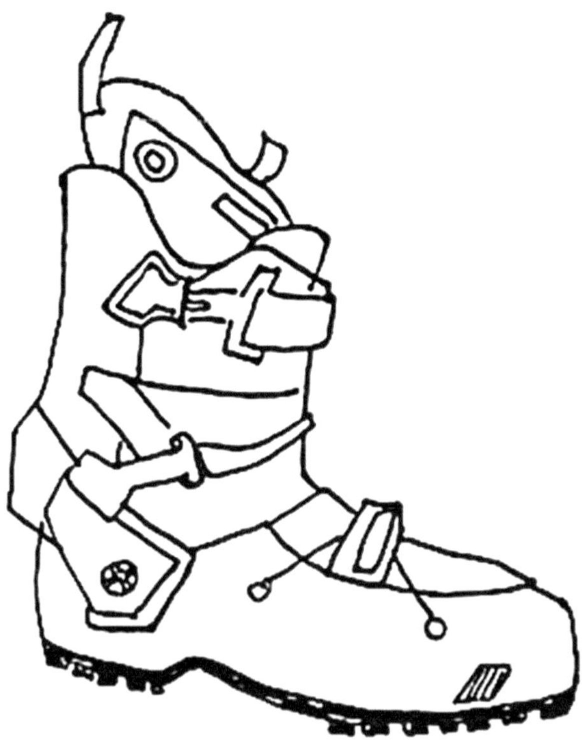

Fig. 4.2 Ski Boot

4.6.1 *Blisters*

Blisters are fluid-filled lesions that form in response to intense friction or pressure, often seen in winter sports due to the rigid structure of the winter sports gear [13]. Activities like skiing, snowboarding, hockey, and skating involve repetitive movements and force distribution which generates shear forces between the epidermis and dermis, ultimately causing separation and fluid accumulation [19]. Friction blisters are most common, and they as a result of forces that separate epidermal cells at the level of the stratum spinosum [14]. The blisters can then fill with fluid due to hydrostatic pressure, and this can cause them to become tender [14]. Blisters typically present as tense, fluid-filled vesicles over erythematous skin [19]. They are most frequently found on the palms of the hands, heels, toes, and lateral aspects of the feet [13]. In more severe cases, blisters may evolve into erosions if the roof ruptures, exposing the dermis and increasing the risk of infection [14]. Hemorrhagic blisters with a blood-tinged fluid content due to dermal capillary involvement may also form in cases of intense trauma. The diagnosis of blisters is clinical, based on the appearance and location of the lesions [14]. The history of recent physical activity involving specific winter gear or footwear helps the clinician in identifying the mechanical origin. Management of blisters includes drainage of large blisters with sterile techniques while preserving the roof to protect the underlying skin. Protective dressings like hydrocolloid patches provide cushioning and promote healing [13, 14]. Preventative strategies are key, such as ensuring properly fitted gear, using moisture-wicking socks, and applying friction-reducing pads or blister prevention tape [19]. Winter athletes should be educated on appropriate footwear adjustments and early symptom management to maintain performance and prevent secondary infection.

References

1. (SIA) SIA. Nearly 10 percent of U.S. population participated in winter sports last season. SGB Media or Snowsports Industries America; 2023. [Available from: https://sgbonline.com/report-nearly-10-percent-of-u-s-population-participated-in-winter-sports-last-season/.
2. Moehrle M. Outdoor sports and skin cancer. Clin Dermatol. 2008;26(1):12–5.
3. Rigel DS, Rigel EG, Rigel AC. Effects of altitude and latitude on ambient UVB radiation. J Am Acad Dermatol. 1999;40(1):114–6.
4. Buller DB, Andersen PA, Walkosz BJ, Scott MD, Maloy JA, Dignan MB, Cutter GR. Compliance with sunscreen advice in a survey of adults engaged in outdoor winter recreation at high-elevation ski areas. J Am Acad Dermatol. 2012;66(1):63–70.
5. NHS. Hypothermia: NHS; 2023 [Available from: https://www.nhs.uk/conditions/hypothermia/.
6. Michaud RG. Cochrane library's summary of review on manipulative treatment misleading, cheats readers. J Am Osteopath Assoc. 2006;106(7):426–7.
7. Giesbrecht GG, Wilkerson JA. Hypothermia, frostbite and other cold injuries: prevention, survival, rescue, and treatment. The Mountaineers Books; 2006.
8. Handford C, Buxton P, Russell K, Imray CE, McIntosh SE, Freer L, et al. Frostbite: a practical approach to hospital management. Extrem Physiol Med. 2014;3:7.

9. Hallam MJ, Cubison T, Dheansa B, Imray C. Managing frostbite. Bmj. 2010;341:c5864.
10. Pons-Guiraud A. Dry skin in dermatology: a complex physiopathology. J Eur Acad Dermatol Venereol. 2007;21(Suppl 2):1–4.
11. Augustin M, Wilsmann-Theis D, Körber A, Kerscher M, Itschert G, Dippel M, Staubach P. Diagnosis and treatment of xerosis cutis – a position paper. J Dtsch Dermatol Ges. 2019;17(Suppl 7):3–33.
12. Engebretsen KA, Johansen JD, Kezic S, Linneberg A, Thyssen JP. The effect of environmental humidity and temperature on skin barrier function and dermatitis. J Eur Acad Dermatol Venereol. 2016;30(2):223–49.
13. Pujalte GGA, Costa LMC, Clapp AD, Presutti RJ, Sluzevich JC. More than skin deep: dermatologic conditions in athletes. Sports Health. 2023;15(1):74–85.
14. Pecci M, Comeau D, Chawla V. Skin conditions in the athlete. Am J Sports Med. 2009;37(2):406–18.
15. Paradise SL, Hu YE. Infectious dermatoses in sport: a review of diagnosis, management, and return-to-play recommendations. Curr Sports Med Rep. 2021;20(2):92–103.
16. Adams BB. Dermatologic disorders of the athlete. Sports Med. 2002;32(5):309–21.
17. Rihn JA, Michaels MG, Harner CD. Community-acquired methicillin-resistant staphylococcus aureus: an emerging problem in the athletic population. Am J Sports Med. 2005;33(12):1924–9.
18. Tlougan BE, Mancini AJ, Mandell JA, Cohen DE, Sanchez MR. Skin conditions in figure skaters, ice-hockey players and speed skaters: part II – cold-induced, infectious and inflammatory dermatoses. Sports Med. 2011;41(11):967–84.
19. Tlougan BE, Mancini AJ, Mandell JA, Cohen DE, Sanchez MR. Skin conditions in figure skaters, ice-hockey players and speed skaters: part I – mechanical dermatoses. Sports Med. 2011;41(9):709–19.
20. Meyer K, Pappas A, Dunn K, Cula GO, Seo I, Ruvolo E, Batchvarova N. Evaluation of seasonal changes in facial skin with and without acne. J Drugs Dermatol. 2015;14(6):593–601.
21. Reunala T, Salmi TT, Hervonen K. Dermatitis herpetiformis: pathognomonic transglutaminase IgA deposits in the skin and excellent prognosis on a gluten-free diet. Acta Derm Venereol. 2015;95(8):917–22.
22. Wang Y, Yang B, Zhou G, Zhang F. Two cases of dermatitis herpetiformis successfully treated with tetracycline and niacinamide. Acta Dermatovenerol Croat. 2018;26(3):273–5.

Chapter 5
Mountaineering Sports

Ryan Scheinkman, Christina Barrett, Alexia Vignau, Rachel Cohen, Philippe Jean-Pierre, Lea Tordjman, Anika Pulumati, Kayla Mashoudy, Daniel Green, and Keyvan Nouri

5.1 Introduction

Mountaineering sports encompass a broad range of outdoor activities including hiking, rock climbing, and alpine sports (covered in the winter sports chapter). Hiking can range from short day-hikes that often require minimal equipment (e.g. hiking shoes) to multiday treks that require large packs and equipment that can lead to injury formation. Rock climbing can be performed on artificially constructed courses or on natural surfaces with climbers using various types and amounts of safety equipment. The sport of rock climbing is a popular recreational activity that is predicted to have approximately 25 million participants [1]. Some of the types of climbing that pose various levels of health risks to climbers, include sport climbing, traditional climbing, top rope climbing, lead climbing, bouldering, and free climbing [2]. Top rope climbing involves the use of a rope suspended from an anchor point at the top of the climbing surface that the climber attaches a harness to with the other end of the rope attached to a belay system, which involves either another individual (belayer) or mechanical system that creates counter pressure on the rope that can slow a climber's descent in the case of a fall or when descending a climbing surface thus minimizing fall injury risk to a climber [2]. By contrast lead climbing involves a climber scaling a climbing surface without a rope above them requiring the climber to anchor themselves at various points along the climb increasing the risk of injury from falls [2]. Free climbing and bouldering pose additional safety

R. Scheinkman (✉) · C. Barrett · A. Vignau · R. Cohen · P. Jean-Pierre · L. Tordjman
A. Pulumati · K. Mashoudy · D. Green · K. Nouri
Dr. Phillip Frost Department of Dermatology and Cutaneous Surgery, University of Miami, Miami, FL, USA
e-mail: scheinkman@med.miami.edu; christina.barrett@miami.edu; axv200@med.miami.edu; rachelcohen@med.miami.edu; philanator@med.miami.edu; lat91@med.miami.edu; kmashoudy@med.miami.edu; dag258@med.miami.edu; knouri@med.miami.edu

K. Nouri (ed.), *Sport-Related Skin Conditions*,
https://doi.org/10.1007/978-3-031-90444-8_5

and health risks to climbers as climbers forgo safety equipment in the form of harnesses and ropes in these types of climbing [2].

Sport climbing involves the use of premade anchors in indoor rock courses or outdoor courses and can involve either top rope or lead climbing [2]. Traditional climbing involves the climber placing anchor points along the climb and can pose injury risks from temporary anchor's failing [2]. Health challenges posed by mountaineering are well documented, such as: injuries from falls, sunburns from ultraviolet exposure, and frostbite from exposure to cold temperatures [3, 4]. Mountaineering sports provide many challenges dermatological insults for its participants, such as: plant dermatitis, animal envenomation, falls from large heights, and soft tissue infections. Hiking and rock-climbing present climbers with environmental exposures to prolonged sun exposure and extremes of temperature that can be a detriment to their dermatological health. The importance of consoling participants in identifying hazards associated with each sport (e.g. venomous/poisonous plants and insects) and the use of protective clothing and equipment (e.g. UV blocking clothing, helmets) could help to prevent dermatological conditions and injuries. Informing patients that will be going on prolonged hikes or climbs about what to stock in their first aid kits could help patients to temporarily treat conditions encountered in the backcountry, while awaiting formal medical care.

5.2 Dermatophytes

Fungal infections of the feet (tinea pedis) and toenails (onychomycosis) are of potential concern for hikers and climbers, especially when in moist environments or if toenails are traumatized while hiking and climbing [5, 6]. Patients with tinea pedis can present with intertriginous pruritic, peeling, and fissuring dermatitis with the plantar surface of the toes exhibiting white scale and erythema and can generally be treated with topical imidazoles [5]. Oral administration of terbinafine, itraconazole, fluconazole, or griseofulvin can also be considered, especially in patients that fail topical treatments [5]. Causative organisms for Tinea Pedis dermatophyte infections include the following fungi species: *Trichophyton rubrum* (most common causative organism), *Epidermophyton floccosum, Trichophyton interdigitale,* and *Tricholosporum violaceum* [5]. Onychomycosis (tinea unguium) presents as nails with discoloration and increased thickness and is generally caused by the following fungal species: *Trichophyton* rubrum (most common cause), *Trichophyton mentagrophytes, Epidermophyton floccosum,* and *Candida albicans*. Oral antifungals (specifically terbinafine, itraconazole, fluconazole) have been found to be effective treatments for onychomycosis. Preventative measures include not sharing shoes, washing feet daily (with soap and water), and keeping one's feet dry by frequently changing socks and allowing footwear to dry if they become wet [5, 6]. Images of onychomycosis and tinea pedis can be seen in the appendix.

5.3 Plant Dermatitis

Plant dermatitis includes a multitude of skin conditions including mechanical irritant, chemical irritant, contact allergic, phytophotodermatitis, and contact urticaria dermatitis depending on the mechanism of exposure and reaction [7]. Mechanical irritants are plant structures that traumatize the skin, such as the glochid structures of some Cacti species that act as barbs that penetrate the skin and plant thorns [7, 8]. These structures can act as a delivery vehicle for chemical irritants or a potential nidus for infection (e.g. sporotrichosis a condition caused by the fungus Sporothrix schenckii present in the subtropics and tropics that can result and pustular and ulcerative lesions that begin as nodular or papular formations from lymphocutaneous involvement often introduced through traumatic inoculation from thorns that can be treated with itraconazole) [7, 9, 10]. Additionally, failure to remove cacti glochids can lead to granuloma formation [11]. Using a combination of tweezers and glue has been found to be an effective method of removing glochids [10]. Chemical irritants include the alkaloid Capsaicin produced by members of the Solanaceae family that trigger burning sensation from interactions neuronal vanilloid receptors, Diterpene esters produced by the Euphorbiaceae family that can cause bullae (with pain, edema, and erythema) from activating protein kinase C, and Protoanemonin produced by Ranunculaceae family causing pain, edema, erythema, bullae, and potential hyperpigmentation due to interactions with disulfide bonds [7]. Phytophotodermatitis are triggered by compounds activated by ultraviolet light exposure that can cause symptoms ranging from erythema to desquamation (e.g. furanocoumarins produced by the Rutacea family) [7]. Contact urticaria, a Type 1 hypersensitivity reaction, can be induced by Stinging nettles (part of the family Urticaceae family) that have structures called trichomes cutaneously introduce acetylcholine, histamine, and formic acid causing urticarial rash, pruritic, and erythema [7].

Hikers and climbers exposed to plants of the *Toxicodendron* genus (e.g. poison ivy and poison oak) can experience Type 4 hypersensitivity allergic contact dermatitis reactions generally due to exposure to the triggering compound Urushiol produced by these plants (Fig. 5.1) [7, 12]. In addition to being counseled on wearing clothing that prevents skin contact with these plants in areas where they are endemic, hikers should be counseled on their appearance to help avoid exposures. Toxicodendron *radicans* (Eastern Poison Ivy) and *T. pubescens* (Eastern Poison Oak) are endemic to Eastern North America and with Eastern Poison Ivy resembling vines with groupings of three teardrop shaped leaves versus Eastern Poison Oak species having groupings of green berries with groupings of three hairy oakleaf shaped leaves growing in small shrubs [13].

Toxicodendron *rydbergii* (Rydberg's poison ivy) is dispersed throughout North America (with the exception of the southeastern United States) resembles a shrub with three leaf groupings and yellow berries [13]. Toxicodendron vernix (poison sumac) is endemic to swampy environments in eastern North America and grows as trees or shrubs with small fruits with more front like leaf clusters with greater

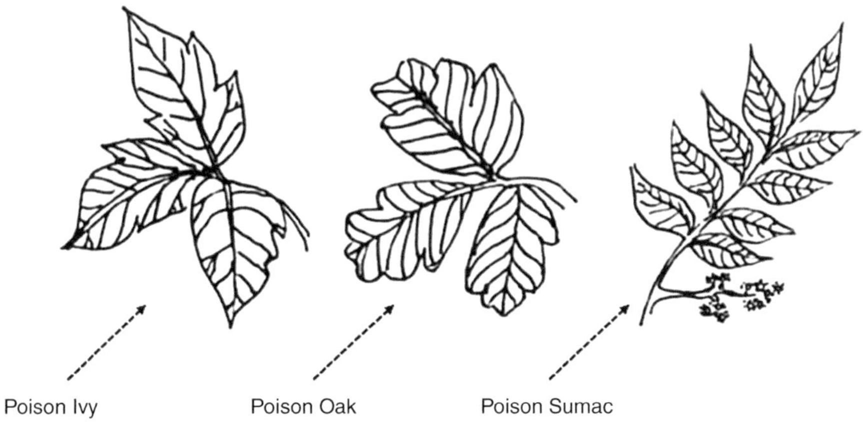

Fig. 5.1 Members of the Toxicodendron Genus

numbers of leaves per stem than the abovementioned Toxicodendron species (i.e. 7 to 13 leaves) [13]. Symptoms can include erythema, pruritic, edema, and papulovesicular eruptions that generally self-resolves but management should include washing contacted areas with soap and water and removing exposed clothing (topical antihistamines can be used to manage pruritic symptoms and in severe cases, prednisone [13].

5.4 Animal Envenomation, Bites, and Stings

Animal bites and stings pose risks for envenomation and nidi for infection for hikers and climbers in addition to the trauma caused by such bites, with signs of cutaneous infection described above and vector borne illness in the subsequent section. Multiple species of arthropods pose risks for biting, stinging, and envenomation for hikers [14]. Members of the insect order Hymenoptera includes include many species of stinging ants, bees, wasps, and hornets [14, 15]. Fire ants (e.g. *Solenopsis richteri* and *Solenopsis invicta*) can affect hikers in multiple US states, the Caribbean, China, Australia, and New Zealand that can aggressively swarm individuals if they come in contact with their nests each can deliver multiple stings by biting victims with their mandibles and delivering venom through a stinger on their abdomens, which deliver a venom that is mostly composed mostly of a water insoluble alkaloid that causes sterile pustules to form [14, 15]. Patients often report pain and pruritis from the stings and cutaneous reactions ranging from formations of wheels around sting area, pustule formation, and large local reactions with multiple pustules overlaying erythema and swelling [14, 15]. Topical antihistamines can for symptomatic relief with patient consoling on leaving pustules intact and cleaning broken pustules with soap and water [14, 15]. Bees (members of Apoidea family) have detachable stingers that detach and should be removed from the skin that cause pain, erythema, and swelling [14]. By contrast, wasps (members of Vespidae family) can sting multiple times [14]. The venoms in Hymenoptera species can act as allergens in some individuals triggering reactions ranging from urticarial rashes to anaphylaxis, in which case patients should be given epinephrine [14, 15].

Centipede (members of class Chilopoda) bites can inject venom (containing metalloproteases, histamine, serotonin) that present with pain, erythema, and swelling surrounding puncture sites that can be treated symptomatically with NSAIDs (Fig. 5.2) [14]. Different millipede species (members of class Diplopoda) can spray caustic secretions (containing hydrogen cyanide, hydrochloric acid, alkaloids, benzoquinones, hydroquinones, and phenols) from micropores that can cause hyperpigmentation (from benzoquinones) or caustic skin reactions (e.g. pain, pruritic, erythema, edema, and blisters) that should be washed with soap and water as well as treated with topical antibiotics [14, 16]. Caterpillars (members of Lepidoptera) can cause erythema, burning pain, swelling, papules, and vesicles from contact with their bristle-like setae, that act as ducts for secretory glands and cells that produce poison (e.g. containing hyaluronidase, histamine, and phospholipase A) can detach into the skin [17]. Tape can be used to extract setae from the skin and the affected area can be treated with topical isopropyl alcohol, ice compresses, and analgesia for pain [17]. Mosquito bites can present with pruritic urticarial wheals and papules around bite sites that can be treated topically with ice compresses and corticosteroids for symptomatic relief [14, 18].

Arachnids, including scorpions, spiders, ticks, and chiggers can harm hikers through their bites and stings [14]. Scorpion stings (from specialized tail structure) in most species produce mainly localized pain that can be managed with analgesia, ice compresses, removing stinger, and cleaning the site with soap and water [14]. Ticks are mentioned in the next section. The *Loxosceles reclusa* spider (Brown Recluse) present in the southern and central United States have bites that range from being painless to sharp in nature that cause hemorrhagic blister formation or tissue necrosis from hemolytic enzymes present in their venom [14]. Treatment for brown recluse bites for milder presentation includes potential tetanus prophylaxis, wound cleaning, and ice compresses, but can require debridement and skin grafting in the case of tissue necroses [14]. Chiggers (members of the Thrombiculidae family) are red mite larvae present in forests and grasses that feed on skin that can result in a

Fig. 5.2 Centipede

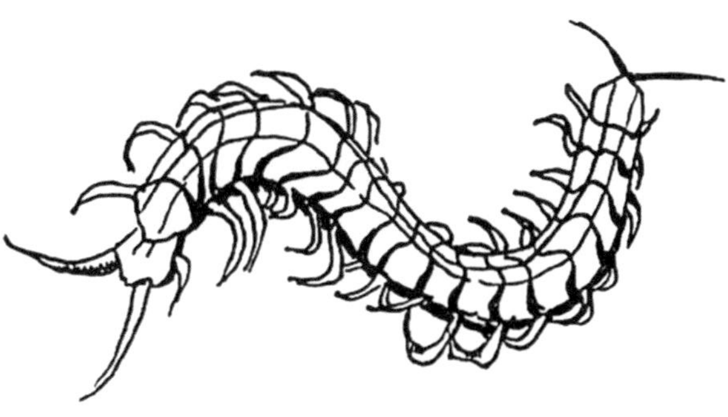

delayed pruritic reaction from their saliva and can be identified as pinpoint red specks that can be removed by showering with symptomatic treatment for pruritis consisting of antihistamines and topical corticosteroids [14].

5.5 Vector-Borne Illnesses

Multiple invertebrate arthropod species encountered by hikers serve as vectors for illness that have cutaneous manifestations [19–21]. Members of the *Ixodes*, *Amblyomma*, *Rhipicephalus*, and *Dermacentor* genera cause multitude of tick-borne illnesses with dermatological findings [21]. Lyme disease caused by the Borrelia *burgdorferi* bacteria, primarily spread by *Ixodes* (e.g. *Ixodes scapularis*) ticks, often presets with the targetoid erythema migrans rash on the limbs and face with occasional associated pruritic symptoms and can be treated with doxycycline (Fig. 5.3) [21]. Although traditionally associated with geographic distribution in the Northeastern United States, Lyme disease cases have been reported as far west as California and as far south as at least Florida [22–24]. Rocky Mountain Spotted fever caused by the *Rickettsia rickettsii* bacteria spread mostly by *Dermacentor* ticks (most commonly in the southeastern and midwestern United States) often presents initially as a papular rash that transitions to pruritic petechiae spreading initially distally from the wrists and ankles to the limbs and trunk over time and can also be treated with doxycycline or chloramphenicol in more serious cases [21, 25]. Tularemia (caused by *Francisella tularensis* and presenting with deep ulcerations at

Fig. 5.3 Deer tick (Ixodes scapularis)

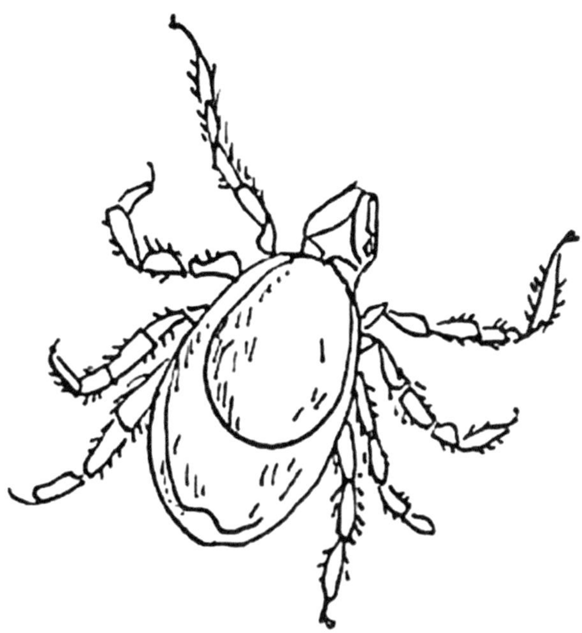

the bite site) and Ehrlichiosis (caused by *Ehrlichia canis* and presenting with an erythematous rash) are additional tick-borne illnesses that can be treated with Streptomycin and Doxycycline, respectively [21]. Hikers in regions endemic to ticks should perform regular full body checks for attached ticks, remove attached ticks as quickly as possible with curved tweezers, and wash site with antibacterial soap to minimize infection risk [21].

Mosquito species of the *Aedes* genera (e.g. *Aedes aegypti* and *A. albopictus)* are known vectors of various infections, including the Chikungunya virus, which can present with cutaneous findings, including maculopapular rash, aphthous ulcers, vesicle and bullae formation among other skin manifestations and has been reported in hikers (e.g. case reported in Florida) [19, 26]. Dengue fever, another mosquito-borne viral illness, presents with cutaneous findings, including morbilliform rashes and hemorrhagic lesions presenting a risk for hikers and climbers particularly in subtropical and tropical locations [27–29]. Plasmodial species (e.g. *P. Falciparum, P. Vivax*, etc.) transmitted by the *Anopheles* mosquito can cause a multitude of cutaneous findings in malaria patients that could be exposed through hiking and climbing in tropical or subtropical regions, including angioedema, gangrene, purpura fulminans, acral skin necrosis, urticaria, and thrombocytopenia petechiae [30, 31]. Hikers spending time in areas of endemic mosquito-borne illness can use medical prophylaxis to minimize potential for disease, such as the antimalarials Atovaquone-proguanil, Doxycycline, Mefloquine, Primaquine, Tafenoquine, Chloroquine, and hydroxychloroquine that provide varying degrees of protection against different plasmodial species in different geographic locations [32].

However, hikers using doxycycline as chemoprophylaxis should be made aware of the potential side effect of increased photosensitivity and should be counseled accordingly about wearing sun protective clothing and sunscreen [33]. Leishmaniasis is a disease caused by the obligate intracellular Leishmania protozoa transmitted by the sandfly (e.g. *Phlebotomus perniciosus*) in the tropics and can present cutaneously with ulcers with hemorrhagic crusts, lymphadenitis, and potential satellite lesions [20, 34–36]. Leishmaniasis treatments include sodium stibogluconate, itraconazole, ketoconazole, and amphotericin B [34]. Hikers can use arthropod repellent sprays on their hikes, such as those containing N,N-diethyl-3-methylbenzamide (DEET), to minimize arthropod vector-borne disease [37]. Chaga's disease is caused by the parasite *Trypanosoma cruzi*, which can be present in the feces of kissing bugs (present in southern areas of North America, Central, and South America) that can be transmitted to humans through contamination of bites that can present as papules or vesiculobullous lesions with areas of parasite entry presenting as chagomas (localized erethema, swelling) with firstline therapy being benznidazole or nifurtimox [14, 38]. These diseases are further summarized in Table 5.1.

Table 5.1 Vector-borne illnesses associated with mountaineering sports

Disease/Condition	Symptoms and physical exam findings	Treatment recommendations
Lyme disease	Targetoid erythema migrans rash on limbs and face with occasional pruritic symptoms	Doxycycline
Rocky mountain spotted fever	Papular rash that transitions to pruritic petechiae from wrists/ankles to limbs	Doxycycline or chloramphenicol
Tularemia	Deep ulcerations at bite site	Streptomycin and Doxycycline
Ehrlichiosis	Erythematous rash	Streptomycin and Doxycycline
Leishmaniasis	Ulcers with hemorrhagic crusts, lymphadenitis, and potential satellite lesions	Sodium stibogluconate, itraconazole, ketoconazole, and amphotericin B
Chaga's disease	Papules or vesiculobullous lesions with areas of parasite entry	Benznidazole or nifurtimox

5.6 Cutaneous Injuries & Wounds

Mountaineering poses risks of injury to its participants from a variety of factors, including equipment failure that can result in falls, injuries caused directly by contact with equipment, injuries from falling objects, fall injuries from issues with belaying, and injuries to ligaments from excessive strain from gripping rock faces [39, 40]. Cutaneous injuries from rock climbing include skin splitting on fingertips (from chalk and wear from climbing), abrasions, puncture wounds, and avulsions [39, 41]. Additionally, finger nail fractures can occur during climbing as reported as a single case during bouldering at the 2010 Open National Rock Climbing Championships in Iran in addition to a single contusion case during a lead climbing fall [42]. Skin contusions occur during competition bouldering, lead climbing, and speed climbing with 13 of the 18 acute medical issues treated for the 443 climbers participating in the 2005 World Championships in Rock Climbing in Munich being skin contusions (8 bouldering, 2 lead climbing, and 3 speed climbing) [43].

Physical stress and injuries caused by rock climbing have been found to result in dermatological foot changes observed by health professionals in a cohort of 53 participating climbers in a one month period in 2021 at the Cereza Wall climbing wall in Plasencia with 62% of the climbers found to have bursitis of the first digit, 51.3% of the climbers exhibiting hyperkeratosis of the distal end of the first digit, 21.6% of climbers exhibiting hyperkeratosis dorsum of the toes, and 15% exhibiting nail changes (e.g. subungual hematoma, onychomycosis, and other onychodystrophies) [44]. Hand and wrist are susceptible to injuries from the torque applied to them during climbing, contact with equipment, and falls with 155 climbers (28%) reporting hand or wrist injuries 545 surveys created by Logan et al. of hand and wrist injuries ever sustained completed by the Climbers' Club of Great Britain [45]. They found that lacerations and abrasions were the second most common injury reported (15% of the total injuries) after tendon injuries, with rope burns accounting for 9% of the injuries, and crush injuries accounting for 4% of the injuries [45]. Permanent skin changes caused by climbing injuries have been reported, such as nine cases of scars caused by injuries reported by climbers (1962 participants with 699 injuries) participating in a retrospective internet survey pertaining to acute sport climbing injuries conducted between 2002 and 2006 [16].

Climbers compared to non-climbers that sustain injuries from falls from cliffs have been found to have greater amounts of soft tissue injuries for climbers from lacerations and contusions due to the closer proximity to rock faces with a retrospective search of injuries obtained from falls from cliffs between 2006 to 2016 in the trauma center of the University of Kentucky Hospital yielding 68% (27 climbers) of the 40 climbers with fall injuries having external soft tissue injuries reported compared 50% (56 non-climbers) of the 111 non-climbers that sustained fall injuries from cliffs [47]. Nelson et al. reviewed 846 cases and Buzzacott et al. reviewed 884 cases of rock climbing injuries reported by emergency departments in the National Electronic Injury Surveillance System between 1990-2007 and 2008-2016 respectively to determine types and locations of injuries obtained during rock climbing as well as demographic information of the rock climbers (e.g. gender) [39, 40]. Nelson et al. and Buzzacott et al. both grouped injuries related to superficial wounds as lacerations (comprised of punctures and avulsions) and soft tissue (composed of abrasions, contusions, crushing injuries, and hematomas) with Nelson et al. finding that lacerations and soft tissue injuries accounted for 17.1% and 16.9% of the injuries sustained during rock climbing reported by the emergency departments studied [39, 40]. Buzzacott et al. found that lacerations and soft tissue injuries each individually accounted for 11% of injuries sustained during rock climbing in their cohort [40]. Nelson et al. and Buzzacott et al. both found that falls accounted for the majority of the injuries reported by their cohorts, 77.5% and 60% respectively as well as contacting items during climbing being more likely to result in lacerations than other types of injuries (e.g. sprains, fractures, soft tissue injuries) [39, 40]. Nelson et al. found that contact with objects resulted in laceration 5.26 times than other injuries, being struck by objects resulted in lacerations 4.19 times than other types of injuries, lacerations were the most common head injurie caused by objects hitting the head, men were more likely to sustain lacerations than woman (odds ratio = 1.65), climbers under the age of 19 were more likely than climbers over the age of 20 to sustain lacerations (odds ratio = 1.99), heads and legs were more likely than other body parts to sustain lacerations (odds ratio = 5.1), and the proportion of lacerations compared to other injury modalities decreased from the start and end of the study period from 56.4% to 11.3% [39]. Buzzacott et al. noted that 42% of the lacerations reported in their cohort occurred in the knee or lower leg and contact with objects resulted in laceration injuries 4.7 times more than other types of injuries (e.g. fracture, sprain soft tissue injuries) [40].

In terms of outdoor injuries obtained at national parks, Bowie et al. over a 3 and half year period surveyed 220 injured climbers with 451 injuries at the Yosemite Medical Clinic in Yosemite National Park to determine types and causes of injuries finding 66% were due to falls, superficial (subcutaneous and skin) injuries broadly accounted for 50% of injuries, abrasions accounted for 25% of the injuries (111 total), contusions accounted for 15% of the injuries (66 total), lacerations accounted for 14% of the injuries (64 total), and most of the patients presented with one severe injury (e.g. fracture) with associated minor injuries (e.g. abrasions) [48]. Addiss et al. analyzed 127 injuries relating to climbing incidents reported by the Safety and Occupational Health Management department of the United States National Park service between 1981 and 1982 finding that 75% of the injuries were related to falls, 69% occurred during ascension of the cliff faces, and that three of the climbers reported having lacerations, abrasions, or milder fractures compared to 29 climbers that reported having multiple fractures [49].

McDonald et al. used an internet survey of climbers over the age of 18 years old that climbed at least four times in America that sustained an injuries while climbing over a year to analyze injury patterns finding that 29 of the 975 were from lacerations with six of the lacerations from indoor climbing, seven of the lacerations from outdoor bouldering, nine of the lacerations from outdoor sport climbing, and seven from traditional outdoor climbing [50]. Gerdes et al. also used a retrospective internet survey to determine the three most severe injuries self-reported by the 1887 participating climbers that reported 2472 injuries finding that 57.6% of all the injuries were in upper extremities lacerations (accounting for 12.1% of the total injuries) more commonly occurred in lower extremities (24.6% of lacerations) followed by fingers (18.7%), heads (15.1%), and hands (14.2%) [51].

Schöffl et al. found that finger injuries accounted for the majority (52%, 474 total) of the 911 injuries reported by 836 climbers participating in a prospective survey of climbing injuries Klinikum Bamberg hospital in Germany between 2009 and 2012 reporting one case of a finger contusion [52]. They juxtaposed the results of this study with their previous study of 604 injuries by climbing patients reported between 1998-2001, where there were 247 finger injuries, including: five of the finger injuries as non-specific soft tissue injuries, five cases of Dupuytren's disease one case of finger cellulitis, and one case of a finger contusion [52–54]. They found that the dermatologically relevant Dupuytren's disease was the eighth most common injury (30 cases, 3.3% of the total conditions reported) in their more recent study and that skin abrasions were the fifth most common source of injury in their previous study (34 cases, 5.6% of the total conditions reported) [52–54]. In another study conducted by Schöffl et al. prospectively between 2007–2011 of all the participants (515,337 registered visits) at a specific indoor rock gym in Germany, there were thirty reported climbing injuries with three of the climbers suffering from contusions from belaying mistakes, one climber receiving a laceration from a climbing error, one belayer receiving rope burns, and another climber reporting contusions for unspecified reasons [55]. Rooks et al. reported that 50% of the 39 climbers participating in a one-month climber survey in 1993 reported a history of laceration or pulled muscle [56]. Braybrook et al. in their analysis of over 17,000 hikers reported that blisters (and ankle sprains) represented the most frequent types of injuries among hikers with the lower limbs accounting for the most affected anatomical site [57]. These results highlight how the mechanics of climbing predispose climbers to cutaneous hand injuries and the mechanics of hiking predispose hikers to lower limb injuries.

5.7 Environmental Effects on Skin

Mountaineering exposes participants to a variety of environmental factors that can significantly impact cutaneous health. Among these, extreme cold poses some of the most serious dermatological challenges. Frostbite, a condition occurring when skin is exposed to very low temperatures leading to ice crystals formation within cells, is a major concern for those engaging in high-altitude or winter climbing and hiking. This ultimately results in cellular damage, inflammation, and thrombosis in the affected tissues. Climbers and hikes are especially susceptible to frostbite on their extremities, particularly the fingers, toes, ears, and nose, and have a heightened risk of developing this condition when exposed to cold, wind, and moisture for prolonged periods of time. By understanding and mitigating these environmental risks, climbers can protect their skin health and enjoy the sport more safely.

Frostbite can be classified into two categories: superficial and deep. Superficial frostbite involves the epidermis and subcutaneous tissues, while deep frostbite affects deeper structures, including tendons, bones, and muscles [58]. The initial management of frostbite focuses on preventing further damage by avoiding thawing and refreezing cycles. Once the individual is in a controlled environment where refreezing is unlikely, rapid rewarming is crucial and is typically achieved by immersing the affected body part in a water bath maintained at 40–42 °C [58]. Additionally, tetanus toxoid should be administered, and the injured area should be immobilized to prevent further injury [58]. There is some debate regarding the optimal management of frostbite blisters, with differing opinions on whether to debride or leave them intact [58]. A different study focusing on alpine climbers revealed an alarming annual frostbite incidence rate of over 33%, with the majority of cases being minor frostbite injuries involving the hands [59]. This high incidence emphasizes this pervasive risk of cold injury among climbers, particularly in alpine environments where temperatures can plummet unexpectedly and drastically. Moreover, another study examining hand and wrist injuries among rock climbers administered questionnaires to members of The Climbers' Club of Great Britain [45]. Interestingly, frostbite accounted for only 1% of all injuries among more frequently encountered issues like tendon injuries and abrasions [45]. Despite its relatively lower incidence in this study, frostbite represents a significant concern due to the severe consequences it can entail.

Hypothermia poses another significant risk to rock climbers, especially those engaging in high-altitude climbs where environmental conditions can be severe and unpredictable. It presents when the body's core temperature is below 35 °C, resulting in impaired muscular coordination, decreased cerebral function, and potentially life-threatening consequences [60]. Factors contributing to the onset of hypothermia in climbers include poor clothing choices, inadequate physical conditioning, overexertion, fatigue, hypoxia, and dehydration. In high-altitude climbing, for every 1000 feet gained in elevation, the temperature drops by approximately 3.5 °F [60]. At 32 °F, extremities receive only 10% of their normal blood flow due to vasoconstriction and this significant reduction in blood flow increases the risk of hypothermia and other cold-related injuries [60]. A significant percentage of mountaineers and wilderness travelers rescued in alpine environments are found to be hypothermic, suggesting the need for climbers to carry adequate gear and make thorough risk assessments before embarking on their climbs [3]. Proper clothing and preparedness are imperative to prevent hypothermia, especially for climbers who might have to stay outdoors overnight. In addition, a study involving Sierra Nevada climbers found that 201 climbers sustained 215 injuries, with hypothermia being a culprit in many cases [60]. Of the injuries resulting from judgmental errors, acute mountain sickness and hypothermia were documented in 68 and 13 patients, respectively [60]. Hypothermia was associated with over 10% of the injuries occurring during the descent, demonstrating the increased risk as climbers become fatigued and environmental conditions worsen. Furthermore, 18 climbers displayed signs and symptoms of hypothermia, further emphasizing its prevalence among this population [60]. The insidious onset of hypothermia, often exacerbated by altitude-related factors such as acute mountain sickness, makes it a very dangerous condition. Symptoms may include shivering, confusion, slurred speech, and loss of coordination, and may develop gradually [60].

It is apparent that sun exposure is one of the most critical factors impacting the skin health of climbers [4]. Despite the evident risks, there are very few studies that specifically address the dermatological implications of sun exposure among this population. This gap in research is likely due to the unique nature of the sport, the transient and often remote locations of climbing activities, and the difficulty in consistently measuring and monitoring environmental exposures and their effects on skin health among this group. In a cross-sectional study conducted to quantify sun exposure risk and evaluate sun exposure habits, protection practices, and attitudes among outdoor rock climbers, 48.4% of climbers reported more than 90 days of sun exposure and 63.6% spent three or more hours per day in the sun during the previous climbing season [4]. Notably, 65.9% of participants experienced at least one sunburn, and 20.7% reported three or more sunburn events during this period [4]. The most common sun protection measures among the climbers was sunscreen with SPF $\geq$ 15 (49.3%) and sunglasses (47%). Long-sleeved shirts, long trousers (21.2%), hats or caps (31.8%), and avoiding midday sun (35.5%) were less commonly employed [4]. Only 14.3% of participants reported reapplying sunscreen at least every two hours, despite frequent sun exposure. Barriers to sunscreen use included irritation to the eyes, greasy feel on the fingers, and forgetting to apply it [4]. Regarding attitudes towards sun exposure further compounded these risks, with 50.7% of participants expressing enjoyment in sunbathing and 48.3% wanting to tan [4]. Although over 80% agreed on the importance of sunscreen due to skin cancer risks, these attitudes suggest a disconnect between knowledge and behavior [4]. This study highlights the need for improved sun protection strategies among rock climbers and potentially other populations that participate in outdoor sports regularly [4].

5.8 Miscellaneous Dermatologic Complications

Rock climbers have been reported to exhibit unique dermatologic changes associated with Paget-Schroetter syndrome, also known as upper extremity deep venous thrombosis (UE-DVT) [61]. Symptoms may include swelling, discoloration, and the small bruise-like lesions, known as burst capillaries, in the affected arm, although it typically presents as nonspecific shoulder pain. This condition is believed to result from the subclavian vein being compressed between the clavicle and first rib during climbing, risking the potential (sub-) total occlusion of the axillary-subclavian venous system. While its incidence is low, Paget-Schroetter syndrome is expected to become increasingly significant due to rising participation in climbing and bouldering sports [61]. Dermatologists should recognize these signs and promptly refer affected patients to vascular specialists, as early diagnosis and intervention are vital to prevent serious complications such as pulmonary embolism [62].

Vijayaraghavan et al. described a case of a female climber who developed a Morel-Lavallée lesion following a rock-climbing fall [63]. These closed traumatic injuries involve the internal degloving of soft tissues from underlying fascial layers, forming a cavity in the prefascial plane that can accumulate fluid, usually blood [64]. A significant risk associated with persistent Morel-Lavallée lesions is skin necrosis, which may occur from compromised blood flow and pressure within the fluid collection, potentially causing tissue ischemia if left untreated [63].

Dupuytren's contracture (DC) is a condition characterized by the formation of fibrous bands in the palmar fascia, leading to progressive flexion deformities of the fingers. Dermatologists frequently encounter DC during consultations, as patients may present with concerns related to a subcutaneous nodule [65]. The rising popularity of rock climbing, coupled with its repetitive and intense grip requirements, predisposes climbers to develop this condition. In a prospective study by Lutter et al., older rock climbers experienced a higher incidence of degenerative conditions, with 10% reporting Dupuytren's disease [66]. Logan et al. found that 19.5% of 1100 climbers developed Dupuytren's disease, with those affected experiencing an earlier onset compared to the general population, indicating a potential link between climbing intensity and the onset of DC [67]. Degreef et al. reported the case of a middle-aged rock climber treated for DC with collagenase injection, who suffered a grade III rupture of the A2 pulley and a grade I injury of the A1 pulley two months post-injection [68]. Collectively, these studies highlight the significant risk of DC in rock climbers and the potential for complications in treatment, despite the condition's typically benign nature.

Zbeda et al. described a rare case of acute septic carpal tunnel syndrome in an indoor rock climber, presenting with severe hand pain, erythema, and progressive numbness. The complication developed four days after an abrasion on the hand sustained during a climbing session. The case highlights the potential for common cutaneous injuries to progress to serious complications and emphasizes the importance of proper hygiene of indoor climbing walls, especially as the popularity of climbing continues to increase [69]. Black heels, or calcaneal petechiae/talon noir, are asymptomatic superficial cutaneous hemorrhages caused by shear forces that rupture of the vasculature, typically seen in athletes involved in sports like tennis and gymnastics [70]. Tammaro et al. reported these superficial lesions in a rock climber, noting their atypical localization on the palmar arch and medial border of the feet, likely attributable to the unique design of climbing shoes [71]. Dermatoscopic evaluation shows a brown and homogeneous pattern without melanin pigmentation, facilitating differentiation from other potentially concerning acral pigmented lesions.

A study by Buda et al. assessed the prevalence of dermatologic conditions among rock climbers, demonstrating that nail diseases affected 65.3% of the 211 athletes surveyed. The most frequently reported nail conditions were onychodystrophy (51.4%), which included onychogryphosis and onycholysis, onychomycosis (12.5%), subungual hematoma (8.3%), and onychocryptosis, or ingrown toenail (4.2%). Men and competitive climbers were significantly more prone to nail disorders, with higher incidence rates correlating with climbing difficulty. Additionally, footwear type, particularly the asymmetrical and smaller climbing shoes commonly worn by climbers, was identified as a contributing factor [72].

References

1. Quick guide: what is sport climbing?: Olympics; [Available from: https://olympics.com/en/news/quick-guide-what-is-sport-climbing].
2. Paige TE, Fiore DC, Houston JD. Injury in traditional and sport rock climbing. Wilderness Environ Med. 1998;9(1):2–7.
3. Smith LO. Alpine climbing: injuries and illness. Phys Med Rehabil Clin N Am. 2006;17(3):633–44.
4. Gutiérrez-Manzanedo JV, González-Montesinos JL, Aguilera-Arjona J, Rodríguez-Martínez A, Vaz-Pardal C, España-Romero V, et al. Ultraviolet sun exposure and sun protection behaviors in outdoor rock climbers. Photochem Photobiol Sci. 2023;22(12):2817–26.
5. Nigam PK, Syed HA, Saleh D. Tinea Pedis [Available from: https://www.ncbi.nlm.nih.gov/books/NBK470421/#:~:text=Tinea%20pedis%20is%20a%20fungal,mild%20soap%20and%20warm%20water].
6. Bodman MA, Syed HA, Krishnamurthy K. Onychomycosis [Available from: https://www.ncbi.nlm.nih.gov/books/NBK441853/].
7. Diedrich V, Zweerink K, Elder B. Plant dermatitis. Emerg Med Clin North Am. 2024;42(3):613–38.
8. Odat TA, Al-Tawara MJ, Hammouri EH. Prickly pear spine keratoconjunctivitis. Middle East Afr J Ophthalmol. 2014;21(1):61–5.
9. Ramos-e-Silva M, Vasconcelos C, Carneiro S, Cestari T. Sporotrichosis. Clin Dermatol. 2007;25(2):181–7.
10. Martinez TT, Jerome M, Barry RC, Jaeger R, Xander JG. Removal of cactus spines from the skin. A comparative evaluation of several methods. Am J Dis Child. 1987;141(12):1291–2.
11. Winer LH, Zeilenga RH. Cactus granulomas of the skin; report of a case. AMA Arch Derm. 1955;72(6):566–9.
12. Fisher AA. Poison ivy/oak/sumac. Part II: specific features. Cutis. 1996;58(1):22–4.
13. Lofgran T, Mahabal GD. Toxicodendron Toxicity [Available from: https://www.ncbi.nlm.nih.gov/books/NBK557866/].

14. Powers J, McDowell RH. Insect Bites [Available from: https://www.ncbi.nlm.nih.gov/books/NBK537235/].
15. Kruse B, Anderson J, Simon LV. Fire Ant Bites [Available from: https://www.ncbi.nlm.nih.gov/books/NBK470576/].
16. Lofgran T, Warrington SJ. Millipede Envenomation [Available from: https://www.ncbi.nlm.nih.gov/books/NBK557454/#:~:text=Millipedes%20are%20unable%20to%20inject,their%20sides%20to%20deter%20predators].
17. Goldman BS, Lee VR, Bragg BN. Butterfly, Moth, and Caterpillar Envenomation [Available from: https://www.ncbi.nlm.nih.gov/books/NBK539851/].
18. Seda J, Horrall S. Mosquito Bites [Available from: https://www.ncbi.nlm.nih.gov/books/NBK539915/].
19. Kumar R, Sharma MK, Jain SK, Yadav SK, Singhal AK. Cutaneous manifestations of Chikungunya fever: observations from an outbreak at a tertiary care hospital in Southeast Rajasthan, India. Indian Dermatol Online J. 2017;8(5):336–42.
20. de Freitas MT, Maia C. Phlebotomus perniciosus. Trends Parasitol. 2024;40(7):649–50.
21. Haddad V Jr, Haddad MR, Santos M, Cardoso JLC. Skin manifestations of tick bites in humans. An Bras Dermatol. 2018;93(2):251–5.
22. Eisen L, Eisen RJ. Changes in the geographic distribution of the blacklegged tick, Ixodes scapularis, in the United States. Ticks Tick Borne Dis. 2023;14(6):102233.
23. Campagna J, Lavoie PE, Birnbaum NS, Furman DP. Lyme disease in northern California. West J Med. 1983;139(3):319–23.
24. Clark KL, Leydet B, Hartman S. Lyme borreliosis in human patients in Florida and Georgia, USA. Int J Med Sci. 2013;10(7):915–31.
25. Braun DS, Greenberg I, Pagadala M. Rocky mountain spotted fever masquerading as gastroenteritis: a common but overlooked clinical presentation. Cureus. 2021;13(4):e14438.
26. Ali AA, Bajric B, Isache CL, Maharaj RP. Mosquito borne illness in a Floridian hiker. Am J Emerg Med. 2021;45(681):e1–2.
27. Thomas EA, John M, Kanish B. Mucocutaneous manifestations of Dengue fever. Indian J Dermatol. 2010;55(1):79–85.
28. Liu J, Tian X, Deng Y, Du Z, Liang T, Hao Y, Zhang D. Risk factors associated with Dengue virus infection in Guangdong Province: a community-based case-control study. Int J Environ Res Public Health. 2019;16(4):617.
29. Chen WJ. Dengue outbreaks and the geographic distribution of dengue vectors in Taiwan: a 20-year epidemiological analysis. Biom J. 2018;41(5):283–9.
30. Farkouh CS, Abdi P, Amatul-Hadi F, Anthony MR, Ali Khan Q, Manja K, et al. Cutaneous manifestations of Malaria and their prognostic windows: a narrative review. Cureus. 2023;15(7):e41706.
31. Hay SI, Guerra CA, Tatem AJ, Noor AM, Snow RW. The global distribution and population at risk of malaria: past, present, and future. Lancet Infect Dis. 2004;4(6):327–36.
32. DeVos E, Dunn N. Malaria Prophylaxis [Available from: https://www.ncbi.nlm.nih.gov/books/NBK551639/].
33. Goetze S, Hiernickel C, Elsner P. Phototoxicity of doxycycline: a systematic review on clinical manifestations, frequency, cofactors, and prevention. Skin Pharmacol Physiol. 2017;30(2):76–80.
34. Enk CD, Gardlo K, Hochberg M, Ingber A, Ruzicka T. Cutaneous leishmaniasis. Hautarzt. 2003;54(6):506–12.
35. Benallal KE, Garni R, Harrat Z, Volf P, Dvorak V. Phlebotomine sand flies (Diptera: Psychodidae) of the Maghreb region: a systematic review of distribution, morphology, and role in the transmission of the pathogens. PLoS Negl Trop Dis. 2022;16(1):e0009952.
36. de Vries HJC, Schallig HD. Cutaneous Leishmaniasis: a 2022 updated narrative review into diagnosis and management developments. Am J Clin Dermatol. 2022;23(6):823–40.
37. Nguyen QD, Vu MN, Hebert AA. Insect repellents: an updated review for the clinician. J Am Acad Dermatol. 2023;88(1):123–30.

38. Meymandi S, Hernandez S, Park S, Sanchez DR, Forsyth C. Treatment of Chagas disease in the United States. Curr Treat Options Infect Dis. 2018;10(3):373–88.
39. Nelson NG, McKenzie LB. Rock climbing injuries treated in emergency departments in the U.S., 1990-2007. Am J Prev Med. 2009;37(3):195–200.
40. Buzzacott P, Schöffl I, Chimiak J, Schöffl V. Rock climbing injuries treated in us emergency departments, 2008-2016. Wilderness Environ Med. 2019;30(2):121–8.
41. Wyatt JP, McNaughton GW, Grant PT. A prospective study of rock climbing injuries. Br J Sports Med. 1996;30(2):148–50.
42. Hosaini SA, Atri AE, Kavosi A. Injuries at the Iranian championship in indoor rock climbing. Wilderness Environ Med. 2013;24(2):167–8.
43. Schöffl VR, Kuepper T. Injuries at the 2005 World championships in rock climbing. Wilderness Environ Med. 2006;17(3):187–90.
44. Cobos-Moreno P, Astasio-Picado Á, Gómez-Martín B. Epidemiological study of foot injuries in the practice of sport climbing. Int J Environ Res Public Health. 2022;19(7):4302.
45. Logan AJ, Makwana N, Mason G, Dias J. Acute hand and wrist injuries in experienced rock climbers. Br J Sports Med. 2004;38(5):545–8.
46. Neuhof A, Hennig FF, Schöffl I, Schöffl V. Injury risk evaluation in sport climbing. Int J Sports Med. 2011;32(10):794–800.
47. Bernard M, Wright R, Anderson H, Bernard A. Wilderness falls: an analysis and comparison of rock climbers and nonclimbers. J Surg Res. 2019;234:149–54.
48. Bowie WS, Hunt TK, Allen HA Jr. Rock-climbing injuries in Yosemite National Park. West J Med. 1988;149(2):172–7.
49. Addiss DG, Baker SP. Mountaineering and rock-climbing injuries in US national parks. Ann Emerg Med. 1989;18(9):975–9.
50. McDonald JW, Henrie AM, Teramoto M, Medina E, Willick SE. Descriptive epidemiology, medical evaluation, and outcomes of rock climbing injuries. Wilderness Environ Med. 2017;28(3):185–96.
51. Gerdes EM, Hafner JW, Aldag JC. Injury patterns and safety practices of rock climbers. J Trauma. 2006;61(6):1517–25.
52. Schöffl V, Popp D, Küpper T, Schöffl I. Injury trends in rock climbers: evaluation of a case series of 911 injuries between 2009 and 2012. Wilderness Environ Med. 2015;26(1):62–7.
53. Schöffl V, Hochholzer T, Winkelmann H, Strecker W. Differentialdiagnose von fingerschmerzen bei sportkletterern. Deutsche Zeitschrift für Sportmedizin. 2003;54:38–43.
54. Schöffl V, Hochholzer T, Winkelmann HP, Strecker W. Pulley injuries in rock climbers. Wilderness Environ Med. 2003;14(2):94–100.
55. Schöffl VR, Hoffmann G, Küpper T. Acute injury risk and severity in indoor climbing-a prospective analysis of 515,337 indoor climbing wall visits in 5 years. Wilderness Environ Med. 2013;24(3):187–94.
56. Rooks MD, Johnston RB, Ensor CD, Mclntosh B, James S. Injury patterns in recreational rock climbers. Am J Sports Med. 1995;23(6):683–5.
57. Braybrook PJ, Tohira H, Birnie T, Brink D, Finn J, Buzzacott P. Types and anatomical locations of injuries among mountain bikers and hikers: a systematic review. PLoS One. 2023;18(8):e0285614.
58. Biem J, Koehncke N, Classen D, Dosman J. Out of the cold: management of hypothermia and frostbite. CMAJ. 2003;168(3):305–11.
59. Harirchi I, Arvin A, Vash JH, Zafarmand V. Frostbite: incidence and predisposing factors in mountaineers. Br J Sports Med. 2005;39(12):898–901. discussion
60. McLennan JG, Ungersma J. Mountaineering accidents in the Sierra Nevada. Am J Sports Med. 1983;11(3):160–3.
61. Lutter C, Monasterio E, Schöffl V. Rock climbing-related subclavian vein thrombosis. BMJ Case Rep. 2015; bcr2015212021.
62. Arko FR, Harris EJ, Zarins CK, Ct O. Vascular complications in high-performance athletes. J Vasc Surg. 2001;33(5):935–42.

63. Vijayaraghavan N, Lee J. Atypical presentation of left knee swelling in a recreational rock-climbing athlete. Curr Sports Med Rep. 2023;22(4):115–6.
64. Singh R, Rymer B, Youssef B, Lim J. The Morel-Lavallée lesion and its management: a review of the literature. J Orthop. 2018;15(4):917–21.
65. Amadio CR, Magalhães BM, Yazawa F, Simone K. Dupuytren's disease: what dermatologists need to know. An Bras Dermatol. 2018;93(5):773–4.
66. Lutter C, Hotfiel T, Tischer T, Lenz R, Schöffl V. Evaluation of rock climbing related injuries in older athletes. Wilderness Environ Med. 2019;30(4):362–8.
67. Logan AJ, Mason G, Dias J, Makwana N. Can rock climbing lead to Dupuytren's disease? Br J Sports Med. 2005;39(9):639–44.
68. Degreef I, Kellens S. Pulley rupture in rock climber after collagenase treatment for Dupuytren contracture. J Hand Surg Asian Pac. 2022;27(1):187–90.
69. Zbeda RM, Rabinovich RV, Vialonga M, Seigerman DA. Acute septic carpal tunnel syndrome in a rock climber. J Orthop Case Rep. 2021;11(4):100–3.
70. Crissey JT, Peachey JC. Calcaneal petechiae. Arch Dermatol. 1961;83:501.
71. Tammaro A, Magri F, Moliterni E, Parisella FR, Mondello M, Persechino S. An uncommon localization of black heels in a free climbing instructor. Int Wound J. 2018;15(2):313–5.
72. Buda R, Di Caprio F, Bedetti L, Mosca M, Giannini S. Foot overuse diseases in rock climbing: an epidemiologic study. J Am Podiatr Med Assoc. 2013;103(2):113–20.

Chapter 6
Racket Sports and Volleyball

Rachel Papavasilopoulos, Ryan Scheinkman, Sophie Bilik, Alexia Vignau, Isabella Guanche, Rachel Cohen, and Keyvan Nouri

6.1 Introduction

Racket sports include tennis, racquetball, squash, pickleball, and badminton. These sports are enjoyed both competitively and recreationally by diverse age groups and skill levels, attracting hundreds of millions of players worldwide. Though the rules and mechanics of these sports differ widely, they all share the same basic principles and equipment. While the health benefits of racket sports are well-recognized, these activities also pose specific dermatological risks. Documented skin issues related to racket sports cover a wide range of conditions, from contact dermatitis (i.e. due to exposure to materials in rackets, grips, and gloves) to mechanical associated conditions (e.g. blisters, calluses, and abrasions). The repetitive motions and intense grip required in racket sports increase susceptibility to friction-based injuries, particularly on the hands, forearms, and feet [1]. Additionally, extended play outdoors exposes athletes to ultraviolet (UV) radiation, while indoor court players might encounter ventilation issues and heightening exposure to perspiration-related skin conditions [2]. Racket sports primarily take place outdoors, with exceptions like badminton and squash being indoor sports. This outdoor setting leaves athletes exposed to prolonged periods of sun exposure during play. The UV radiation levels experienced by outdoor sports players often exceed the daily recommended exposure limits, significantly increasing their risk for sunburn, chronic photodamage, and skin cancers such as melanoma or squamous cell carcinoma [2]. Despite these

R. Papavasilopoulos · R. Scheinkman (✉) · S. Bilik · A. Vignau · I. Guanche · R. Cohen
K. Nouri
Dr. Phillip Frost Department of Dermatology and Cutaneous Surgery, University of Miami, Miami, FL, USA
e-mail: rkp73@miami.edu; scheinkman@med.miami.edu; smb545@miami.edu; axv200@med.miami.edu; idg18@med.miami.edu; rachelcohen@med.miami.edu; knouri@med.miami.edu

K. Nouri (ed.), *Sport-Related Skin Conditions*,
https://doi.org/10.1007/978-3-031-90444-8_6

risks, many athletes fail to adopt adequate sun protective behaviors. Regular application of broad-spectrum sunscreen, use of UPF-rated protective clothing, hats, and seeking shade during breaks can mitigate these risks, yet education and awareness campaigns are necessary to encourage these preventative measures [2].

In addition to UV exposure, the high temperatures common during outdoor matches exacerbate the effects of heat on the skin. Prolonged physical activity in such conditions makes the impact of heat increasingly relevant to dermatologic conditions [3]. High humidity further complicates matters, leading to excessive sweat production. This sweat creates slippery grips and occlusive conditions, often resulting in friction-based injuries such as blisters and calluses on the hands and feet [4]. In order to mitigate this issue, players may choose to use absorbent grips or other anti-slip materials to maintain control of their rackets. However, these products often contain synthetic ingredients that can act as irritants, increasing the risk of contact dermatitis [5]. Beyond the effects of synthetics, the combination of humidity, sweat, and occlusion creates a favorable environment for dermatoses such as acne mechanica, intertrigo, and tinea infections, which are commonly seen in players. The physical demands of racket sports further compound the risks to athletes. These activities involve repetitive, high-impact movements, such as quick directional changes, rapid acceleration and deceleration, and powerful, repetitive swing motions. This repetitive mechanical stress places significant strain on players' extremities, particularly their wrists, elbows, knees and ankles [6]. Such movements heighten the risk for both acute and chronic injuries, including tendinitis and stress fractures. Badminton, squash, and racquetball have been shown to pose higher risks than other racket sports for injuries such as lacerations, sprains, and fractures. This is likely due to frequent collisions with equipment, abrupt movements, or falls during competitive play [6].

Volleyball encompasses both indoor and beach disciplines, each presenting unique challenges to athletes' skin health. Indoor volleyball, played on hardwood or synthetic courts, involves six players per team executing rapid movements, diving maneuvers, and explosive jumps. Beach volleyball, contested on sand courts typically in pairs, exposes athletes to additional environmental elements while demanding similar athletic skills. The physical demands of volleyball create distinctive patterns of skin stress and trauma. Players repeatedly perform explosive movements, including jumping, diving, and lateral transitions, while maintaining constant contact with either court surfaces or sand. These movements, combined with specialized equipment requirements such as knee pads, athletic tape, and protective gear, create unique conditions that affect skin integrity and health. Position specialization in volleyball, from setters to defensive specialists, further contributes to specific patterns of dermatological conditions based on the predominant movements and responsibilities of each role. The dermatological implications of volleyball extend beyond mere mechanical trauma. Indoor facilities create distinct microclimates with controlled temperature and humidity, yet often present challenges with ventilation and surface friction. Beach volleyball environments expose athletes to ultraviolet radiation, sand friction, and variable weather conditions, each contributing to specific dermatological concerns. These environmental factors, combined with the sport's physical demands, create a complex interplay of conditions that affect athlete health and performance.

6.2 Infectious Racket Sport Dermatoses

6.2.1 Tinea and Dermatophyte Infection

Tinea versicolor, or pityriasis versicolor, is a benign, noncontagious fungal infection of the skin. Caused by an overgrowth of the yeast *Malassezia* [7]. Tinea versicolor presents as hyperpigmented or hypopigmented macules often located around the trunk and extremities [7]. These macules can sometimes be accompanied by mild itching and fine scaling superimposed on the lesions. Some patients also report progression from well-demarcated macules into larger, connected patches of dyspigmentation over time [8]. *Malassezia* is harmless in its yeast form but becomes problematic when transformed into its mycelial form. Though the exact mechanisms that trigger this transformation are not fully understood, several environmental factors increase the odds of developing this condition [8]. These environmental factors are common in racket sports and predispose this population to developing tinea versicolor and other tinea dermatophyte infections. As *Malassezia* is a lipophilic yeast, the use of oily lotions and sunscreens, as well as increased sweat production, creates a rich environment for the yeast to thrive and grow. More significantly, racket sports games are often lengthy, resulting in players frequently exercising in humid, sweat-prone conditions for extended periods predisposing athletes to fungal skin infections [7]. Other Tinea and dermatophyte infections are discussed in greater detail in Sect. 13.7.

First-line treatments for this condition include topical washes and are proven to be highly effective for curing this condition. Ketoconazole 2.5% shampoo, cream, or gel form and selenium sulfide are two well-known treatments for tinea versicolor [8]. For more severe cases, physicians may consider prescribing itraconazole or fluconazole; however, this is uncommon and may pose risks related to potential side effects such as GI problems, headaches, and fatigue. Patients may also take extra care to prevent recurrence by increasing the frequency of towel switching, outfit changes, and post-workout showers [7].

6.2.2 Intertrigo

Intertrigo is an inflammatory condition often resulting from opposing skin surfaces and folds that rub together. This is often induced by mechanical factors and can cause erosion and maceration. Secondary infections with bacterial, viral, or fungal agents can also worsen symptoms [5]. Infectious agents can include gram-negative bacteria and gram-positive bacteria, but *Candida* superinfection is the most common [9]. Diagnosis can usually be made from the history, presentation, and physical exam alone. The presence of secondary infection can be determined by clinical examination, and confirmation can be obtained by examining skin scrapings under a microscope following the application of potassium hydroxide solution, and the presence of hyphae confirms dermatophytic lesions [10]. A wood's lamp evaluation and cultures of skin scrapings can also help diagnose causative pathogens or malignant suspicions [5].

Intertrigo can present as red eroded patches on skin that affect warm, moist areas. Commonly affected locations include intertriginous areas, including inframammary folds, groin, axillae, interdigital regions, and abdominal folds [10]. Symptoms include itching, burning, stinging, and erythema, all of which may be exacerbated by continued rubbing and friction in these areas. Therefore, athletic accessories including the racket handle and the movements required in racketball sports, may contribute to the incidence of intertrigo among racketball players. Risk factors include poor hygiene, closed-toes or ill-fitting shoes, tight-fitting clothes, and hyperhidrosis. Primary treatment includes preventing or eliminating friction in high-contact areas. Showering soon after training and keeping skin cool and dry using absorbent and breathable clothing is also recommended. Nylon and synthetic fibers can exacerbate this condition. Topical or oral antibiotics or antifungal coverage or topical anti-inflammatories are recommended in the absence of secondary infections due to the risk of infection exacerbation [9]. Long-term use of high-potency steroids also has an increased risk of skin thinning, atrophy, and telangiectasias at the site of application [4]. Miconazole powder can also be used in flare-prone areas but is less effective for managing active disease.

6.3 Contact Dermatoses and Equipment-Related Conditions in Racket Sport Players

6.3.1 Allergic Contact Dermatitis

Repeated and prolonged exposure to irritants commonly found in tennis equipment can result in allergic contact dermatitis, also known as "racket-grip irritation." Patients may present with well-demarcated erythematous plaques with pruritic vesicles, accompanied by edema and excoriations due to scratching [11]. Materials such as leather, polyester, paraffins, latex, aluminum chloride hexahydrate, and neoprene make up the vast majority of tennis grips, which are used to cover the handle of the racket for extra cushioning [12]. Oftentimes, players may not be able to initially determine the cause of the dermatitis due to the typical delayed Type IV hypersensitivity response. Due to the frequent nature of regripping rackets, a patient may have a difficult time immediately determining what ingredients triggered the reaction and may only identify it upon re-exposure. Athletes may go years without adverse reactions to similar equipment and may overlook potential allergens [13]. Additionally, the likelihood of developing ACD is increased with mechanical stress, sweating, and elevated temperature [13]. Minor abrasions on the hands from the repetitive nature of racket sports further expose players to the aforementioned irritants and increase the likelihood of an allergic reaction [14]. Similar reactions occur from other components of racket sports equipment, tennis balls, are largely composed of an internal rubber base surrounded by latex. The felt fibers wear down quickly, exposing players to the latex-bound core [15]. For patients with latex allergies, this can easily result in widespread ACD. Squash, racquetball, and padel balls contain similar materials, with some, such as squash balls, lacking a protective outer layer.

Certain footwear has also been implicated in contact dermatitis cases. Ethyl butyl thiourea, a synthetic compound commonly used in neoprene production, was identified as the cause of a series of athletic shoe dermatitis cases [14]. This synthetic is used in the inner soles of various athletic shoes, not limited to a single brand. Patients sensitized to this agent are likely to encounter it again in other neoprene-containing products, making avoidance challenging [14]. Foot dermatitis may persist despite the immediate removal of the offending allergen. As with hand dermatitis, abrasions on the feet are common in racket sports, further exposing patients to potentially harmful substances [16]. Identification and removal of the offending agent is the most effective treatment for contact dermatitis. Thorough patient interviews and clear documentation of sports equipment used can expedite irritant identification. Patch testing is the gold standard for diagnosis but may not be necessary if the causative agent is identified and avoided.

6.3.2 Acne Mechanica

Athletes are at particular risk for acne mechanica, especially those with an already existing predisposition to acne [17]. Acne mechanica, also known as friction acne or acne traumatica, is considered a complication of acne vulgaris rather than a distinct type of acne. For individuals with a history of acne vulgaris, acne mechanica manifests as a secondary effect of an already present acne condition. It tends to worsen due to repeated exposure to external mechanical factors like friction, occlusion, and heat [18]. The condition initially presents as acneiform eruptions in areas exposed to irritation and may progress to more severe nodules and cysts over time, particularly if the source of mechanical stress is not removed [19]. These eruptions occur in locations where hair follicles are concentrated, including the buttocks, back, inner thighs, chest, and shoulders [17]. Athletic accessories like headbands and wristbands are commonly used in a variety of racket sports to prevent sweat from reaching the eyes and hands during play. These absorbent and towel-like materials have been shown to trigger acne mechanica due to their occlusive and abrasive nature on the skin [17]. Accessories like these create a warm and humid environment with limited airflow, allowing oils and sweat to build up beneath them.

Similarly, tight-fitting clothing, such as sports bras, increases the incidence of this form of acne on the back and chest, especially in female athletes.

An important consideration is secondary scarring associated with this condition. Lesions often appear in areas of the body less commonly thought to be affected by acne, but which are prone to scarring. Early and proactive treatment of this issue is crucial in the prevention of new lesions and further scarring [17]. Typical acne vulgaris treatments are effective for treating acne mechanica. Topical therapies, including benzoyl peroxide washes, salicylic acid, and azelaic acid, are considered first-line and effective treatments for this condition [19]. For more severe disease progression, integration of oral antibiotic therapy, particularly doxycycline and minocycline, can be especially effective. In patients with underlying hormonal acne exacerbated by the above mechanical stress, treatments such as isotretinoin (either oral or topical), as well as spironolactone or oral contraceptives, are recommended [18]. Though medical intervention is often needed, it is important to advise patients to avoid tight-fitting athletic wear and to ensure frequent changing of sweatbands to reduce the odds of recurrence and increased severity of the condition [17].

6.4 Mechanical Trauma and Position-Specific Injuries in Racket Sport Players

6.4.1 Subungual Hematoma

Subungual hematoma, more commonly known as "Tennis Toe," is a nail bed bruise resulting from a traumatic injury. These hematomas may occur from wearing tight-fitting sneakers or from repeated trauma to the front of the shoe, as commonly seen in tennis players [20]. Injuries to the delicate vasculature of the nail bed result in hematoma formation under the nail plate. As blood pools in this confined space, a purple or black discoloration forms, typically covering over 50% of the nail bed [21]. Subungual hematomas are frequently accompanied by severe, throbbing pain and inflammation, which can be especially problematic for athletes, as contact with the area is difficult to avoid [22]. Though pain subsides relatively quickly, recovery of the nail may take anywhere from six to nine months as regrowth occurs slowly. In more severe cases, damage to the nail matrix may prevent regrowth altogether [20]. Physicians may decide to perform a minor trephination procedure to alleviate symptoms more rapidly. This procedure involves careful insertion of a needle into the hematoma area, ensuring avoidance of the nail matrix and sensitive areas. Excess blood is drained, and patients quickly report resolution of their symptoms [21]. To prevent recurrence of this condition, recommendations for better-fitting shoes should be made. Furthermore, incorporating cushioning pads, like toe caps, within athletic shoes can be an effective strategy to minimize trauma resulting from the repetitive stopping, pivoting, and quick directional changes essential in racket sports. These pads help absorb shock, protecting the feet from pressure-related injury and lowering the risk of further damage while supporting the healing process [23].

6.4.2 *Talon Noir*

Calcaneal petechiae, also known as talon noir ('black heel'), is an asymptomatic, benign trauma-induced hemorrhagic lesions of the epidermis of the heel. They present as a darkening of skin on the posterolateral or posterior aspect of the heel (Fig. 6.1) [24]. Talon noir lesions present as acute onset lesions with intraepidermal hemorrhage, and can vary in color, number, size, and location. Lesions can present with a brown, red, red-brown, or black coloration. Common pigmentation patterns include homogenous, globular, or parallel ridges [25]. Tache noire ('black palm') is an equivalent diagnosis that occurs on the palm and can occur on the hands of athletes engaged in racket sports [26]. Both talon noir and tache noir lesions result from repeated trauma or shearing forces that can be present in racket sports [26].

Movements that can precipitate the bleeding include jumping, twisting, or sudden stopping on the affected area. The repeated pounding or lateral shearing forces cause a rupture of fragile blood vessels, resulting in microhemorrhages and extravasation of blood cells through sweat ducts, into the epidermis [25]. Diagnosis of talon

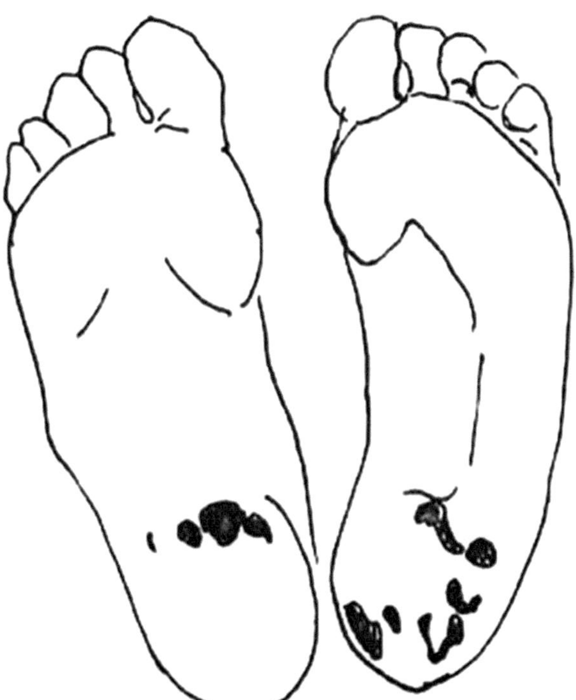

Fig. 6.1 Taon noir

noir and tache noir can be done with scarification of the lesion with a scalpel followed by evaluation with dermoscopy or sent for histologic analysis. Diagnostic confirmation is given by histopathology, which may reveal presence of blood in the stratum corneum, hyperkeratosis, and extravasated erythrocytes. Differential diagnoses may include the presence of melanocytic proliferation, therefore, close inspection is critical for ruling out malignancy. No treatment is necessary for calcaneal petechiae, and these lesions tend to resolve spontaneously [27].

6.5 Hair-Related Conditions and Environmental Dermatoses in Racket Sport Players

6.5.1 Traction Alopecia

Traction alopecia is a form of hair loss that occurs from continuous and repetitive tension on the hair roots [28]. Traction alopecia occurs across all races and ethnic groups but is most common in patients of color. The largest risk factor for developing this condition is wearing tight, high-tension hairstyles for extended periods, including ponytails, buns, locs, and braids [28]. Athletes, especially those with longer hair, often wear their hair in these styles during exercise for prolonged durations. Patients with tighter curl patterns are particularly susceptible, especially when hair is worn tightly [28]. This hair loss most often manifests along the frontotemporal hairline [28]. Classic dermoscopic findings include pinpoint yellow and black dots, short vellus hairs (fringe sign), and tapering hairs. Hair casts, which are white cylinders wrapped around the base of the hair shaft, help differentiate this form of alopecia from others [29]. Traction folliculitis, characterized by perifollicular erythema and pustules around irritated strands, is also associated with this condition [29]. Patients may report stinging and burning pain in the areas of hair loss. Hair related conditions are summarized in Table 6.1.

However, those with early disease progression may be asymptomatic or report only mild, short-lasting pain and redness [28]. Traction alopecia falls under both non-scarring and scarring alopecia, categorized by its progression and likelihood of reversibility [29]. Early identification and treatment are crucial to prevent disease progression. If left untreated, hair loss becomes irreversible, which can impact

Table 6.1 Hair-related conditions and environmental dermatoses associated with Racket Sports and Volleyball

Disease/condition	Symptoms and physical exam findings	Treatment recommendations
Traction alopecia	Hair loss along the frontotemporal hairline	Reducing tight hairstyles, gentle hair ties, topical corticosteroids and ILK injections
Frictional alopecia	Hair loss on the lower legs or around the scalp	Reducing headbands or tight socks

patients' well-being and may only be treatable through hair transplantation [28]. Removing the offending hairstyle is the primary treatment for this condition and is particularly beneficial in early stages when hair loss and irritation are first noticed [28]. For athletes, this may be challenging, as looser hairstyles may interfere with activity. Alternatives such as gentle hair ties and low-tension ponytails or buns may help accommodate both needs. Topical corticosteroids and ILK injections into prominent patches of hair loss are proven to trigger regrowth. Typical alopecia regimens, including topical or oral minoxidil, applied or taken daily, can prevent further hair loss and stimulate growth over time [28].

6.5.2 Frictional Alopecia

Frictional alopecia is a non-scarring subtype of alopecia that occurs following repeated mechanical trauma. Frictional alopecia can occur on any hair-bearing surface of the body that experiences repetitive contact or trauma. In racketball athletes, this condition may occur on the lower legs and may occur secondary to friction due to footwear, socks, or both. In patients with an older onset age of alopecia, alopecia may also be secondary to age-associated dropout of hair follicles [28]. This is often an asymptomatic condition but sometimes associated with pruritis that could be found incidentally upon physical examination and this condition can persist for many years even with removal of the source of friction. Skin biopsies can be performed for diagnostic purposes. Biopsies of frictional alopecia do not show any pathologic changes and there is no inflammatory component. Arterial insufficiency is a possible differential but can be ruled out by ultrasound doppler and evaluation of ankle brachial pressure index [29].

6.6 Environmental Effects on Volleyball Athletes

The volleyball environment presents distinct challenges for skin health, with significant differences between indoor and beach settings. Indoor volleyball facilities create unique microclimates that significantly impact skin health and disease development. Temperature typically ranges from 18 to 30 °C, with relative humidity varying between 40% and 80%, creating conditions that can promote various dermatological conditions. The artificial playing surfaces, characterized by specific friction coefficients between 0.5 and 0.7, contribute to distinct patterns of mechanical trauma [30]. Indoor lighting and air circulation patterns further influence the development and progression of skin conditions, particularly in facilities with suboptimal ventilation systems. Beach volleyball environments present an entirely different set of challenges, with athletes experiencing direct UV exposure ranging from 2 to 6 hours daily during competition and training [30]. Sand temperatures can reach 45 °C, creating significant thermal stress on the skin, particularly during extended playing sessions. Wind exposure, varying from gentle breezes to strong gusts up to 30 mph, combines with high humidity levels (60–100%) to create unique challenges for skin barrier function and wound healing [30].

The impact of these environmental factors manifests differently across playing positions. Liberos and defensive specialists, who spend significantly more time in contact with the playing surface, show the highest rates of friction-related injuries, with floor burns affecting 35–45% of these players during a competitive season [31]. The repeated court contact, combined with equipment interfaces, creates distinct patterns of skin trauma that require specific preventive strategies [32]. Setters face unique challenges related to repeated ball contact and digital trauma, with 25–30% experiencing hand and finger conditions during their competitive careers [31]. The combination of repetitive mechanical stress and equipment friction patterns creates a distinct profile of skin conditions specific to the setting position [5]. These conditions often become chronic without proper preventive measures and early intervention. Outside hitters and middle blockers experience different patterns of skin trauma related to their vertical jumping and landing patterns. Impact-related conditions affect 20–25% of outside hitters, while network-related conditions affect 15–20% of middle blockers [31].

The combination of jumping mechanics, lateral movement patterns, and equipment interface creates position-specific risk factors that require targeted prevention strategies. Environmental prevention strategies must be tailored to the specific demands of indoor and beach volleyball. Indoor facility management plays a crucial role in skin health maintenance, with optimal conditions requiring careful control of temperature, humidity, and ventilation. Successful indoor prevention programs maintain temperatures between 20 and 22 °C and humidity levels between 40% and 60%, while ensuring adequate air circulation throughout the playing area. Regular surface maintenance and cleaning protocols further reduce the risk of skin conditions related to court contact [31]. Beach volleyball requires comprehensive sun protection strategies, with research indicating that regular use of broad-spectrum SPF 30+ sunscreen, combined with UPF-rated clothing and scheduled shade breaks, significantly reduces the risk of acute and chronic sun damage [3]. Sand-related protection strategies focus on foot conditioning, surface temperature monitoring, and proper maintenance of sand depth and quality. These measures have shown significant effectiveness in reducing the incidence of sand-related skin trauma and infections.

6.7 Infectious Conditions and Wound Care in Volleyball Athletes

The unique environmental conditions and physical demands of volleyball create distinct patterns of infectious skin conditions that affect both indoor and beach athletes. These infections, ranging from superficial fungal colonization to deep bacterial infections, require specific understanding and management approaches within the context of volleyball-specific exposures and trauma patterns. Fungal infections, particularly tinea pedis, represent a significant concern in the volleyball population, affecting 15–25% of indoor players and up to 35% of beach volleyball athletes [30]. The increased prevalence in beach players is attributed to the combination of barefoot play, sand exposure, and public beach facility use. The causative organisms, predominantly Trichophyton rubrum and T. mentagrophytes, thrive in the warm, moist environment created by athletic footwear during indoor training. Beach players face additional risks from contaminated sand and shared shower facilities, creating a more complex prevention challenge [30]. Bacterial infections present unique challenges in the volleyball environment, with pitted keratolysis showing distinct prevalence patterns between indoor and beach players. Indoor court players demonstrate an 18–22% prevalence rate, while beach players show higher rates of 25–30%, likely due to increased foot exposure to moisture and sand [34]. This condition, caused by Corynebacterium species, particularly affects performance due to its impact on weight-bearing areas during jumping and quick directional changes. The bacterial colonization patterns show position-specific variations, with defensive specialists showing higher rates due to increased court contact time.

Viral infections, particularly herpes gladiatorum, present significant concerns in the volleyball community, with distinct transmission patterns between indoor and beach environments. Indoor players show outbreak rates of 3–7% in collegiate teams, particularly during tournament play when close contact during blocking and defensive maneuvers are most intense [35]. Beach volleyball players, while experiencing lower rates of herpes gladiatorum (2–4%), face an increased risk of herpes labialis due to sun exposure and environmental stress. The transmission patterns reflect the different nature of player contact in each discipline, with indoor players experiencing more upper body contact during blocking and beach players facing increased risk during sand-based defensive moves.

Wound care in volleyball presents unique challenges due to the specific nature of injuries and environmental exposures. Indoor players commonly experience friction wounds and abrasions from court contact, while beach players face additional challenges from sand contamination and environmental exposure. The management of these wounds requires consideration of both the immediate playing environment and the potential for infection with sport-specific pathogens. Studies have shown that wound healing rates differ significantly between indoor and beach players, with beach volleyball athletes showing delayed healing times due to sand exposure and environmental factors [30]. The prevention and management of infectious conditions in volleyball requires a comprehensive approach that addresses both individual and team-wide factors. Indoor facilities must maintain proper ventilation and surface cleaning protocols, while beach volleyball venues require regular sand maintenance and potential testing for bacterial contamination. Personal hygiene protocols must be adapted to the specific demands of each discipline, with particular attention to foot care and wound management in beach volleyball athletes.

6.8 Mechanical Trauma and Position-Specific Injuries in Volleyball Athletes

Mechanical trauma in volleyball presents distinct patterns based on playing position, environment, and specific movement demands. The repetitive nature of volleyball movements, combined with surface contact and equipment use, creates unique patterns of acute and chronic skin conditions that significantly impact player performance and health. Friction blisters represent one of the most common acute mechanical injuries in volleyball, affecting up to 40% of competitive players during a typical season [31]. The prevalence increases during tournament play, where multiple matches per day create cumulative stress on the skin. Setters show a particular predisposition to finger and hand blisters due to repeated ball contact, while defensive specialists commonly develop blisters on knees and elbows from court contact. Beach volleyball players demonstrate different blister patterns, with foot blisters predominating due to sand friction and temperature effects. The development of these blisters shows strong correlation with playing intensity, environmental conditions, and individual susceptibility factors [36].

Setter's knuckle, a characteristic condition affecting the proximal interphalangeal joints, particularly of the second and third fingers, represents a position-specific injury pattern unique to volleyball. Recent studies indicate that up to 25% of setters develop this condition during their career, with higher rates observed in those who train more than 15 hours per week [35]. The repetitive ball contact during setting motions creates distinct patterns of mechanical stress that can lead to both acute inflammation and chronic structural changes. Beach volleyball setters show slightly lower prevalence rates, possibly due to the different ball dynamics in sand volleyball, but often present with more severe cases due to the combined effects of sun exposure and sand friction [35]. Floor burns and abrasions constitute another significant category of mechanical trauma, particularly affecting defensive specialists and liberos. Indoor players experience these injuries on exposed skin areas during diving and sliding movements. The introduction of modern playing surfaces has altered the pattern and severity of these injuries, though they remain a consistent concern. Beach volleyball players face unique challenges with sand abrasions, which affect 50–60% of players and show different healing patterns due to environmental exposure [30].

Digital nerve compression and chronic stress changes represent significant concerns for volleyball athletes, particularly setters and outside hitters who experience repeated ball contact. The condition affects approximately 15% of players, with symptoms ranging from temporary numbness to chronic sensory changes [37]. The development of these conditions shows strong correlation with cumulative exposure time and technique factors. Beach volleyball players demonstrate lower rates of digital nerve compression but higher rates of general hand trauma due to sand impact and environmental exposure [38]. Talon noir and hyperkeratosis of the feet present distinct patterns between indoor and beach volleyball players. Indoor players commonly develop Talon noir affecting approximately 10% of athletes, particularly those playing on harder surfaces, while hyperkeratosis develops in up to 45% of competitive players as an adaptive response to repeated mechanical stress [5]. Beach volleyball players show higher rates of plantar surface changes, with sand-induced hyperkeratosis. These conditions often coexist with other foot-related issues, creating complex patterns of mechanical adaptation and injury.

6.9 Contact Dermatoses and Equipment-Related Conditions in Volleyball Athletes

6.9.1 Contact Dermatoses

Contact dermatoses represent a significant challenge in volleyball, affecting an estimated 15–30% of players during competitive seasons. The extensive use of protective equipment, combined with the intense physical nature of the sport, creates unique conditions that predispose athletes to both irritant and allergic contact dermatitis. Equipment-related dermatoses primarily manifest in two distinct forms, with irritant contact dermatitis (ICD) accounting for approximately 80% of cases among volleyball players, while allergic contact dermatitis presents more complex diagnostic and management challenges [5]. Knee pad-related dermatitis emerges as one of the most prevalent equipment-related conditions, affecting up to 25% of professional players during a season [32]. The condition shows distinct patterns between positions, with liberos and defensive specialists demonstrating the highest rates due to increased floor contact and defensive movements. The mechanical friction combined with sweating creates an optimal environment for barrier disruption, while repetitive movements specific to volleyball, such as diving and sliding, further exacerbate the condition [39]. Players with pre-existing skin barrier dysfunction show increased susceptibility to these conditions, highlighting the importance of preventive measures in vulnerable athletes.

Allergic contact dermatitis, while less common than ICD, presents more challenging management issues in volleyball players. Recent studies have identified several common allergens in volleyball equipment, with rubber accelerators in knee pads and elastic components accounting for 40% of cases [32]. Chromates in leather equipment contribute to 15% of cases, textile dyes in uniforms and protective gear account for 25%, and neoprene and other synthetic materials represent 20% of cases [32]. The chronic nature of ACD often requires more comprehensive management strategies, including allergen identification and equipment modification. Beach volleyball players show lower rates of ACD due to reduced equipment use but face unique challenges with sunscreen and sand guard-related reactions. Athletic tape use creates another distinct category of contact dermatoses, affecting 10–15% of regular users [40]. The condition occurs more frequently with finger and ankle taping compared to other applications, with increased risk during tournament play when tape use is more prolonged and frequent. Both mechanical factors (tension-related skin damage, moisture trapping, and friction during dynamic movements) and chemical factors (adhesive component sensitivity, interaction with sweat and skin products, and cumulative irritant effects) contribute to the development of tape-related dermatitis. Beach volleyball players face additional challenges with tape adherence and skin irritation due to sand exposure and increased sweating.

6.9.2 Acne Mechanica

Equipment-related acne mechanica presents a unique challenge in volleyball, particularly affecting areas where protective equipment creates occlusion and friction against the skin. This condition is observed in up to 30% of players, with higher rates during intense training periods and in humid conditions [41]. The combination of mechanical friction, heat, and moisture creates an ideal environment for the development of this condition, particularly under knee pads and other protective equipment. Prevention strategies focus on moisture management, equipment cleaning, and proper fitting of protective gear. Current management strategies emphasize a multi-faceted approach incorporating equipment modification, skin barrier protection, environmental controls, and training modifications. The use of hypoallergenic materials, proper fitting and adjustment of equipment, and regular replacement of worn items form the cornerstone of prevention [41]. Additionally, the implementation of pre-activity barrier creams, moisture management strategies, and post-activity skin care routines has shown promising results in reducing the incidence and severity of contact dermatoses in volleyball players [42].

6.10 Hair-Related Conditions and Environmental Dermatoses in Volleyball Athletes

Hair-related dermatoses represent a significant but often overlooked category of conditions affecting volleyball players, particularly female athletes who frequently style their hair for competition. These conditions impact both player comfort and performance while potentially leading to long-term complications if not properly managed [43]. The unique demands of volleyball, including rapid head movements, tight hairstyling requirements, and environmental exposures, create distinct patterns of hair and scalp conditions that require specific preventive and management strategies. Traction alopecia emerges as one of the most prevalent hair-related conditions in volleyball players, affecting approximately 20–30% of female athletes who regularly wear tight hairstyles during competition and training [44]. The condition primarily affects the frontal hairline and temporal regions where hair is pulled most tightly for securing in ponytails or buns. Studies have shown that the risk increases significantly in players who maintain tight hairstyles for extended periods, such as during tournament play or two-a-day training sessions [45]. The combination of tight styling and physical activity-induced sweating creates particularly challenging conditions for hair and scalp health. Beach volleyball players face additional challenges due to the combined effects of sun exposure, sand, and salt water on hair integrity.

Frictional alopecia presents unique challenges in volleyball players who frequently wear headbands or other protective gear that causes repeated friction against the scalp. Higher rates of frictional alopecia are observed in those who wear protective headgear for extended periods [46]. The mechanical trauma from repeated friction, combined with moisture accumulation, can lead to progressive hair loss in affected areas, particularly along the hairline and areas of equipment contact. Indoor players show different patterns of frictional alopecia compared to beach players, likely due to differences in protective equipment use and environmental exposures [30]. Scalp folliculitis represents a significant concern among volleyball players. The condition is exacerbated by the combination of sweating, tight hairstyles, and occlusive headgear commonly used in the sport. The warm, moist environment created during intense physical activity provides ideal conditions for bacterial proliferation, leading to follicular inflammation and potential secondary infections [47]. Recent research has highlighted the importance of proper scalp hygiene and equipment cleaning protocols in preventing this condition. Beach volleyball players demonstrate higher rates of folliculitis during summer months, possibly due to increased sweating and sand exposure.

Environmental factors create distinct challenges for hair and scalp health in volleyball players. Beach volleyball athletes face particular challenges with UV-related damage to both hair and scalp. The combination of intense physical activity, sweating, and extended sun exposure creates particular challenges for maintaining scalp health. Indoor players commonly develop seborrheic dermatitis (affecting 10–20% of players) and other scalp conditions related to the enclosed environment and intense physical activity [48]. Tinea capitis, while less common in adult athletes, remains a concern particularly in youth volleyball players [49]. The sharing of protective headgear and close physical contact during play can facilitate the transmission of dermatophyte infections. The condition requires particular attention due to its potential for transmission within teams and the necessity for systemic treatment. The risk appears higher in environments with high humidity and shared equipment use [49].

6.11 Miscellaneous Dermatoses in Volleyball Athletes

Solar erythema and miliaria represent significant dermatological challenges in volleyball, particularly affecting beach volleyball athletes and indoor players in warm environments. These conditions, while often considered minor, can significantly impact player performance and long-term skin health when occurring in the context of competitive volleyball's unique demands. Solar erythema presents a particular challenge for beach volleyball athletes, with studies indicating that up to 60% of players experience significant sunburn episodes during a competitive season despite awareness of sun protection measures. The nature of beach volleyball creates exceptional sun exposure challenges, as players must maintain performance during times with peak UV index, while engaging in intense physical activity that compromises sunscreen effectiveness through sweating and sand contact. Research has demonstrated that beach volleyball players receive 20–30% more UV exposure than other beach athletes due to the vertical nature of the sport, ball tracking requirements, and the reflective properties of sand, which can reflect up to 25% of UV radiation [30].

The management of solar erythema in volleyball requires a comprehensive approach that extends beyond basic sun protection measures. Beach volleyball athletes face particular challenges with sunscreen maintenance during competition, as the combination of sweating, sand contact, and repeated diving movements significantly reduces sunscreen effectiveness. Studies have shown that standard sunscreen application protocols, typically recommending reapplication every two hours, prove inadequate in volleyball-specific conditions where players may lose up to 50% of their sun protection within thirty minutes of intense play [50]. Miliaria presents distinct patterns in volleyball athletes, affecting both indoor and beach players but manifesting differently based on the playing environment. The condition particularly affects areas of equipment contact, where occlusion combines with intense physical activity to create ideal conditions for sweat duct obstruction. Beach volleyball players demonstrate different patterns of miliaria, with prevalence rates of 45–50% during peak season, often complicated by sand friction and environmental humidity [51]. The relationship between protective equipment and miliaria development shows sport-specific patterns in volleyball. The combination of compression from protective equipment, repetitive movement patterns, and sustained elevation in local skin temperature creates particularly challenging conditions for sweat gland function. Beach volleyball players, while using less protective equipment, show higher rates of miliaria crystallina in exposed areas, likely due to the combined effects of sun exposure, sweating, and sand friction [31].

References

1. Bylak J, Hutchinson MR. Common sports injuries in young tennis players. Sports Med. 1998;26(2):119–32.
2. Snyder A, Valdebran M, Terrero D, Amber KT, Kelly KM. Solar ultraviolet exposure in individuals who perform outdoor sport activities. Sports Med Open. 2020;6(1):42.
3. Kliniec K, Tota M, Zalesińska A, Łyko M, Jankowska-Konsur A. Skin cancer risk, sun-protection knowledge and behavior in athletes—a narrative review. Cancers (Basel). 2023;15(13):3498.
4. Sheary B. Steroid withdrawal effects following long-term topical corticosteroid use. Dermatitis. 2018;29(4):213–8.
5. Emer J, Sivek R, Marciniak B. Sports dermatology: part 1 of 2 traumatic or mechanical injuries, inflammatory conditions, and exacerbations of pre-existing conditions. J Clin Aesthet Dermatol. 2015;8(4):31–43.

6. Nhan DT, Klyce W, Lee RJ. Epidemiological patterns of alternative racquet-sport injuries in the United States, 1997–2016. Orthop J Sports Med. 2018;6(7):2325967118786237. https://doi.org/10.1177/2325967118786237.
7. Mayo Clinic. Tinea versicolor—Symptoms & causes. Mayo Clinic [Internet]. [cited 2024 Nov 13]. Available from: https://www.mayoclinic.org/diseases-conditions/tinea-versicolor.
8. Karray M, McKinney WP. Tinea versicolor. [Updated 2024 Feb 12]. In: StatPearls [Internet]. Treasure Island (FL): StatPearls Publishing; 2024 Jan–. Available from: https://www.ncbi.nlm.nih.gov/books/NBK482500/.
9. Pujalte GG, Costa LMC, Clapp AD, Presutti RJ, Sluzevich JC. More than skin deep: dermatologic conditions in athletes. Sports Health. 2022;15(1):74–85.
10. Romanelli M, Voegeli D, Colboc H, Bassetto F, Janowska A, Scarpa C, Meaume S. The diagnosis, management and prevention of intertrigo in adults: a review. J Wound Care. 2023;32(7):411–20.
11. Helm TN. Allergic contact dermatitis. Medscape [Internet] 2024 Jul 2 [cited 2024 Nov 13]. Available from: https://emedicine.medscape.com/article/1049216-clinical.
12. HMP Global Learning Network. Sports gear-associated contact dermatitis. HMP Global Learning Network [Internet]. [cited 2024 Nov 13]. Available from: https://www.hmpglobal-learningnetwork.com/site/thederm.
13. Hamm R. Atypical wounds: Contact dermatitis. AccessMedicine Network [Internet]. 2020 [cited 2024 Nov 13]. Available from: https://www.accessmedicinenetwork.com/posts/59086-atypical-wounds-contact-dermatitis.
14. Litchman G, Nair PA, Atwater AR, et al. Contact dermatitis. [Updated 2023 Sep 4]. In: StatPearls [Internet]. Treasure Island (FL): StatPearls Publishing; 2024 Jan–. Available from: https://www.ncbi.nlm.nih.gov/books/NBK459230/.
15. Allergy & Asthma Network. Latex-free sports equipment [Internet]. [cited 2024 Nov 13]. Available from: https://allergyasthmanetwork.org/images/Allergies/latex-free-sports-equipment.pdf.
16. Howard MM. The best Yonex badminton rackets. SportsRec [Internet] 2018 Dec 11 [cited 2024 Nov 13]. Available from: https://www.sportsrec.com/6665968/the-best-yonex-badminton-rackets.
17. Torjesen I Acne mechanica caused by skin-skin friction Dermatology Times 2019 M;40(5).
18. Eichenfield DZ, Sprague J, Eichenfield LF. Management of acne vulgaris: a review. JAMA. 2021;326(20):2055–67.
19. Mills OH, Kligman A. Acne Mechanica. Arch Dermatol. 1975;111(4):481–3. https://doi.org/10.1001/archderm.1975.01630160071007.
20. American Osteopathic College of Dermatology. Subungual hematoma. AOCD [Internet]. [cited 2024 Nov 13]. Available from: https://www.aocd.org/page/SubungualHematoma.
21. Streitz M. How to do nail trephination. In: Merck manuals professional edition [Internet]. San Antonio: San Antonio Uniformed Services Health Education Consortium; 2023 Apr [cited 2024 Nov 13]. Available from: https://www.merckmanuals.com/professional/injuries-poisoning/how-to-do-skin-soft-tissue-and-minor-surgical-procedures/how-to-do-nail-trephination.
22. Pingel C, McDowell C. Subungual hematoma drainage. StatPearls [Internet]. Treasure Island (FL): StatPearls Publishing; 2024 [updated 2023 July 25; cited 2024 Nov 13]. Available from: https://www.ncbi.nlm.nih.gov/books/NBK482508.
23. Helmsa A, et al. Surgical pearl: prompt treatment of subungual hematoma by decompression. J Am Acad Dermatol. 2000;42(3):508–9.
24. Primary Care Dermatology Society. Talon noir. Primary Care Dermatol Soc [Internet] 2021 Nov 19 [cited 2024 Nov 13]. Available from: https://www.pcds.org.uk/clinical-guidance/talon-noir.
25. Calcaneal petechiae. DermNet [Internet]. 2024 May 23 [cited 2024 Nov 13]. Available from: https://dermnetnz.org/topics/calcaneal-petechiae.
26. Choudhury S, Mandal A. Talon noir: a case report and literature review. Cureus. 2023;15(3):e35905. https://doi.org/10.7759/cureus.35905.

27. Filho F, Quaresma M, Paolini K, Rocha N, Kac B, Azulay-Abulafia L. Talon noir: Dermoscopy-assisted differential diagnosis of pigmented lesions. Surg Cosmet Dermatol. 2013;5(2):123–5.
28. Zhao J, Cohen PR. Frictional alopecia of the distal legs: case series and review. Dermatol Online J. 2016;22(8)
29. Arora G, Khandpur S, Bansal A, Shetty B, Aggarwal S, Saha S, et al. Current understanding of frictional dermatoses: a review. Indian J Dermatol Venereol Leprol. 2022;89:170–88.
30. Rallis E, Tertipi N, Sfyri E, Kefala V. Prevalence of skin injuries in beach volleyball athletes in Greece. J Clin Med. 2024;13(7):1452.
31. Aagaard H, Scavenius M, Jørgensen U. An epidemiological analysis of the injury pattern in indoor and in beach volleyball. Int J Sports Med. 1997;18(3):217–21.
32. Corazza M, Minghetti S, Benetti S, Marchetti N, Borghi A, Virgili A. Allergic contact dermatitis in a volleyball player due to protective adhesive taping. Eur J Dermatol. 2011;21(3):430–1.
33. Carr PC, Cropley TG. Sports dermatology: skin disease in athletes. Clin Sports Med. 2019;38(4):597–618.
34. Brandão J, Valério E, Weiskerger C, Veríssimo C, Sarioglou K, Novak Babič M, et al. Strategies for monitoring microbial life in beach sand for protection of public health. Int J Environ Res Public Health. 2023;20(9):6100.
35. Baugh CM, Weintraub GS, Gregory AJ, Djoko A, Dompier TP, Kerr ZY. Descriptive epidemiology of injuries sustained in National Collegiate Athletic Association men's and women's volleyball, 2013–2014 to 2014–2015. Sports Health. 2018;10(1):60–9.
36. Brennan FH Jr. Managing blisters in competitive athletes. Curr Sports Med Rep. 2002;1(6):319–22.
37. Gitkind AI, Zhao P, Oh-Park MY, Fast A. Median palmar cutaneous nerve injury in a volleyball player. Am J Phys Med Rehabil. 2009;88(4):272–4.
38. Toth C. Peripheral nerve injuries attributable to sport and recreation. Neurol Clin. 2008;26(1):89–113.
39. Rajkumar J, Chandan N, Lio P, Shi V. The skin barrier and moisturization: function, disruption, and mechanisms of repair. Skin Pharmacol Physiol. 2023;36(4):174–85.
40. Hamnerius N, Dahlin J, Bruze M, Nilsson K, Sukakul T, Svedman C. Colophonium-related allergic contact dermatitis caused by medical adhesive tape used to prevent skin lesions in soldiers. Acta Derm Venereol. 2023;103:adv18428.
41. Liebich C, Wegin VV, Marquart C, Schubert I, von Bruehl ML, Halle M, et al. Skin diseases in elite athletes. Int J Sports Med. 2021;42(14):1297–304.
42. Beam JW, Buckley B, Holcomb WR, Ciocca M. National athletic trainers' association position statement: management of acute skin trauma. J Athl Train. 2016;51(12):1053–70.
43. Vano-Galvan S. Hair and scalp-related disorders are a trending topic in dermatology, with a significant increase in number of consultations in the last decade. J Eur Acad Dermatol Venereol. 2023;37(1):16–7.
44. Pulickal JK, Kaliyadan F. Traction alopecia. StatPearls [Internet]. Treasure Island (FL): StatPearls Publishing; 2024 [updated 2024 Feb 12; cited 2024 Nov 13]. Available from: https://www.ncbi.nlm.nih.gov/books/NBK470434/.
45. Larrondo J, McMichael AJ. Traction alopecia. JAMA Dermatol. 2023;159(6):676.
46. Liu C, Abbas F, Seehra J. Headgear-induced temporary pressure alopecia. J Orthod. 2019;46(4):335–42.
47. Lugović-Mihić L, Barisić F, Bulat V, Buljan M, Situm M, Bradić L, et al. Differential diagnosis of the scalp hair folliculitis. Acta Clin Croat. 2011;50(3):395–402.
48. Adams BB, Kindred C. Common and uncommon hair and nail problems in sports. Cutis. 2005;75(5):269–75.
49. Winokur RC, Dexter WW. Fungal infections and parasitic infestations in sports: expedient identification and treatment. Phys Sportsmed. 2004;32(10):23–33.
50. Görig T, Apfelbacher C, Drewitz KP, Reimers AK, Breitbart EW, Diehl K. Sunburn and sun protection during recreational outdoor sport in summer: findings from the German general population aged 16–65 years. Photodermatol Photoimmunol Photomed. 2023;39(6):589–97.
51. Nichols AW. Heat-related illness in sports and exercise. Curr Rev Musculoskelet Med. 2014;7(4):355–65.

Chapter 7
Bat-&-Ball Sports

Kristiana Barbato, Ryan Scheinkman, Yasmine Mohseni, Alexia Vignau, Edward Brotgandel, Rachel Cohen, and Keyvan Nouri

7.1 Introduction

Every year, over 80 million Americans enjoy bat-and-ball sports like baseball, softball, and cricket [1]. Given cricket is the second most popular sport in the world, understanding the associated health conditions and proper healthcare involving these sports is critical [1]. Baseball, softball, and cricket are a group of sports that utilize similar equipment like a bat, ball, catcher's glove, and helmet. These sports require bat-and-ball contact with the goal of hitting the ball far enough to give players enough time to reach home base. Compared to baseball, softball uses a larger ball, smaller field, and is a more female-dominated sport. In cricket, only the batsman and players near the batsman are allowed to wear protective gear like padding and helmets [2]. In both sports, males wear a cup to protect the groin from impact and the catcher typically has additional protective clothing like a face shield, throat guard, chest protector, and shin guard [3, 4]. All of these sports are considered limited contact sports, however the repetitive actions and acceleration and deceleration required during these sports makes players prone to friction-related and traumatic dermatological conditions [5]. Additionally, in baseball all players wear gloves creating a moist, warm environment and enabling the development of opportunistic dermatological conditions such as fungal and bacterial infections.

K. Barbato · R. Scheinkman (✉) · Y. Mohseni · A. Vignau · E. Brotgandel · R. Cohen
K. Nouri
Dr. Phillip Frost Department of Dermatology and Cutaneous Surgery, University of Miami, Miami, FL, USA
e-mail: kxb1437@med.miami.edu; scheinkman@med.miami.edu; yxm823@med.miami.edu; axv200@med.miami.edu; exb1079@med.miami.edu; rachelcohen@med.miami.edu; knouri@med.miami.edu

K. Nouri (ed.), *Sport-Related Skin Conditions*,
https://doi.org/10.1007/978-3-031-90444-8_7

7.2 Infectious Dermatoses

7.2.1 Bacterial Infections

The most common forms of cutaneous trauma that occur from baseball and softball injuries are contusions, abrasions, lacerations, or hematomas [1]. The aforementioned skin traumas are a potential concern for bacterial infections as open wounds provide pathogens an opportunity to enter the body and replicate. Cutaneous injuries preceding bacterial infections may lead to impetigo, cellulitis, or folliculitis. Patients with impetigo may present with either the bullous or non-bullous form. More commonly seen, non-bullous impetigo presents as small pustules which become yellowish-brown crusted plaques. It is typically caused by *Staphylococcus aureus* or *Staphylococcus pyogenes* [6]. These lesions develop in areas of traumatized skin often seen in baseball, softball, and cricket. Comparatively, bullous impetigo lesions are large bullae caused by *S. aureus*. Although impetigo is originally considered a mild infection, it may progress into more virulent infections, such as acute rheumatic fever, if not addressed properly [6]. Effective treatment options for impetigo include topical antibiotics, such as mupirocin, or oral antibiotics, such as amoxicillin [7].

Another bacterial infection that batting sports players are prone to is cellulitis. Patients with cellulitis may present with an acute infection with erythema, swelling, and tenderness surrounding a skin trauma [8]. Patients may also present with fever, tachycardia, and pain. The infection is most often caused by exposure to beta-hemolytic *Streptococcus*. A meta-analysis utilizing a Mantel-Haenszel fixed-effects model compared the treatment options available for cellulitis. From the data that was analyzed, they were unable to conclude a definitive most effective antibiotic option [9]. However, oral cephalosporin or oral penicillin can be used to treat cellulitis [9]. Prevention of cellulitis in these athletes includes maintaining dry skin and ensuring proper wound care for ulcerations [10].

Headgear often worn by baseball, softball, and cricket players predisposes them to hair follicle infections. Folliculitis may present as small, follicular papules or pustules, often caused by *S. aureus* or *Streptococcus* [11]. Folliculitis can maturate and form an abscess, leading to the formation of furuncles. Otherwise known as boils, furuncles are caused by bacterial infections to the hair follicle that have matured into erythematous nodules [11]. Treatment for folliculitis is dependent on the type of infection [12]. For example, staphylococcal folliculitis can be treated first-line with cephalexin in addition to proper wound care. If MRSA is suspected, treatment with trimethoprim-sulfamethoxazole is advised [12].

7.2.2 Dermatophyte Infections

Common fungal infections seen in bat-and-ball sports include *Tinea pedis* and *tinea cruris*, which are located on the feet and groin respectively. The tinea fungi are not obligate parasites and can survive outside of the host for some time, typically in warm, moist environments [12]. The protective gear such as stiff footwear and groin cups used in baseball and cricket offer the proper breeding ground for these infections. Additionally, the shared communal locker rooms provide opportunities for the fungi to spread. *Tinea* infections are caused by either *Microsporum*, *Epidermophyton*, or *Trichonphyton* infections, also known as dermatophytes [13]. Patients with *tinea pedis* present with scaling in interdigital spaces and the bottom of the foot (Fig. 7.1) [13]. Whereas, patients with *tinea cruris* present with an erythematous rash with a scaly edge around the groin [13]. When diagnosing tinea of *Microsporum* origin, the use of a Wood's light (barium silicate containing 9% nickel oxide lamp with wavelength of greater than 365 nm) in dark room causes the hairs to shine bright green [13]. Treatment of *tinea* infections typically include topical allylamines, such as terbinafine 1% cream, twice daily for 4–6 weeks. More severe cases may require oral terbinafine (250 mg daily for 2 weeks) in addition to the aforementioned topical agent [1]. To prevent *tinea pedis* it is important for athletes to wear moisture-absorbing socks and keep feet dry.

Tinea versicolor is caused by the fungal species *Malassezia* where the patient presents with scaly hypopigmented or hyperpigmented macules or patches [14]. Darker skin tones often present with hypopigmented lesions whereas lighter skin tones present with hyperpigmented lesions [14]. Lesions usually affect sebum rich areas of the body such as the neck, shoulder, trunk, and upper arms [14]. The occurrence of *tinea versicolor* is prevalent in hot and humid climates, often where these sports take place [14]. A potassium hydroxide test that reveals short hyphae mixed with spore clusters confirms a positive diagnosis [14]. Additionally, under a Wood's

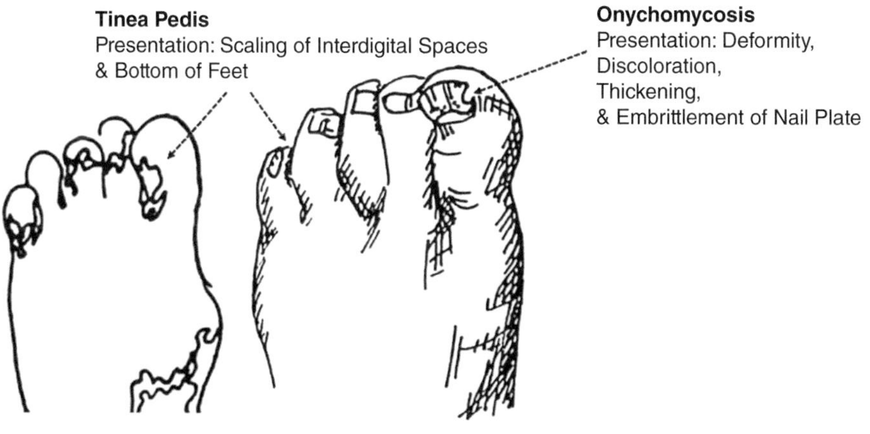

Fig. 7.1 Dermatophytic Infections of the Feet

ultraviolet lamp, the infection portrays a yellowish-orange hue [12]. Typically, a seven day course of a topical antifungal, such as a topical azole or terbinafine, is appropriate for patients [12]. For severe and recurrent cases, an oral antifungal may be used [14]. For athletes who experience recurrent cases of *tinea versicolor*, prophylactic treatment of oral itraconazole twice daily one day per month is deemed efficacious in preventing relapses [15].

Tinea unguium, also known as onychomycosis, is seen in softball, baseball, and cricket players due to trauma to their nails. One study noted that athletes are 2.5-fold more likely to develop this fungal infection with the toenails being seven times more commonly affected [16]. Another study conducted in 2017 surveyed athletic trainers of all 30 Major League Baseball (MLB) teams. Of those who responded, nail problems, like onychomycosis, were listed as the third most common condition after blisters and contact dermatitis [16]. The high incidence of this fungal infection can be traced back to footwear creating a warm environment, making these players more susceptible to infection. The common causative pathogens of onychomycosis are *Trichophyton rubrum* and *Trichonphyton mentagrophytes* (presenting with thickening, embrittlement, discoloration, and deformity of nail plate) [16]. A potassium hydroxide test of stained nail clippings with septate hyphae indicates a positive diagnosis of *Trichophyton* spp. [1]. However, a periodic acid Schiff (PAS) or Gomori methenamine silver (GMS) staining has proven to be more sensitive in identifying this infection [17]. Treatment of onychomycosis is difficult due to the location of the infection. The nail barrier presents a challenge for drug penetration, making recurrent infections common [16]. Oral terbinafine has demonstrated efficacy in treating onychomycosis [16]. Due to the difficulty of treatment, prevention of onychomycosis is important. Bat-and-ball sport players should ensure short toenail length is maintained and that clothing, especially socks, are properly washed.

7.2.3 Viral Infections

Verrucae encompass a wide variety of benign skin growths resulting from dermal infection by the human papillomavirus (HPV) family. These skin lesions present as hyperkeratotic verrucous papules consisting of stratified squamous epithelium. These lesions can be further defined by their specific presentation and location, including common warts (verruca vulgaris), plantar warts (verruca plantaris), and filiform warts [18]. While extremely common in the general population, their prevalence may be increased in batting sports athletes. While the obvious skin-to-skin contact between teammates can spread HPV to cause verrucae infection, there is also significant evidence demonstrating that viruses that can spread through non-sexual contact are able to remain stable on fomites, although it is unknown if the fomites can spread infection through free capsids of the virion or those inside of infected keratinocytes [19]. Regardless, this ability to remain stable and be transmitted through micro-abrasions increases the likelihood that players are infected through the routine sharing of equipment. Additionally, the induction of micro-abrasions through the use of shared equipment such as bats, balls, gloves, and mitts further increases the chances of infection. Beyond the person-to-person transmission of HPV resulting in verrucae, the odds of self-inoculation are high in areas of abrasion even without the sharing of equipment. This results in the common finding of verrucae presenting in groups as opposed to isolated lesions [20]. An existing plantar wart can spread to other locations on the foot due to micro-abrasions that occur as a result of repetitive foot movement during the playing of batting sports.

Treatment options include topicals such as salicylic acid (sold as Compound W), imiquimod, 5-fluoruracil, and squaric acid diphenylcyclopropenone [21]. Further treatment of recalcitrant lesions includes procedures such as cryotherapy and curettage and intralesional injection with *Candida* antigen or bleomycin [22]. Treatment can be challenging, and verrucous lesions frequently recur after treatment. Therefore, prevention of verrucous infections is ideal and can be achieved through similar tactics to the prevention of any infectious dermatosis. Limiting sharing of equipment, minimizing abrasions in infected areas, and covering of existing lesions can help to prevent the spread between players and to new locations on already-infected individuals.

7.3 Allergic Contact Dermatitis & Friction-Related Dermatoses

7.3.1 Allergic Contact Dermatitis

The close contact of a variety of potential antigens to batting sports athletes' skin can result in the development of allergic contact dermatitis (ACD) from a variety of causes. ACD is a delayed hypersensitivity reaction mediated by sensitized T-lymphocytes that presents as an inflammatory skin reaction after contact of an offending antigen with skin [23]. Batting sports athletes are often exposed to many common contact allergens and this repetitive exposure can result in the sensitization that upon subsequent re-exposure results in the presentation of the reaction as a dermatitis. Often the identification of the antigen can be determined from the location of the dermatitis. Colophony, also known as rosin, is a known common contact allergen that is used as a sticky substance by pitchers in baseball and softball to help increase grip on balls to gain a competitive advantage. Contact dermatitis conditions are summarized in Table 7.1.

Rosin-induced allergic contact dermatitis often presents on palms of throwing hands, and unilateral presentation is an indicator of such an etiology [24]. Similar dermatoses can present from hand contact to other allergens, such as lanolin used as softening agents in mitts or organic compounds such as quinones and phenols found in the wood of wooden bats. Interestingly, fields seeded with *Soliva pterosperma* (also known as jo-jo weed and lawnweed) are commonly found on sporting grounds in New Zealand and Australia. The diagnosis of bindii (jo-jo) dermatitis can be

Table 7.1 Allergic contact dermatitis & friction-related dermatoses associated with Bat-and-Ball Sports

Disease/ Condition	Symptoms and physical exam findings	Treatment recommendations
Allergic Contact Dermatitis	Unilateral inflammation on the palms of throwing hands	Removal of allergenic trigger or use barrier protection. Topical corticosteroids to assist in resolution
Friction Bullae	Lesions on throwing hands or dominant batting hand	Drain blisters if symptomatic. Wet dressings for deroofed lesions
Athlete's Nodules	Skin-colored intradermal lesions on body parts not protected with equipment	Keratolytic topicals or excision of bothersome lesions for hyperkeratotic lesions
Calluses	Hyperkeratotic lesions on palms or fingers	Water soaks, keratolytic topicals, paring with pumice stones
Acne Mechanica	Scattered inflammatory papules and pustules in areas of friction, occlusion, or pressure	Similar to acne vulgaris treatments (topical washes, antibiotics, and retinoids). Optional photodynamic therapy and laser treatments

made based on a clinical history [25]. Treatment of allergic contact dermatitis begins with removal of the allergenic trigger or use of barrier protection to prevent contact. The use of topical corticosteroids can assist in the resolution of active dermatitis. If the specific antigen is not known, allergen testing including patch testing and open-application tests can be employed to elucidate the exact allergen for future avoidance [23].

7.3.2 *Friction Bullae*

Bat-and-ball sports, like any other physical activity, requires movements that induce friction, and these abrasive events can result in the presentation of friction dermatoses. Friction bullae are one such condition. These lesions present due to shearing forces that create separations in the epidermis at the layer of the stratum spinosum. This desquamation often fills with fluid due to hydrostatic pressures, creating an uncomfortable pressure sensation [26]. The presentations of friction bullae often vary depending on the role of the player and their actions. Pitchers and throwers often develop lesions on their throwing hands, while batters develop lesions on their dominant batting hand. Lesions on the feet often develop in running players and is worse with ill-fitting shoes that produce unintended pressure points in areas such as the achilles tendon or the toes. Diagnosis can be made with a physical examination and clinical history, though lesions in traditionally non-abrasive areas can merit further workup to rule out an underlying bullous condition. Prevention of friction bullae can be achieved with proper-fitting equipment and through extra padding, such as by wearing batting gloves or low-friction bandages over heels [27]. These lesions are often self-resolving, though symptomatic pain relief can be provided with draining of blisters while keeping the roof of the lesion intact to prevent subsequent infection. For lesions that have deroofed, wet dressings are the ideal method of treatment, with hydrocolloid and other gel-based dressings providing a moist environment that encourages drainage and healing while protecting from outside contamination [28].

A friction dermatosis specific to pitching players is called baseball pitcher's friction dermatitis. This condition is the result of a combination of friction experienced during the pitching motion and an atopic background of the patient [29]. This diagnosis can be made after excluding simple irritant or allergic components, though it can be managed similarly with topical corticosteroids and limitation of future irritation. Patients can be asked to attempt to modify their motion to limit further insult to the skin. Though if not feasible, a similar effect can be obtained with barrier padding such as stockings or sleeves to limit friction [29].

7.3.3 Athlete's Nodules

Athlete's nodules are connective tissue nevi related to sports activities, often through the friction from gripping an object or from worn equipment. Also called collagenomas, these skin-colored intradermal lesions are the result of chronic friction. Diagnosis can be made clinically, though biopsy can confirm the diagnosis with histopathology showing simple hypertrophy of the epidermis and dermis. The lesions regress over time when the offending action is removed. In the context of batting sports athletes, these can present on the hands of batters without proper protection such as batting gloves. For catching and running players, ill-fitting mitts, cleats, and shin guards can induce presentation of such lesions on the legs and feet. Patients should be recommended thicker protective equipment such as batting gloves and well-fitting equipment. For more hyperkeratotic lesions, treatment with keratolytic topicals can be indicated with the option of curettage or excision of more bothersome lesions [30, 31].

7.3.4 Calluses

Calluses are similar hyperkeratotic lesions derived from repetitive pressure and friction, though they can be differentiated by well-demarcated borders. On histology, they appear as a thickening of the stratum corneum. Batting players often present with these lesions on their palms where the bat is gripped, while pitchers often develop lesions on their fingers where the ball is gripped. Diagnosis can be made with a physical examination while the patient grips the bat or ball as they do during play to confirm overlay of the object and lesion. Differential diagnoses such as corns and verrucous lesions can be excluded with the absence of a hyperkeratotic core or capillary presentation on dermoscopy. While benign and often intentionally kept by players as a protection from further trauma, the lesions can be painful when bullae do form and can inhibit functionality or gripping ability. These firm lesions can be gently softened with water soaks, keratolytic topicals, and paring with pumice stones as tolerated. Lesions can be prevented from reforming with thicker padded batting gloves and frequent moisturizer use [32]. One case report demonstrated how calluses can present similarly to melanocytic lesions when exogenous coloration occurs from pine tar, frequently used in baseball to improve grip on balls and bats [33]. Dermoscopy and clinical history taking was essential in the ruling out of a more insidious process and needs to be considered when treating suspected batting sports athletes.

7.3.5 Acne Mechanica

Sports-induced acne, also known as acne mechanica, is a condition that presents similarly to acne vulgaris with scattered inflammatory papules and pustules. While it can be difficult to differentiate from an exacerbation of acne vulgaris with a simple physical examination, acne mechanica presents in areas of friction, occlusion, and pressure [34]. These often present in areas where protective equipment is worn, such as under helmets (particularly on the forehead, cheeks, and chin) of batters and masks (on the periphery of the face) in umpires and catchers. In more serious presentations, acne mechanica can progress to acne keloidalis nuchae, typically on the occipital region [35]. The condition often self-improves over periods of abstaining from wearing the offending equipment, such as during the offseason. Prevention can be achieved through removal of helmets and masks when not necessary and management with frequent skin cleansing, particularly after play. Treatment modalities are similar to acne vulgaris with topical washes including benzoyl peroxide, antibiotics (topical and oral), and retinoids (topical and oral) [36]. Refractory presentations can be treated further with photodynamic therapy and laser treatments, and acne keloidalis nuchae can potentially benefit from intralesional steroid injections [1, 37].

7.4 Skin Lesions Related to Trauma

7.4.1 Talon Noir and Tache Noir

The common actions of abrupt acceleration and deceleration, as well as sliding and diving to bases in baseball make players especially prone to traumatic skin lesions such as abrasions and hemorrhagic lesions. One form of hemorrhagic lesions seen in batting sports is Talon noir or calcaneal petechiae or "black heel", which is a superficial cutaneous hemorrhage in the papillary dermis resulting in multiple small punctate lesions on the convex part of the heel. This condition is a result of repetitive shearing of the epidermis over the rete arteriosum of the papillary dermis [38]. This lesion is observed in various sports that involve repetitive and abrupt starting and stopping motions of the feet and heels such as basketball, football, and baseball. Tache noir is a similar lesion observed on the thenar eminence of the hand, often seen in fielders and catchers due to the repetitive force of the baseball hitting this aspect of the hand [1]. The diagnosis of both talon noir and black palms can be confirmed via shave biopsy and histology in which benzidine stain shows the presence of hemoglobin deposits. Alternatively, dermatoscopy alone can be used to observe features that distinguish talon noir from melanocytic lesions such as red-black homogenous pigmentation with peripheral red-block globules outside of the main lesion [38]. Both talon noir and tache noir are asymptomatic and benign and typically should not prevent players from engaging in their sport. Given there is some clinical resemblance to malignant melanoma it is crucial to differentiate these lesions using the diagnostic methods above.

7.4.2 Post Traumatic Port Wine Stain (Fegeler Syndrome)

Post Traumatic Port Wine Stain (PTPWS) is an acquired condition that can be observed secondary to blunt trauma in batting sports. Port Wine Stains (PWS) are vascular malformations consisting of abnormally dilated capillaries in the middle to superficial dermis. The capillary dilations and ectasias tend to expand with time, leading to a visible expansion of the cutaneous lesion. Port wine stains present as a unilateral erythematous patch and are typically congenital in nature. Although acquired cases are rare, numerous cases of port wine stains secondary to trauma have been documented, and interestingly, a systematic review of the literature has reported that 30% of acquired port wine stains are secondary to sports trauma [39]. The exact cause of these lesions is still unknown; however, their etiology has been hypothesized to be related to alterations in autonomic innervation and neural modulation of blood vessel tone. Some studies have found decreased nerve density in the blood vessels of a PWS lesion compared to normal skin. It is believed that this decreased nerve density is related to dysfunctional regulation of capillary dilation seen in PWS [39]. Current treatment for acquired PTPWS centers around laser therapy, with the most frequently used being pulsed dye lasers and photodynamic therapy. Treatment typically requires multiple sessions and can be spaced months apart.

7.4.3 Athletes Toenail

Batting sport athletes are also prone to various nail-related lesions because of repetitive trauma to the feet and toes as well as ill-fitting cleats. One such lesion is a subungual hematoma which is a hemorrhagic lesion located beneath the nail plate within the nail bed and is a result of repetitive anterior force of the toe against shoes and cleats. This can often occur with repetitive sliding to bases in batters. Subungual hematomas are often painful and can be relieved with rest and foot soaking. If needed a trephination procedure can be performed involving insertion of a small hole and drainage of the subungual blood to provide relief [1]. To prevent subungual lesions, it is suggested that players tightly lace their cleats to prevent forward sliding of the feet during activity. It is also suggested to keep toenails cut as short and close to the skin as possible to prevent subsequent trauma.

References

1. Farhadian JA, Tlougan BE, Adams BB, et al. Skin conditions of baseball, cricket, and softball players. Sports Med. 2013;43:575–89. https://doi.org/10.1007/s40279-013-0022-4. PMID: 23456491. https://link-springer-com.access.library.miami.edu/article/10.1007/s40279-013-0022-4.
2. Diffen. Baseball vs Cricket. Diffen. 2024. https://www.diffen.com/difference/Baseball_vs_Cricket.
3. Sports Law Blogger. Do baseball players own cups? Sports Law Blogger. 2024. https://sportslawblogger.com/do-baseball-players-own-cups.html.
4. DGE Cricket. Cricket abdominal guard: what it is & how a Cricket player can use an abdominal guard. DGE Cricket. 2024. https://dgecricket.com.au/cricket-abdominal-guard-what-it-is-how-a-cricket-player-can-use-an-abdominal-guard/?srsltid=AfmBOopi-3BmwvI02uCq3bzRuszMM_V0TJgK9dBZSigyNG6vovU42yOF.
5. MLB. Slide Rule. MLB.com. 2024. https://www.mlb.com/glossary/rules/slide-rule.
6. D'Cunha NM, Peterson GM, Baby KE, Thomas J. Impetigo: a need for new therapies in a world of increasing antimicrobial resistance. J Clin Pharm Ther. 2018;43(1):150–3. https://doi.org/10.1111/jcpt.12639.
7. American Academy of Family Physicians. Medical and legal aspects of the family physician's role in sports. Am Fam Physician. 2007;75:859–64. https://www.aafp.org/pubs/afp/issues/2007/0315/p859.html.
8. Hendricks S, Du Toit S. Prevalence and risk factors for injury in South African professional Rugby players: a prospective study. Clin J Sport Med. 2011;21:130–7. https://doi.org/10.1111/j.1529-8019.2011.01398.x.
9. Brindle R, Williams OM, Barton E, Featherstone P. Assessment of antibiotic treatment of cellulitis and erysipelas: a systematic review and meta-analysis. JAMA Dermatol. 2019;155(9):1033–40. https://doi.org/10.1001/jamadermatol.2019.0884.
10. Raff AB, Kroshinsky D. Cellulitis: a review. JAMA. 2016;316(3):325–37. https://doi.org/10.1001/jama.2016.8825.
11. Adams BB. Sports-related skin infections. Expert Rev Dermat. 2006;1(1):3–6. https://doi.org/10.1586/17469872.1.1.3.
12. Pujalte GGA, Costa LMC, Clapp AD, Presutti RJ, Sluzevich JC. More than skin deep: dermatologic conditions in athletes. Sports Health. 2023;15(1):74–85. https://doi.org/10.1177/19417381211065026.

13. Harris R, Cook D. Physical activity and risk of colorectal cancer: a meta-analysis of prospective studies. BMJ. 2012;345:e4380. https://doi.org/10.1136/bmj.e4380.
14. Leung AK, Barankin B, Lam JM, Leong KF, Hon KL. Tinea versicolor: an updated review. Drugs Context. 2022;11:2022-9-2. https://doi.org/10.7573/dic.2022-9-2. PMID: 36452877; PMCID: PMC9677953.
15. Faergemann J, Gupta AK, Al Mofadi A, Abanami A, Shareaah AA, Marynissen G. Efficacy of itraconazole in the prophylactic treatment of Pityriasis (Tinea) versicolor. Arch Dermatol. 2002;138(1):69–73. https://doi.org/10.1001/archderm.138.1.69.
16. Daggett C, Brodell RT, Daniel CR, et al. Onychomycosis in athletes. Am J Clin Dermatol. 2019;20:691–8. https://doi.org/10.1007/s40257-019-00448-4.
17. Barak O, Asarch A, Horn T. PAS is optimal for diagnosing onychomycosis. J Cutan Pathol. 2010;37(10):1038–40. https://doi.org/10.1111/j.1600-0560.2010.01545.x. Epub 2010 Apr 12. PMID: 20412344.
18. Verma KK, Burningham KM, Tyring SK. Innovation in Warts and Molluscum: an updated comprehensive review. Dermatol Clin. 2025;43(1):95–102. https://doi.org/10.1016/j.det.2024.08.007. Epub 2024 Sep 10. PMID: 39542567.
19. Ryndock EJ, Meyers C. A risk for non-sexual transmission of human papillomavirus? Expert Rev Anti-Infect Ther. 2014;12(10):1165–70. https://doi.org/10.1586/14787210.2014.959497.
20. McLaughlin JS, Shafritz AB. Cutaneous warts. J Hand Surg Am. 2011;36(2):343–4. https://doi.org/10.1016/j.jhsa.2010.11.036. PMID: 21276900.
21. Kwok CS, Gibbs S, Bennett C, Holland R, Abbott R. Topical treatments for cutaneous warts. Cochrane Database Syst Rev. 2012;2012(9):CD001781. https://doi.org/10.1002/14651858.CD001781.pub3. PMID: 22972052; PMCID: PMC8101088.
22. Rush J, Dinulos JG. Childhood skin and soft tissue infections: new discoveries and guidelines regarding the management of bacterial soft tissue infections, molluscum contagiosum, and warts. Curr Opin Pediatr. 2016;28(2):250–7. https://doi.org/10.1097/MOP.0000000000000334. PMID: 26900921.
23. Weston WL, Bruckner A. Allergic contact dermatitis. Pediatr Clin N Am. 2000;47(4):897–907, vii. https://doi.org/10.1016/s0031-3955(05)70247-9. PMID: 10943264.
24. Lievonen S, Pesonen M, Suomela S. Allergic contact dermatitis caused by colophonium in resin creams. Contact Derm. 2024;91(1):70–2. https://doi.org/10.1111/cod.14545. Epub 2024 Mar 15. PMID: 38487934.
25. Commens CA, Bartlett BH, McGeoch AH, Kossard S. Bindii (jo-jo) dermatitis the clinical and histopathological spectrum. Australas J Dermatol. 1982;23(3):110–5. https://doi.org/10.1111/j.1440-0960.1982.tb00740.x. PMID: 6763862.
26. Knapik JJ, Reynolds KL, Duplantis KL, Jones BH. Friction blisters. Pathophysiology, prevention and treatment. Sports Med. 1995;20(3):136–47. https://doi.org/10.2165/00007256-199520030-00002. PMID: 8570998.
27. Worthing RM, Percy RL, Joslin JD. Prevention of friction blisters in outdoor pursuits: a systematic review. Wilderness Environ Med. 2017;28(2):139–49. https://doi.org/10.1016/j.wem.2017.03.007. PMID: 28602272.
28. Barnes HR. Wound care: fact and fiction about hydrocolloid dressings. J Gerontol Nurs. 1993;19(6):23–6. https://doi.org/10.3928/0098-9134-19930601-08. PMID: 8509607.
29. Inui S, Yamamoto S, Ikegami R, Ozawa K, Itami S, Yoshikawa K. Baseball pitcher's friction dermatitis. Contact Derm. 2002;47(3):176–7. https://doi.org/10.1034/j.1600-0536.2002.470308_13.x. PMID: 12492562.
30. Cohen PR, Eliezri YD, Silvers DN. Athlete's nodules: sports-related connective tissue nevi of the collagen type (collagenomas). Cutis. 1992;50(2):131–5. PMID: 1511619.
31. Uchiyama M, Tsuboi R, Mitsuhashi Y. Athlete's nodule. J Dermatol. 2009;36(11):608–11. https://doi.org/10.1111/j.1346-8138.2009.00718.x. PMID: 19878395.
32. Mailler EA, Adams BB. The wear and tear of 26.2: dermatological injuries reported on marathon day. Br J Sports Med. 2004;38(4):498–501. https://doi.org/10.1136/bjsm.2004.011874. PMID: 15273194; PMCID: PMC1724877.

33. Donaldson M, Chamlin SL, Vivar KL. Pine tar callus: a mimicker of a melanocytic lesion. Pediatr Dermatol. 2019;36(3):379–80. https://doi.org/10.1111/pde.13773. Epub 2019 Feb 27. PMID: 30809830.
34. Emer J, Sivek R, Marciniak B. Sports dermatology: part 1 of 2 traumatic or mechanical injuries, inflammatory conditions, and exacerbations of pre-existing conditions. J Clin Aesthet Dermatol. 2015;8(4):31–43. PMID: 26060516; PMCID: PMC4456799.
35. Knable AL Jr, Hanke CW, Gonin R. Prevalence of acne keloidalis nuchae in football players. J Am Acad Dermatol. 1997;37(4):570–4. https://doi.org/10.1016/s0190-9622(97)70173-7. PMID: 9344195.
36. Marks R. Acne and its management beyond the age of 35 years. Am J Clin Dermatol. 2004;5(6):459–62. https://doi.org/10.2165/00128071-200405060-00011. PMID: 15663343.
37. Pozo DD, Usatine RP, Heath CR. Moving beyond traditional methods for treatment of acne Keloidalis Nuchae. Cutis. 2024;114(3):88–9. https://doi.org/10.12788/cutis.1083. PMID: 39413321.
38. Urbina F, León L, Sudy E. Black heel, talon noir or calcaneal petechiae? Australas J Dermatol. 2008;49(3):148–51. https://doi.org/10.1111/j.1440-0960.2008.00454.x. PMID: 18638222.
39. Adams BB, Lucky AW. Acquired port-wine stains and antecedent trauma: case report and review of the literature. Arch Dermatol. 2000;136(7):897–9. https://doi.org/10.1001/archderm.136.7.897. PMID: 10890992.

Chapter 8
Football (American, Association, and Rugby)

Lea Tordjman, Kristen Dean, Rachel Summers, Ryan Scheinkman, Sarah Antonevich, Alexia Vignau, Samuel San Antonio, Rachel Cohen, Peter Velthuis, and Keyvan Nouri

8.1 Introduction

American football, rugby, and soccer (association football) are some of the most physically demanding and widely played sports around the world, each involving intense physical activity, frequent player-to-player contact, and shared locker room spaces. While these sports vary in rules, playing style, and level of contact, they have many common dermatologic risks stemming from environmental exposures such as sunlight, bodily contact, increased sweating, and surface-player interaction [1]. The high-intensity and high-contact nature of these sports exposes athletes to unique dermatologic conditions that need to be identified and treated for both prevention and management in medicine. Each of these sports are unique in the types and frequencies of dermatologic conditions the players experience. For example, in football, the use of extensive protective gear (helmets, shoulder pads, and gloves) and the high-contact nature of the sport contribute to a range of skin-related issues, ranging from helmet-related dermatoses to highly-infectious conditions [2]. Football fields are often made from natural grass or a synthetic turf surface, both of which introduce unique risks through skin contact, abrasions, and environmental exposure.

Rugby, on the other hand, involves less protective equipment when compared to football. This exposes the athlete's skin to more direct contact with other players

L. Tordjman · K. Dean · R. Summers · R. Scheinkman (✉) · S. Antonevich · A. Vignau
S. S. Antonio · R. Cohen · K. Nouri
Dr. Phillip Frost Department of Dermatology and Cutaneous Surgery, University of Miami, Miami, FL, USA
e-mail: lat91@med.miami.edu; kkd45@med.miami.edu; scheinkman@med.miami.edu; sma347@med.miami.edu; axv200@med.miami.edu; sxs3273@miami.edu; rachelcohen@med.miami.edu; knouri@med.miami.edu

P. Velthuis
Department of Dermatology, Erasmus University, Rotterdam, The Netherlands
e-mail: peter@drvelthuis.nl

K. Nouri (ed.), *Sport-Related Skin Conditions*,
https://doi.org/10.1007/978-3-031-90444-8_8

and the ground. This sport's focus on continuous play, frequent tackles, and scrums means that athletes are often exposed to a high degree of friction and forceful contact, predisposing them to more mechanical skin injuries like cuts, abrasions, and cellulitis [3]. Rugby fields are typically natural grass, which increases the risk of environmental allergens and potential bacterial or fungal exposure. Soccer has even less protective equipment (shin guards and gloves for goalies) compared to the other two sports. It is more known for occasional slide tackles, and player-to-player contact. The lack of protection in soccer directly exposes the skin to the field surface and other players. This increases the risk for many potential skin conditions including blisters, friction dermatitis, and sun-related skin damage from prolonged outdoor exposure [4, 5].

Despite their technical differences, American football, rugby, and soccer share many risk factors for sports-induced dermatologic conditions. Environmental exposures, such as UV radiation, are a primary concern for athletes who are typically practicing and competing for long hours outdoors. This can lead to acute and long-term skin damage [1]. Pressure-induced conditions are often seen in these athletes due to repetitive mechanical forces on specific body areas. For example, the bony prominences in the feet and hands contribute to blisters, calluses, and potential pressure ulcers [1, 6]. The continuous contact with protective equipment in football or high-impact scrums in rugby highlights the role of direct pressure in predisposing athletes to these types of skin conditions.

Additionally, inflammatory skin reactions such as acne and cellulitis are common in all three sports, and they are often triggered by environmental factors or friction from equipment [7]. Inflammation can occur due to sweating, exposure to allergens, or bacterial contamination, and is exacerbated by factors such as turf contact or contact with other players. Lastly, player-surface interaction is a notable contributor to dermatologic conditions across these three specific sports. This common interaction between player skin and field surface adds another layer of dermatologic vulnerability. For example, due to the large amount of tackling and sliding on grass and artificial turf, these athletes see an increased risk of friction dermatitis or "turf burn" [8]. In natural grass, soil contaminants or bacterial exposure can lead to heightened risk of infections. More details about skin conditions from ultraviolet radiation exposure during outdoor play and from exposure to extremes temperature are discussed in Chaps. 5 and 4, respectively.

8.2 Equipment Related Dermatologic Conditions

8.2.1 Helmet-Related Dermatoses

Acneiform eruptions, colloquially referred to as "helmet acne", refer to a spectrum of acne-like conditions that are particularly prevalent among athletes who use helmets during training or competition. These eruptions arise from a combination of occlusion, sweat, and friction (i.e. acne mechanica), which promote follicular obstruction and bacterial colonization (discussed in greater detail in Sect. 8.4). American football and rugby players are especially at risk due to the frequent use of protective gear, such as tight-fitting helmets and scrum caps, respectively, that can trap heat and moisture against the skin (Fig. 8.1). These lesions typically present as erythematous papules, pustules, and comedones concentrated in areas of headgear contact, such as the forehead, chin, and hairline. Over time, repeated mechanical irritation can worsen inflammation, leading to persistent or severe acneiform lesions. Diagnosis is primarily clinical, based on lesion morphology and location relative to helmet use. Treatment and management are discussed in greater detail in Sect. 8.4 but involves optimizing hygiene practices, such as cleansing the skin immediately after helmet removal and using antimicrobial washes containing benzoyl peroxide or salicylic acid [9]. In more severe cases, topical or systemic retinoids and antibiotics may be indicated. Athletes are advised to ensure proper helmet fit and consider using moisture-wicking helmet liners to reduce occlusion and sweat accumulation.

Acne keloidalis nuchae (AKN) is a chronic inflammatory condition affecting the back of the neck, frequently seen in male athletes who wear helmets with tight straps or padding that rub against the posterior scalp (also discussed in greater detail in Sect. 8.4). This condition is characterized by follicular-based papules and pustules that coalesce into hypertrophic scars or keloid-like plaques over time. Clinically, AKN presents with firm, raised lesions that are often pruritic or tender. Advanced cases may result in disfiguring scars that interfere with helmet fit and performance. Risk factors for AKN include short, closely shaved haircuts, frequent sweating, and mechanical friction from helmets. Rugby and football players are particularly vulnerable due to the prolonged use of headgear during play. Diagnosis is clinical and can be confirmed through biopsy, which reveals perifollicular inflammation and fibrosis. Treatment (discussed in greater detail Sect. 8.4) focuses on reducing friction and inflammation. Topical corticosteroids, retinoids, and antibiotic washes are first-line therapies, while intralesional corticosteroids may be used for hypertrophic lesions. In severe or refractory cases, surgical excision may be necessary. Preventive measures, including cushioning helmet straps and avoiding closely shaved haircuts, are essential for athletes with a history of AKN.

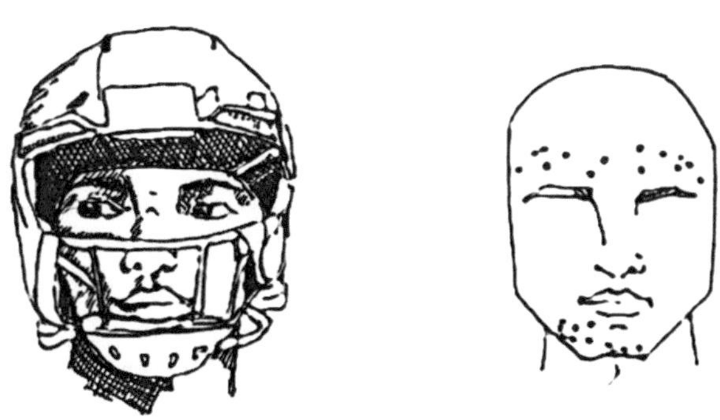

Fig. 8.1 Helmet-induced acneiform eruptions

Forehead dermatitis is a common irritant or allergic contact dermatitis in athletes caused by prolonged helmet use, sweat, and exposure to materials like foam padding or adhesives. Football and rugby players often report redness, scaling, and pruritus in the forehead region where helmets press against the skin [6]. This condition typically presents as erythematous, scaly plaques with possible vesiculation or crusting in severe cases. Chronic exposure can lead to lichenification or hyperpigmentation. Diagnosis involves clinical examination and a history of helmet use. Patch testing may identify specific allergens in helmet materials. Treatment includes topical corticosteroids to reduce inflammation, alongside barrier repair with emollients. Athletes should be encouraged to clean helmet padding regularly and use hypoallergenic liners to minimize irritant exposure. When symptoms persist, switching to helmets made of alternative materials may be necessary [10].

8.2.2 Glove-Associated Dermatoses

Pompholyx, also known as dyshidrotic eczema, is a chronic, vesicular hand dermatitis often seen in athletes who wear gloves for prolonged periods. Rugby players, American football players, and soccer goalkeepers are particularly susceptible due to excessive sweating, prolonged moisture exposure, and repetitive friction inside tight-fitting gloves [11]. This condition typically presents as intensely pruritic vesicles on the palms, lateral fingers, and occasionally the dorsal hands. The vesicles are small and may coalesce into larger bullae, followed by peeling and scaling as they resolve. Secondary infections can occur, leading to erythema and crusting. Diagnosis is clinical, based on the characteristic vesicles and exacerbation linked to glove use. Differential diagnoses include allergic contact dermatitis and tinea manuum, which can be ruled out through patch testing or KOH examination [12]. Treatment focuses on reducing exposure to irritants and allergens. Topical corticosteroids are the mainstay of therapy, particularly during acute flare-ups. Moisturizers and barrier creams can help prevent recurrences. For refractory cases, systemic therapies like oral corticosteroids or immunosuppressants may be considered. Athletes are encouraged to use moisture-wicking gloves and change gloves frequently during play to reduce sweating and irritation [10].

Hand eczema is a multifactorial dermatitis that frequently affects athletes wearing gloves, particularly those exposed to repeated sweating, friction, and potential allergens in glove materials. Football linemen, rugby players, and soccer goalkeepers are at heightened risk due to the prolonged and intense use of gloves during play [9]. Clinically, hand eczema presents as erythematous patches, scaling, and fissuring on the palms and fingers. Chronic exposure may lead to hyperkeratosis and painful cracking, while acute flares can involve vesicles and significant inflammation. Allergic reactions to glove materials, such as latex or rubber additives, may exacerbate symptoms [12]. Diagnosis is clinical but may require patch testing to identify allergens or irritants contributing to the condition. Exclusion of fungal infections is also important, particularly in cases of chronic hyperkeratosis.

Management includes avoiding prolonged glove use and reducing exposure to potential allergens. Topical corticosteroids and emollients are effective for inflammation and barrier repair, respectively. Athletes may benefit from wearing gloves lined with hypoallergenic materials and taking breaks during training to allow the skin to breathe. In severe cases, systemic treatments like cyclosporine or phototherapy may be necessary [6]. Prevention involves keeping hands dry, using absorbent liners, and washing hands with gentle, non-irritating cleansers after glove removal.

8.2.3 Shoe and Foot Dermatoses

Blisters are a common foot condition in athletes caused by repetitive friction and shear forces, often exacerbated by poorly fitting footwear or prolonged activity. Soccer, rugby, and football players are particularly susceptible due to rapid directional changes, intense physical exertion, and long durations in tight athletic footwear [10]. Blisters typically present as fluid-filled vesicles or bullae over pressure-prone areas like the heels, toes, and plantar surfaces. They may be painful, especially if ruptured, and can lead to secondary infections if not properly managed. Diagnosis is clinical, based on the appearance and location of the lesions. Management involves protective measures to prevent further friction, such as using padded or moisture-wicking socks and applying blister dressings or moleskin. Ruptured blisters should be cleaned, dressed, and monitored for signs of infection. Prevention strategies include ensuring proper footwear fit, applying lubricants to reduce friction, and conditioning the feet gradually to athletic activity [6].

Pressure ulcers in athletes result from prolonged pressure or repetitive trauma to specific areas of the feet, often under tight footwear or poorly cushioned cleats. Football linemen and rugby players are particularly vulnerable due to prolonged standing or scrimmaging in restrictive footwear [11].

Lesions present as erythematous, painful areas over bony prominences like the metatarsal heads or heels, which may progress to ulceration if pressure persists. Severe cases can involve deep tissue damage and infection. Diagnosis is clinical, with ulcer grading used to assess severity. Management includes offloading pressure from the affected area using padding, orthotics, or specialized footwear. Dressings that promote a moist wound environment, such as hydrocolloid or foam dressings, can aid healing. Athletes should replace poorly fitting shoes and ensure adequate foot protection during play [12].

Calluses and hyperkeratosis occur due to chronic friction and pressure, commonly affecting athletes' feet, particularly in sports like soccer and rugby that require high-intensity footwork [10].

Lesions present as thickened, yellowish plaques of keratinized skin, often on weight-bearing areas such as the heels, balls of the feet, and toes. While generally asymptomatic, excessive hyperkeratosis can lead to discomfort, cracking, or ulceration. Diagnosis is clinical, based on the characteristic thickened appearance.

Treatment involves regular debridement of calluses and application of keratolytic agents like urea or salicylic acid creams. Properly cushioned footwear and orthotics can redistribute pressure and reduce recurrence. Athletes should be counseled on foot hygiene and the importance of maintaining skin moisture balance [6].

Subungual hematomas result from acute trauma to the toenail, common in sports with repetitive toe impacts, such as soccer and rugby. Tight-fitting shoes and sudden stops or kicks can exacerbate the risk [11]. Lesions appear as dark discoloration under the nail plate, corresponding to pooled blood. Pain and pressure under the nail are common complaints. Diagnosis is clinical, confirmed by the characteristic appearance of discoloration. Treatment involves relieving pressure through nail trephination for symptomatic relief. Preventive measures include wearing properly sized footwear and using protective toe caps. Mild cases may resolve spontaneously with nail growth [12].

8.2.4 Shin Guard and/or Padding Related Dermatoses

Textile dermatitis is a contact dermatitis caused by irritants or allergens in shin guard or padding materials, such as dyes, adhesives, or latex. Soccer and rugby players are particularly susceptible due to prolonged shin guard use and sweating [11]. Lesions present as erythematous, pruritic patches or plaques localized to areas in direct contact with shin guards. Chronic exposure may lead to lichenification or post-inflammatory hyperpigmentation. Diagnosis involves clinical examination and, in some cases, patch testing to identify specific allergens. Management includes topical corticosteroids for inflammation and avoidance of the offending material. Athletes can switch to hypoallergenic shin guards or wear a barrier layer, such as moisture-wicking sleeves, under their gear. Regular cleaning and drying of shin guards are essential to prevent further irritation [6].

Friction dermatitis results from repetitive rubbing of shin guards or padding against the skin, often compounded by sweating and heat. Soccer players, in particular, are prone to this condition due to the tight, prolonged use of shin guards during play [10]. Lesions appear as erythematous patches with possible erosions or crusting in severe cases. Over time, areas of thickened skin may develop. Diagnosis is based on clinical presentation and history of shin guard use. Management involves reducing friction through the use of padded liners or well-fitted shin guards. Topical emollients and barrier creams can help restore the skin's protective function. Athletes should be encouraged to avoid prolonged dampness and clean shin guards regularly to minimize irritation and potential secondary infections [11].

8.3 Infectious Dermatoses

Rugby, football, and soccer are intense high-contact sports that involve frequent physical interaction, shared equipment, and communal facilities. There are all factors that create prime conditions for the spread of infectious diseases among these athletes. Research shows that athletes in contact sports face a greater risk for certain infectious diseases, including those transmitted via skin abrasions, contaminated surfaces, and inadequate hygiene in shared locker room environments [1, 13]. Infectious diseases are of particular concern for these sports teams not only because they affect an individual player's health, but also because of the potential for outbreaks within teams. This can have a large impact on overall team performance and game schedules. Early diagnosis, treatment, and targeted preventive strategies are all essential for medical and coaching staff to minimize these risks.

8.3.1 Bacterial Infections

Bacterial infections represent a significant portion of the infectious disease risks in rugby, football, and soccer, due to the high-contact nature of these sports. Athletes are especially vulnerable to bacterial transmission through skin lesions and abrasions that are commonly encountered on turf or natural grass or even from close body contact with other players. Common bacterial infections seen in these sports include *Staphylococcus aureus and* group A *Streptococcus* species. These can lead to more serious infections such as MRSA (methicillin-resistant Staphylococcus aureus), impetigo, and cellulitis—all of which can spread rapidly if not managed with early identification and appropriate treatment [1, 3, 13]. Bacterial infections not only present immediate health and infectious concerns but also risk becoming chronic if inadequately treated. Increased cleanliness and preventive measures in athletic team environments are essential in limiting bacterial spread, with particular focus on athlete wound care, hygiene, and regular facility sanitation. MRSA is a bacterial infection caused by *Staphylococcus aureus* bacteria that is resistant to many standard antibiotics and therefore more difficult to treat. It is particularly prevalent in high-contact sports where athletes frequently experience skin trauma, close physical interaction, and shared facilities. Rugby, football, and soccer players are at a heightened risk of MRSA transmission due to their specific exposure to turf abrasions, person-to-person contact, and the shared locker rooms and gym equipment [14]. A study in 2016 found that the prevalence of MRSA colonization in athletes in the United States was around 8%, with colonization in collegiate football athletes specifically around 8% as well [15].

Clinically, MRSA infections present as erythematous, indurated nodules or abscesses, often accompanied by central fluctuation and purulent drainage. These lesions can initially resemble folliculitis or furuncles but quickly enlarge and present with pronounced tenderness, warmth, and surrounding cellulitis. Lesions can also develop into painful carbuncles or deeper abscesses. Lastly, untreated infections may extend into subcutaneous tissue layers or even form sinus tracts [6]. Diagnosis of MRSA is based on clinical examination and confirmation with bacterial culture and sensitivity testing from wound swabs or drainage. Molecular testing may also be used to confirm the methicillin resistance. Management includes incision and drainage (I&D) of abscesses when indicated, followed by targeted antibiotic therapy. Antibiotic therapy consists of either TMP-SMX 160–800 mg per oral thrice daily (PO TID) for seven days or Clindamycin 600 mg PO TID for seven days or 300–450 mg QID PO [6]. Athletes are typically advised to refrain from participation until there have been no new lesions for 48 hours, treatment for at least 72 hours, and the lesions are not actively moist or draining [6]. Rigorous wound care and hygiene are essential, and proactive facility sanitation can reduce reinfection and risk of spread.

Erythrasma is a superficial infection with the causal bacteria, *Corynebacterium minutissimum* [11]. This bacteria frequently affects athletes due to the combination of moisture and friction in skin folds from sweating. Skin contact and communal facilities in sports can increase transmission risks, especially in warm and humid conditions. Athletes in sports with tight uniforms or protective gear, such as football and rugby, are particularly vulnerable. A study found that 40% of football players are affected by *erythrasma* and the inguinal region was the most affected [16]. *Erythrasma* presents in athletes as well-demarcated, reddish-brown patches with fine scaling, most commonly in intertriginous regions such as the groin, axillae, and between the toes. Lesions may appear macerated with subtle scaling, progressing to exhibit a slightly wrinkled texture [12]. Unlike fungal infections, *Erythrasma* is often asymptomatic, though mild pruritus or a burning sensation may occur in some cases [9].

Wood's lamp examination aids in the diagnosis of *Erythrasma*, with affected areas fluorescing a coral-red color due to porphyrins produced by the bacteria [12]. KOH preparations can help differentiate *Erythrasma* from fungal infections [16]. Gram staining and cultures, though rarely needed, can confirm the presence of *C. minutissimum*. Topical clindamycin or erythromycin is typically effective for localized infections, while more extensive cases may require oral antibiotics [16]. Prevention for *Erythrasma* includes maintaining dry skin folds and minimizing prolonged moisture exposure, such as by changing out of sweaty gear immediately after practice. Athletes may participate during treatment for *Erythrasma* if lesions are covered to prevent friction-related irritation and potential spread [9].

8.3.2 Viral Infections

Viral infections also pose a significant risk to the athletes playing rugby, American football, and soccer due to exposures commonly arising from close contacts, environmental factors, and shared facilities. These athletes face increased susceptibility to dermatological viral infections due to frequent cuts and abrasions that allow viral entry, as well as from contact with contaminated surfaces such as equipment. For example, *Molluscum contagiosum* and *Verruca vulgaris* (common warts) thrive in moist and warm conditions, making locker rooms and gyms vulnerable for transmission. Viral skin conditions can compromise an athlete's ability to participate in sports due to contagiousness and potential for skin irritation and secondary bacterial infection.

Verruca vulgaris (cutaneous wart), caused by human papillomavirus (HPV), is a common virus that often affects athletes through shared equipment and communal spaces [6]. Approximately 5–30% of children and young adults will have a cutaneous wart at some point, and this can impact their participation in sports [11]. The virus can enter through microabrasions in the skin, common in team sports like football, rugby, and soccer, especially when contact with rough surfaces is frequent. Locker rooms and damp environments can facilitate HPV transmission [11].

The lesions then classically manifest as hyperkeratotic, exophytic papules with a rough, verrucous surface [17]. The warts can display pinpoint black dots within the papule that are due to thrombosed capillaries. They are commonly found on hands, fingers, and knees in athletes due to high contact in those regions. The warts may be tender if located over pressure points or subjected to repeat trauma [11]. It is not uncommon for athletes to present with confluent or multiple warts due to autoinoculation from constant friction and skin contact in sports settings. The diagnosis of *Molluscum contagiosum* is primarily clinical, supported by lesion morphology. Dermoscopic examination may reveal the characteristic thrombosed capillaries which enhances diagnostic accuracy [17]. Histopathologic examination, if conducted, reveals papillomatosis and hyperkeratosis. Treatment options for *Molluscum contagiosum* include cryotherapy, salicylic acid, or laser ablation to decrease lesion burden and reduce the risk of spread [17]. Topical therapies like salicylic acid require adherence over several weeks, while cryotherapy may offer quicker results [6]. Covering lesions and ensuring proper hygiene practices can minimize the risk of spread to other athletes [11]. Athletes can usually return to play as long as lesions are covered to prevent further spread.

8.3.3 Fungal Infections

Fungal infections are another common concern in contact sports due to prolonged exposure to moist environments like locker rooms, gyms, and shared showers. Conditions such as onychomycosis (fungal nail infection) and tinea pedis ("athlete's foot") frequently affect athletes who endure long hours in damp athletic footwear or shared training areas as these contribute to the growth and spread of fungi [1, 6, 9]. Rugby, football, and soccer players are particularly susceptible to tinea dermatophyte infections, which can spread rapidly. To prevent outbreaks amongst teams, regular sanitization, personal hygiene, and proper treatment of fungal infections are essential [1]. Onychomycosis is a fungal infection of the nail bed and plate that is common among athletes exposed to damp environments. Prevalence of toenail infection is seven times more prevalent in athletes than fingernails [18]. Sports like American football, soccer, and rugby which require tight footwear and prolonged moisture exposure from socks and sweating, have heightened risk of nail infections. These sports are also prone to trauma to the foot and toenail due to quick movements which can increase the risk for onychomycosis.

Nails infected with onychomycosis appear thickened, discolored (yellow, white, or brown), and brittle with subungual debris and onycholysis [11]. The distal-lateral type is common and displays thickening and separation from the nail bed, with occasional periungual erythema [18]. Diagnosis of onychomycosis is confirmed with a KOH (potassium hydroxide) preparation, fungal culture, or periodic acid-Schiff (PAS) stain of the athlete's nail clippings [11]. Treatment of onychomycosis involves oral antifungals (terbinafine, oral azole, or griseofulvin) or topical antifungal agents for less severe cases. Regimens can include: Terbinafine: 250 mg table PO daily for 6–12 weeks, Itraconazole: 200 mg table PO daily for 6–12 weeks, Fluconazole: 150 mg table PO weekly until nail is normal or acceptably improved [6]. Athletes can continue play as there are no restrictions from competition, but regular nail care and drying practices are encouraged to prevent reinfection, which occurs about 40–70% of the time [11].

Tinea pedis, often caused by *Trichophyton* species, thrives in warm, moist areas, making it common among athletes who share locker rooms and showers. Rugby football players with constant footgear use are especially vulnerable. One study estimated the prevalence of tinea pedis in athletes to be between 15% and 70% [19]. The simple form of tinea pedis commonly presents in the interdigit space showing maceration, scaling, and fissuring between toes. In the complex form, superinfection often occurs with gram-negative and gram-positive bacteria and presents with pain, macerations, erosions, or crusting [19]. Diagnosis of tinea pedis is made via a KOH prep which reveals segmented hyphae or a fungal culture [6]. Treatment or tinea pedis includes topical antifungals, such as azoles, and drying powders for 4 weeks [6]. Athletes are allowed to continue competing but should keep feet dry, change their socks frequently, and avoid walking barefoot in communal areas to prevent spread [20].

Tinea corporis is caused by dermatophytes like *Trichophyton* or *Microsporum* species [6]. It spreads through skin-to-skin contact and shared equipment which makes it common in sports with physical contact, like rugby, football, and soccer. Lesions of tinea corporis present as annular, erythematous plaques with a scaly, advancing border and central clearing. The lesions may coalesce or expand to form polycyclic patterns [11]. Pruritus can also be seen with tinea corporis. Diagnosis of tinea corporis is confirmed with a 10% or 20% KOH preparation which shows septated fungal hyphae or fungal culture [6]. Topical imidazoles (clotrimazole, ketoconazole, miconazole) or allylamines (terbinafine, naftifine) are the primary treatment for tinea corporis. They are applied TID for 7 days [6]. Athletes should cover lesions during play to reduce transmission risk and refrain from play until infection control is achieved [6].

Tinea versicolor is caused by the yeast *Malassezia* and commonly affects athletes, particularly those in humid environments or with prolonged sweat exposure

[6]. The yeast is part of the skin's normal flora but can become pathogenic under conditions like increased sebaceous activity and excessive sweating, which are typical in high-intensity sports [21]. Athletes in sports like football, rugby, and soccer are particularly susceptible due to frequent sweating and the use of occlusive sportswear, which can promote the growth of *Malassezia*. Lesions of *Tinea versicolor* typically appear as hyper- or hypopigmented macules with fine scaling which can coalesce into larger patches. It is typically found on the trunk, shoulders, and upper arms [6]. In athletes, these lesions may become more extensive in areas where sweating is heaviest. Lesions can exhibit mild erythema but are typically asymptomatic, though some athletes may report mild pruritus, particularly after sweating [6].

Clinical diagnosis of *Tinea versicolor* is aided by Wood's lamp examination in which affected areas fluoresce with a yellow-green hue [21]. Direct microscopy of skin scrapings with potassium hydroxide (KOH) can also be performed and reveal the characteristic "spaghetti and meatballs" appearance of numerous short, stubby hyphae intermixed with clusters of spores [21]. Dermoscopy can assist in identifying the uniform, fine scale pattern typical of *Tinea versicolor* [6] . Treatment of *Tinea versicolor* generally involves topical antifungals such as ketoconazole or selenium sulfide shampoo which are applied to affected areas for 1–2 weeks. For extensive cases, oral antifungals (such as fluconazole) may be indicated [22]. Athletes can typically continue play as long as active lesions are treated and preventive hygiene practices are followed [6]. This includes showering promptly after activity and avoiding occlusive clothing when possible.

8.4 Inflammatory Dermatoses

Inflammatory skin conditions include a range of dermatologic disorders triggered by mechanical, environmental, and immunologic factors [17]. For athletes, these conditions are particularly common due to frequent sweating, prolonged equipment use, and exposure to various external irritants. The physical exertion and environmental factors associated with football, rugby, and soccer in particular, can provoke or exacerbate inflammatory responses in the skin, leading to both acute and chronic presentations [6]. Management of these conditions is essential for maintaining skin integrity, comfort, and performance in athletes (Table 8.1).

8.4.1 Acneiform Dermatitis

Acne is one of the most common inflammatory skin conditions, especially in younger athletes. This population is at a greater risk due to increased sweating and use of occlusive equipment. A study in 2021 found that about 50% of athletes suffer from acne at some point in their lifetime [23]. The rise in sebum production and

Table 8.1 Inflammatory dermatoses associated with football

Disease/ Condition	Symptoms and physical exam findings	Treatment recommendations
Acneiform vulgaris	Polymorphic lesions and clusters of comedones in areas covered by protective gear	Benzoyl peroxide and retinoids. More severe cases may need antibiotics or isotretinoin
Acne Mechanica	Erythematous, follicular-based papules or pustules in areas of repeated friction or pressure	Modifying or reducing frictional sources, topical treatments, moisturizers, and regular cleaning of equipment.
Acne Keloidalis Nuchae	Small, firm papules and pustules at the hairline on the posterior neck	Topical corticosteroids or retinoids, antimicrobial washes, optional intralesional corticosteroid injections, and in more severe cases, surgical excision.
Xerosis	Itchy inflamed patches	Barrier protection
Eczema dermatitis	Erythematous, scaly patches with poorly defined borders	Emollients, topical corticosteroids, and NSAIDs
Contact dermatitis	Erythematous, pruritic plaques	Eliminate exposure to irritant, topical corticosteroids, and emollients
Lichenoid dermatitis	Small, polygonal, flat-topped, violaceous papules	Topical steroids, antihistamines, and avoid primary trigger and friction to affected area

occlusion from gear such as helmets or pads can lead to follicular obstruction and inflammation [6]. Acne in athletes varies from common presentations like *Acne vulgaris* to more sport-specific forms like Acne mechanica and Acne keloidalis nuchae (discussed above), each with distinct triggers and treatments [9]. Acne vulgaris is a common chronic inflammatory skin condition characterized by the blockage and inflammation of pilosebaceous units. It most commonly affects areas like the face, chest, and back [10]. In athletes, factors such as sweating, occlusive sports equipment, and frequent clothing friction can exacerbate acne formation. This condition is particularly prevalent in sports where helmets, pads, or chin straps contribute to prolonged skin occlusion and mechanical irritation. Acne vulgaris presents with polymorphic lesions that include open comedones (blackheads), closed comedones (whiteheads), inflammatory papules, pustules, cysts, and nodules [9]. This is termed nodulocystic acne and can be painful for the players and cause post-inflammatory hyperpigmentation or scarring. Athletes may experience clusters of comedones and inflammatory lesions in areas covered by helmets, shoulder pads, or other protective gear [9].

Acne vulgaris is diagnosed clinically based on the characteristic distribution and variety of lesions across affected areas [9]. The assessment includes a thorough history of triggers, including recent equipment use and skincare regimens. The severity of acne is often categorized as mild, moderate, or severe, which helps guide treatment choices [24]. In athletes, differentiating acne vulgaris from acne mechanica (triggered primarily by mechanical irritation) is important, as management strategies can vary. Management of acne vulgaris in athletes includes topical therapies such as benzoyl peroxide, retinoids (tretinoin, adapalene), and in more severe cases, topical or systemic antibiotics (clindamycin, doxycycline) [6]. For individuals experiencing resistant or severe nodulocystic acne, dermatologists may prescribe isotretinoin, which is a teratogen in pregnancy [6]. Athletes are advised to maintain regular skin cleansing routines, avoid comedogenic skin care products, and consider sweat-wicking gear to reduce skin occlusion. With appropriate management, athletes can continue to participate in sports, but adherence to preventive measures is emphasized to avoid flare-ups.

Acne mechanica is a condition induced by repetitive friction, pressure, and occlusion of the skin [9]. It is frequently seen in athletes due to the extensive use of protective gear and sports equipment [25]. The condition is particularly common in contact sports like football, rugby, and wrestling, where helmets, shoulder pads, or tight uniforms contribute to skin irritation and clogged pores. Acne mechanica is often considered an exacerbation of acne vulgaris but can also occur in individuals without prior acne issues [6]. Lesions in acne mechanica typically include papules, pustules, and nodules localized to areas of repeated friction or pressure [9]. Athletes may experience erythematous, follicular-based papules or pustules in areas such as the forehead, shoulders, and upper back. These lesions often lack comedones, distinguishing them from typical acne vulgaris [6]. Chronic friction can lead to post-inflammatory hyperpigmentation and even scarring in severe cases. Skin affected by acne mechanica may appear dry and inflamed due to repeated physical stress.

Diagnosis is based on a clinical examination and history of sports activities or equipment use associated with friction or pressure, such as helmets or shoulder pads [9]. The distribution of acne lesions along areas of contact with equipment and the absence of comedones can aid in distinguishing acne mechanica from acne vulgaris [6]. Clinicians may also inquire about skincare routines and equipment-cleaning practices to identify potential irritants. Treatment involves modifying or reducing the frictional sources when possible. Topical treatments, such as benzoyl peroxide, salicylic acid, or topical antibiotics, can help manage inflammation [6]. Non-comedogenic moisturizers may be used to protect the skin barrier and minimize irritation. To prevent recurrence, athletes are advised to keep skin clean and dry, use barrier products, and ensure regular cleaning of equipment and clothing. They may continue sports participation but should follow preventive measures to limit flare-ups, such as wearing sweat-wicking undergarments beneath equipment [6].

Acne keloidalis nuchae (AKN) is a chronic inflammatory condition that affects the nape of the neck and is primarily seen in individuals with curly or coarse hair [26]. This condition is often present in athletes who wear helmets, chin straps, or collars, such as football and rugby players, that apply pressure and friction to the posterior neck [26]. The constant friction and mechanical stress can exacerbate AKN. AKN begins with small, firm papules and pustules at the hairline on the posterior neck [26]. Over time, these lesions can form keloidal plaques and raised areas with a smooth, shiny surface. The papules may be erythematous or hyperpigmented and are often accompanied by pruritus and tenderness [26]. In advanced stages, the affected area may show hypertrophic scarring and fibrosis, resulting in hair loss (alopecia) within the plaques and potential keloid formation [26]. Athletes may also report discomfort due to the continuous irritation from sports equipment in the affected area.

The diagnosis of AKN is clinically based on the characteristic distribution along the occipital scalp and posterior neck and the presence of keloid-like papules [26]. A detailed history, including sports equipment use and hair grooming practices is important. A biopsy is rarely needed but can confirm the diagnosis in atypical cases by showing perifollicular inflammation and fibrosis. Management of AKN focuses on reducing inflammation, minimizing mechanical irritation, and addressing scarring. Initial treatments include topical corticosteroids or retinoids to reduce inflammation, and antimicrobial washes to prevent secondary infection [26]. Intralesional corticosteroid injections may be used to treat hypertrophic scars and keloids. In severe cases, surgical excision of the keloid plaques may be considered. Athletes are encouraged to reduce friction in the neck area caused by padding equipment or using barrier creams. Athletes may continue sports participation with protective modifications [26]. AKN often has a chronic, relapsing course, so it is important that athletes adhere to preventative measures. *Cellulitis* caused by *Staphylococcus aureus* and *Streptococcus pyogenes* involving the deep dermis and subcutaneous tissues can, in some circumstances, present as pustules with erythematous base and differentiated from acneiform eruptions from other systemic symptoms and wider spread erythema [11, 27].

8.4.2 Xerosis

Xerosis, or dry skin, is frequently observed in athletes exposed to cold, dry environments, excessive sweating, or those who undergo extensive cleansing routines post-training [28]. This dryness can lead to a compromised skin barrier, predisposing athletes to various types of dermatitis. Dermatitis in athletes encompasses multiple subtypes, including eczema, contact dermatitis, and lichenoid dermatitis. These are each aggravated by repetitive friction, sweating, and allergen exposure. These conditions can manifest in itchy, inflamed patches that affect comfort and performance, underscoring the importance of tailored skincare and barrier protection in athletes [28].

8.4.3 Eczema Dermatitis

Eczema dermatitis, commonly referred to as atopic dermatitis, is a chronic inflammatory skin condition characterized by episodic flare-ups of dry, itchy, and inflamed skin [29]. This condition is especially prevalent among athletes in sports that involve frequent sweating which can exacerbate skin dryness and inflammation. Cold, dry climates or prolonged exposure to sunlight in outdoor sports can also trigger or worsen eczema in predisposed individuals. Eczema dermatitis presents as erythematous, scaly patches with poorly defined borders [29]. Affected areas may develop vesicles in acute flares or lichenified plaques in chronic cases due to repetitive scratching [29]. Athletes commonly experience eczema on the flexural surfaces, such as the antecubital and popliteal fossae, as well as exposed areas like the face, neck, and hands. The skin often appears xerotic and in severe cases may display fissuring. Pruritus is a hallmark symptom that is often exacerbated by sweating and physical activity in sports [29].

Diagnosis of eczema dermatitis is based on the clinical presentation of pruritic, recurrent eczematous lesions, particularly on flexural areas. A personal or family history of atopy (e.g., asthma, allergic rhinitis) is often seen [29]. A thorough assessment of potential irritants and exacerbating factors in the athlete's environment, such as gear or exposure to allergens, can help tailor management.Management of eczema dermatitis includes regular use of emollients to restore the skin barrier, topical corticosteroids to reduce inflammation during flares, and non-steroidal anti-inflammatory agents like calcineurin inhibitors in sensitive areas [29]. For athletes, maintaining optimal skin hydration and using non-irritant cleansers is essential, as well as modifying equipment or gear to reduce friction and heat. Athletes may continue participation but should avoid known triggers and adhere to maintenance therapy to reduce the frequency of flare-ups [6].

8.4.4 Contact Dermatitis

Contact dermatitis is an inflammatory skin condition resulting from exposure to irritants or allergens. In athletes, frequent contact with sports equipment, adhesives, and environmental factors places them at increased risk for this dermatolgic condition [6]. Contact dermatitis is categorized into irritant contact dermatitis (ICD), which occurs when skin is damaged by physical or chemical irritants, and allergic contact dermatitis (ACD), which is an immune-mediated response to specific allergens. Both types are common in athletes involved in contact sports or those who use extensive protective gear, such as shin pads and goalie gloves in soccer [7, 30, 31].

Contact dermatitis presents as erythematous, pruritic plaques with vesiculation in acute cases, and lichenified, scaling patches in chronic exposures. ICD lesions tend to be localized to areas of direct exposure, such as hands or wrists, often from prolonged use of equipment [31]. ACD can present with well-demarcated plaques, often displaying a distribution pattern that mirrors the offending allergen or material (e.g., areas in contact with adhesives or rubber bands). Chronic cases may exhibit hyperkeratosis or fissuring, which can be painful and disruptive to athletic performance [6].

Diagnosis of contact dermatitis is made through clinical history and physical examination, focusing on the distribution and pattern of lesions. Patch testing can confirm ACD by identifying specific allergens responsible for the reaction. For ICD, identifying the irritant through history alone is usually sufficient, as it is often related to frequent or prolonged exposure to sweat, water, or equipment materials in athletes [30]. Treatment of contact dermatitis involves eliminating exposure to the causative irritant or allergen [6]. Topical corticosteroids are commonly prescribed to reduce inflammation and emollients to help repair the skin barrier [6]. Athletes should be advised on protective measures, such as wearing non-allergenic barrier creams or selecting hypoallergenic gear. Return to play is generally unrestricted, but measures to avoid recurrence are essential, as repeated exposures can lead to worsening of symptoms [6].

8.4.5 Lichenoid Dermatitis

Lichenoid dermatitis is a skin condition characterized by inflammation and a distinctive "lichenoid" appearance. It typically presents with flat-topped, violaceous (purple-hued) papules [32]. This condition can arise from various triggers, including medications, infections, and even repetitive trauma. Lichenoid dermatitis is seen in athletes due to the skin's constant exposure to external stressors such as sun, sweat, and mechanical abrasion. Lichenoid dermatitis presents with small, polygonal, flat-topped papules with a violaceous hue, primarily localized to areas of repeated friction or trauma [33]. Lesions may exhibit the Wickham striae, a characteristic pattern of fine, white, lacy lines on the papules' surface [32]. Common sites include the wrists, shins, and lower back, though lesions can appear in any area subject to frequent contact or friction. Pruritus can be significant and scratching can lead to secondary scaling and post-inflammatory hyperpigmentation.

Diagnosis of lichenoid dermatitis is largely clinical and supported by the distinctive appearance of the lesions [33]. A biopsy may be performed if the presentation is atypical, showing dense lymphocytic infiltrate at the dermo-epidermal junction, which is characteristic of lichenoid reactions [33]. History of medication use, recent infections, or known exposure to triggering substances should be assessed, as they may aid in identifying potential causes. Treatment of lichenoid dermatitis focuses on reducing inflammation and alleviating symptoms. Topical corticosteroids can help manage inflammation, and antihistamines may relieve pruritus [32]. Athletes should avoid known triggers and minimize friction or trauma to affected areas. With appropriate management, athletes can continue participation; however, modifications in equipment or protective padding may be recommended to prevent recurrence [33].

References

1. Adams BB. Dermatologic disorders of the athlete. Sports Med. 2002;32(5):309–21.
2. Kirkland R, Adams BB. Dermatological problems in the football player. Int J Dermatol. 2006;45(8):927–32.
3. Okamoto O, Kai Y, Munemoto S, Suzuki R, Akishino K, Hashimoto H. A clinical and statistical analysis of abscess in cellulitis. J Dermatol. 2021;48(8):1162–71.

4. Weston WL, Morelli JG. Dermatitis under soccer shin guards: allergy or contact irritant reaction? Pediatr Dermatol. 2006;23(1):19–20.
5. Aizawa A, Ito A, Masui Y, Sasaki K, Ishimura Y, Numata M, Abe R. A case of allergic contact dermatitis caused by goalkeeper gloves. Contact Derm. 2018;79(2):113–5.
6. Pujalte GGA, Costa LMC, Clapp AD, Presutti RJ, Sluzevich JC. More than skin deep: dermatologic conditions in athletes. Sports Health. 2023;15(1):74–85.
7. Kockentiet B, Adams BB. Contact dermatitis in athletes. J Am Acad Dermatol. 2007;56(6):1048–55.
8. van den Eijnde W, Peppelman M, Weghuis MO, van Erp PE. Psychosensorial assessment of skin damage caused by a sliding on artificial turf: the development and validation of a skin damage area and severity index. J Sci Med Sport. 2014;17(1):18–22.
9. Pecci M, Comeau D, Chawla V. Skin conditions in the athlete. Am J Sports Med. 2009;37(2):406–18.
10. Wolkenstein P, Machovcová A, Szepietowski JC, Tennstedt D, Veraldi S, Delarue A. Acne prevalence and associations with lifestyle: a cross-sectional online survey of adolescents/young adults in 7 European countries. J Eur Acad Dermatol Venereol. 2018;32(2):298–306.
11. Paradise SL, Hu YE. Infectious dermatoses in sport: a review of diagnosis, management, and return-to-play recommendations. Curr Sports Med Rep. 2021;20(2):92–103.
12. Masood M, Heath CR, Usatine RP. Erythrasma. J Fam Pract. 2022;71(10):E13–e4.
13. Begier EM, Frenette K, Barrett NL, Mshar P, Petit S, Boxrud DJ, et al. A high-morbidity outbreak of methicillin-resistant Staphylococcus aureus among players on a college football team, facilitated by cosmetic body shaving and turf burns. Clin Infect Dis. 2004;39(10):1446–53.
14. Redziniak DE, Diduch DR, Turman K, Hart J, Grindstaff TL, MacKnight JM, Mistry DJ. Methicillin-resistant staphylococcus aureus (MRSA) in the Athlete. Int J Sports Med. 2009;30(8):557–62.
15. Karanika S, Kinamon T, Grigoras C, Mylonakis E. Colonization with methicillin-resistant staphylococcus aureus and risk for infection among asymptomatic athletes: a systematic review and metaanalysis. Clin Infect Dis. 2016;63(2):195–204.
16. Zisova L, Valchev V, Kasabov G. Erythrasma in athletes and football players. Wien Med Wochenschr. 2021;171(1–2):24–8.
17. Tlougan BE, Mancini AJ, Mandell JA, Cohen DE, Sanchez MR. Skin conditions in figure skaters, ice-hockey players and speed skaters: part II—cold-induced, infectious and inflammatory dermatoses. Sports Med. 2011;41(11):967–84.
18. Daggett C, Brodell RT, Daniel CR, Jackson J. Onychomycosis in athletes. Am J Clin Dermatol. 2019;20(5):691–8.
19. Field LA, Adams BB. Tinea pedis in athletes. Int J Dermatol. 2008;47(5):485–92.
20. Evans EG, Dodman B, Williamson DM, Brown GJ, Bowen RG. Comparison of terbinafine and clotrimazole in treating tinea pedis. BMJ. 1993;307(6905):645–7.
21. Leung AK, Barankin B, Lam JM, Leong KF, Hon KL. Tinea versicolor: an updated review. Drugs Context. 2022:11.
22. Gupta AK, Lyons DC. Pityriasis versicolor: an update on pharmacological treatment options. Expert Opin Pharmacother. 2014;15(12):1707–13.
23. Liebich C, Wegin VV, Marquart C, Schubert I, von Bruehl ML, Halle M, et al. Skin diseases in elite athletes. Int J Sports Med. 2021;42(14):1297–304.
24. Luebberding S, Kolbe L, Kerscher M. Influence of sportive activity on skin barrier function: a quantitative evaluation of 60 athletes. Int J Dermatol. 2013;52(6):745–9.
25. Mazhar M, Simpson M, Marathe K. Inner thigh friction as a cause of acne mechanica. Pediatr Dermatol. 2019;36(4):546–7.
26. Knable AL Jr, Hanke CW, Gonin R. Prevalence of acne keloidalis nuchae in football players. J Am Acad Dermatol. 1997;37(4):570–4.
27. Raff AB, Kroshinsky D. Cellulitis: a review. JAMA. 2016;316(3):325–37.
28. Pons-Guiraud A. Dry skin in dermatology: a complex physiopathology. J Eur Acad Dermatol Venereol. 2007;21(Suppl 2):1–4.

29. Peters N, Peters AT. Atopic dermatitis. Allergy Asthma Proc. 2019;40(6):433–6.
30. Frewen J, Bergendorff O, Divekar P. Shin-pad dermatitis in a young footballer. Clin Exp Dermatol. 2021;46(7):1379–80.
31. Marzario B, Burrows D, Skotnicki S. Contact dermatitis to personal sporting equipment in youth. J Cutan Med Surg. 2016;20(4):323–6.
32. Payette MJ, Weston G, Humphrey S, Yu J, Holland KE. Lichen planus and other lichenoid dermatoses: kids are not just little people. Clin Dermatol. 2015;33(6):631–43.
33. Magro CM, Crowson AN. Lichenoid and granulomatous dermatitis. Int J Dermatol. 2000;39(2):126–33.

Chapter 9
Basketball

Rahul Aggarwal, Isabella Guanche, Garrett D. Forman, Ryan Scheinkman, Edward Brotgandel, Alexia Vignau, Eli Kasheri, and Keyvan Nouri

9.1 Introduction

A high-intensity sport, basketball is characterized by intense bursts of activity, rapid directional changes, and frequent physical contact between players. During a typical game, athletes engage in repeated episodes of running, jumping, and lateral movement. All the while, players are in close physical proximity to each other. This combination of high-intensity exercise and physical proximity creates a unique environment that can significantly impact players' skin health [1]. There are various sources that can lead to the dermatologic challenges faced by basketball players. High-intensity physical exertion can cause prolonged periods of sweating, which leads to persistent moisture on the skin surface. Prolonged exposure to sweat not only disrupts the skin's natural barrier function but also creates an environment conducive to microbial growth. Furthermore, other risk factors include friction generated between skin, athletic equipment (jerseys and uniforms, protective gear, and shoes), and shared spaces in basketball, which include locker rooms, indoor courts, and exercise facilities. These areas can act as reservoirs for various pathogens that affect the skin. Furthermore, the dynamic nature of the sport exposes players to frequent physical trauma, ranging from minor abrasions to more significant injuries, all of which can compromise skin integrity and predispose athletes to secondary infections [2].

Rahul Aggarwal and Isabella Guanche contributed equally with all other contributors.

R. Aggarwal · I. Guanche · G. D. Forman · R. Scheinkman (✉) · E. Brotgandel · A. Vignau
E. Kasheri · K. Nouri
Dr. Phillip Frost Department of Dermatology and Cutaneous Surgery, University of Miami, Miami, FL, USA
e-mail: rxa1273@med.miami.edu; idg18@med.miami.edu; gxf319@med.miami.edu; scheinkman@med.miami.edu; exb1079@med.miami.edu; axv200@med.miami.edu; elikasheri@med.miami.edu; knouri@med.miami.edu

K. Nouri (ed.), *Sport-Related Skin Conditions*,
https://doi.org/10.1007/978-3-031-90444-8_9

9.2 Perspiration and Moisture-Related Conditions

9.2.1 Intertrigo

Intertrigo is an inflammatory condition affecting flexural surfaces of the body, particularly the groin and underarms, and is characterized by repetitive mechanical friction between adjacent skin surfaces. The condition is exacerbated by moisture accumulation and increased surface temperature, which creates an optimal environment for epidermal maceration and inflammation [3–5]. Basketball athletes are especially vulnerable to intertrigo due to prolonged sweating from intense physical play. Professional basketball jerseys are often made from moisture-wicking, polyester fabrics that enable proper ventilation and cooling of sweat [4]. However, athletes are more susceptible to intertrigo if they play in tight-fitting fabrics, such as compression clothing. Many basketball players play in compression clothing for recovery purposes, which can accumulate sweat even if the material is wicking. Symptoms of intertrigo manifest as a red or red-brown rash, accompanied by intense pruritis, burning sensations, and localized discomfort. Without proper management, intertrigo can progress to secondary bacterial or fungal infections (most commonly *Candida* species), potentially disrupting an athlete's performance and training regimen [5]. In cases of intertrigo with bacterial involvement, examination with a Wood's lamp would reveal a coral-red fluorescence.

Prevention and management strategies are crucial for basketball athletes. Recommended interventions include using absorbent agents like talc-based powders, wearing loose-fitting and moisture-wicking clothing, and maintaining rigorous skin hygiene. A recent study in the Journal of Cosmetic Dermatology highlighted the potential efficacy of topical barrier sprays containing antiseptic and anti-inflammatory agents in managing intertrigo [6]. Athletes should prioritize skin drying and ventilation during practice and game intervals. Furthermore, any subsequent infections should be treated. Treatment agents may include topical clotrimazole or nystatin for fungal infections and topical antibiotics such as mupirocin for non-severe bacterial dermatitis.

9.2.2 Miliaria Rubra

Miliaria rubra is a dermatologic condition characterized by the obstruction of eccrine sweat glands, which disrupts normal sweat extraction and leads to significant skin complications. The pathophysiology involves blockage of sweat ducts, resulting in sweat accumulation within the dermis and epidermis and the formation of inflammatory vesicles beneath the sweat glands [7–9]. This is primarily mediated by cutaneous debris and bacteria such as Staphylococcus epidermidis [8].

Basketball players are prone to excessive sweating, the most common risk factor for miliaria rubra. Like intertrigo, miliaria rubra commonly affects flexural surfaces, in addition to the upper trunk, scalp, and neck. Clinical manifestations include small, inflamed blister-like bumps (2–4 mm) consisting of non-follicular papules and papulovesicles. Athletes typically experience intense itching or prickling sensations, accompanied by background skin erythema [9]. If left unmanaged, the condi tion can progress to pustule formation, potentially compromising an athlete's performance and skin health. Anhidrosis due to obstruction and further bacterial infection may also occur in more severe disease. The development of miliaria rubra is exacerbated by multiple factors as stated before, including synthetic clothing that occludes sweat glands, tight compression wear that limits skin breathing, and prolonged physical exertion in warm, humid indoor environments (if playing in an indoor court). Effective prevention and management strategies focus on mitigating sweat gland obstruction and promoting skin cooling. Athletes should prioritize breathable, synthetic fabrics, take cool baths post-activity, and utilize targeted treatments such as calamine lotion to alleviate discomfort [9, 10]. Furthermore, players should use headbands and bring spare towels when playing to minimize prolonged exposure to sweat. Additionally, mild topical steroids and antiseptics can help manage inflammation and prevent secondary infections, ensuring optimal skin health and athletic performance.

9.2.3 Candidiasis

Candidiasis is an infection caused by *Candida* fungi, characteristically thriving in moist, warm environments. Basketball athletes are particularly susceptible to yeast infections due to frequent close contact, poor hygiene practices, sharing towels and equipment, and potential open wounds from abrasions. The infection predominantly targets high-moisture body regions, such as the groin and underarms, where prolonged sweating and restricted skin ventilation create an optimal environment for fungal proliferation [11, 12].

Clinical manifestations of candidiasis in athletes include localized skin infections, characterized by potential irritation, erythema, and discomfort. "Satellite lesions", which are non-continuous with the primary rash, can commonly be seen due to fungal spread along skin folds. If left unmanaged, the condition can progress to more extensive skin complications and potentially secondary infections that may interrupt training and competitive performance [12]. Prevention and management strategies are crucial for basketball athletes and encompass a comprehensive approach to skin health. Recommended interventions include maintaining rigorous personal hygiene, utilizing antifungal creams, wearing breathable and moisture-wicking clothing, implementing rapid post-activity clothing changes, and applying drying powders in susceptible anatomical regions [13]. Treatment of active candidiasis typically involves application of antifungal creams, such as nystatin, clotrimazole, and miconazole. These treatments are very effective, with complete cure rates of 73–100% [14].

9.2.4 *Pitted Keratolysis*

Pitted keratolysis is a bacterial foot infection characterized by microbial colonization in low-airflow environments. The most vulnerable epidermal layer is the top layer of skin, the stratum corneum. Clinical manifestations of pitted keratolysis include distinctive, craterlike multifocal pits, or malodorous punched-out lesions. The pits may appear white, gray, or brown, and the lesions are often symmetric [15]. The condition is particularly exacerbated by excessive foot sweating and prolonged moisture retention. Basketball athletes are especially vulnerable to this infection due to factors including limited shoe ventilation, prolonged periods in tight basketball shoes, constant foot moisture during gameplay, and repetitive foot impact and friction. Patients often experience malodor, the most common symptom, in addition to pain and pruritus [16].

These symptoms can significantly impact an athlete's comfort and performance, especially since pitted keratolysis commonly occurs in weight-bearing areas. Wood's lamp examination may show coral red fluorescence. However, the diagnosis is clinical. Prevention and management strategies are critical for basketball players and involve a comprehensive approach to foot care. Recommended interventions include topical antibiotics such as clindamycin and erythromycin, antiseptic treatments, moisture-wicking socks, frequent shoe and sock changes, and rigorous foot hygiene protocols. In some cases, prescribed antifungal and antibacterial topical treatments may be necessary to effectively manage and resolve the infection [16].

9.3 Friction-Related Dermatologic Conditions

9.3.1 *Blisters*

Basketball players are especially susceptible to blisters, primarily on their feet, due to the sport's rapid directional changes and pivoting movements. Factors such as improperly fitting shoes and moisture-retaining socks can further increase blister risk among basketball players. These skin lesions form at the stratum spinosum epidermal layer due to repetitive motion and friction that separates cellular structures. As hydrostatic pressure builds, the separated areas fill with plasma-like fluid containing lower protein concentrations [17]. The characteristic symptoms of blisters include reddened skin, localized heat, stinging sensations, and fluid-filled skin bubbles that may appear clear or blood-tinged. Effective prevention and treatment strategies involve wearing moisture-wicking, double-layer socks (including grip socks), ensuring properly fitted shoes, and applying powder or petroleum jelly to friction-prone areas. Wearing loose socks can often cause blisters. Clinical practice suggests that professionally draining large, painful blisters while preserving the blister roof can significantly reduce patient discomfort [18].

9.3.2 Calluses and corns

Calluses and corns are hyperkeratotic lesions, representing the body's natural protective mechanism against mechanical stress. When exposed to repeated friction, the skin thickens as a defensive response. This progressive buildup can lead to discomfort and potentially restrict mobility, particularly in athletes who experience consistent mechanical pressure [19–21]. Basketball athletes are especially prone to calluses due to the sport's repetitive movements, including constant foot-to-shoe friction, frequent jumping, and landing impacts. The gold standard of treatment for calluses includes scalpel debridement with regular application of topical keratolytic, such as salicylic acid [20]. Measures that can be taken outside the clinical setting include wearing properly fitted shoes that reduce friction and minimize foot sliding within the shoe, using proper orthopedic insoles and protective padding to minimize further irritation, soaking the affected area in warm water for 5–10 minutes to soften the skin, filing the callus or corn with a pumice stone, applying moisturizing lotion to maintain skin hydration, and maintaining well-trimmed toenails to prevent skin stress [21].

9.3.3 Chafing

Chafing is a painful skin condition characterized by erythema and pain caused by continuous friction between skin surfaces, clothing, or other materials. This is a condition prevalent in athletes and often occurs in the inner thighs, groin, and axilla. Contrary to common belief, cotton clothing can actually retain moisture and exacerbate chafing, making moisture-wicking fabrics a better preventive choice. Moisture is a primary contributor to chafing, so athletes should take proactive measures to minimize skin dampness [22]. Strategies to prevent chafing include applying moisture-absorbing powders or antiperspirants, wearing breathable, moisture-wicking athletic clothing, using lubricants like petroleum (which also functions as an effective treatment agent), and generally keeping the skin dry. If athletes desire immediate relief, they can apply petroleum jelly to create a protective barrier, talcum powder to reduce friction and absorb moisture [23].

9.3.4 Friction and Shoe Contact Dermatitis

Friction dermatitis is a specific type of irritant dermatitis characterized by an eczematous process triggered by persistent physical friction. Basketball athletes are particularly susceptible to friction dermatitis, with common affected areas including feet from repetitive shoe and sock interactions and hands from continuous basketball handling. The repetitive nature of athletic movements creates an environment where skin can become increasingly vulnerable to this inflammatory response [24]. The condition manifests through characteristic symptoms, including reddened and inflamed skin, localized pain, and increased skin sensitivity in areas subjected to prolonged mechanical stress [25]. Furthermore, if basketball players are playing on a court with asphalt (typical in outdoor settings) instead of polished wood, they are more likely to develop abrasions and friction dermatitis if they fall. In these cases, players should wear knee and leg sleeves, along with protective padding. Management of friction dermatitis requires a comprehensive approach that addresses both symptom relief and underlying friction-related irritation. For friction dermatitis on a player's hands, they can use grip gloves in order to provide protective padding, while minimizing any restrictions on their basketball handling. Other strategies include applying emollients to maintain skin moisture and support healing, using topical corticosteroids for short-term inflammation control, identifying and minimizing sources of repetitive friction, and selecting moisture-wicking, breathable athletic wear [26].

Toe box dermatitis, also known as shoe contact dermatitis, is a complex skin condition that can arise from two primary mechanisms: mechanical friction (irritative dermatitis) or a type IV hypersensitivity allergic reaction to shoe materials such as leather or rubber (allergic contact dermatitis). Basketball athletes are susceptible to both types of irritation. Mechanical friction can result from repetitive movements and friction between toes in narrow shoes. The inside of basketball shoes is usually made from leather, which can cause an allergic reaction. Usually, the rash will be asymmetrical with the volar and dorsal aspects of the feet being affected. Shoe contact dermatitis can be treated with topical corticosteroids and emollients. Antibiotics and antifungals may be needed if there is a suspected infection [27].

9.4 Pressure-Related Dermatologic Conditions

Subungual hematoma is a painful condition characterized by blood accumulation beneath the toenail, typically resulting from acute traumatic injury or repetitive pressure. In basketball, this condition frequently occurs due to the sport's dynamic nature, characterized by sudden stops, rapid directional changes, and high-impact jumping (Fig. 9.1). The repeated vertical compression and lateral forces experienced during basketball movements can cause significant nail bed damage, potentially leading to structural changes, chronic pain, and nail deformities, specifically causing basketball toe [28, 29]. The pathophysiology involves direct trauma to the nail bed, causing blood vessels to rupture and create a blood pooling between the nail plate and underlying soft tissue. The primary symptoms include immediate pain, discoloration of the nail (typically dark red or black), and potential nail separation from the nail bed. Athletes may experience significant discomfort, particularly when pressure is applied to the affected toe.

The condition can range from mild, involving a small blood pocket, to severe, where the entire nail becomes discolored and potentially detached [28]. Basketball

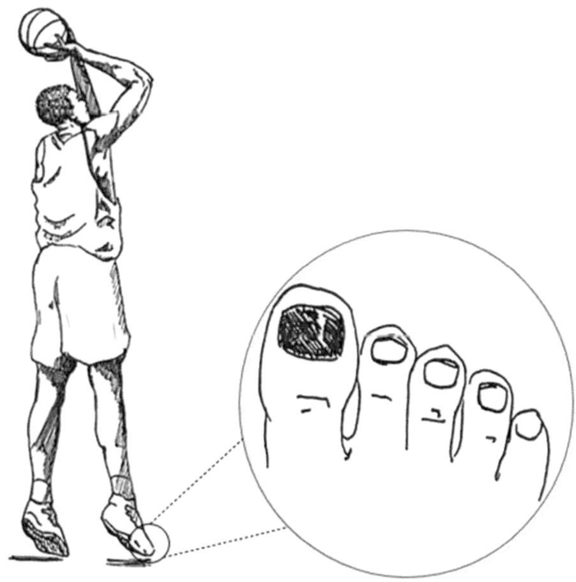

Fig. 9.1 Subungual hematoma from jump shot

players with tight-fitting shoes, those who frequently jump, and athletes with improper shoe sizing are at heightened risk. Preventive measures include wearing properly fitted basketball shoes (with adequate toe box space and shock absorption) and using protective padding. Athletes should also focus on techniques that minimize sudden, high-impact foot movements and use shock-absorbing insoles [29]. Furthermore, regular foot assessments, maintaining nail hygiene, and addressing any early signs of trauma can prevent long-term complications [30]. Management of subungual hematoma primarily includes standard rest, ice, compression, and elevation (RICE) of the affected area. Trephination can generally be performed for acute (<24–48 hours old) injuries and nail bed repair may be performed if the nail or digit is threatened.

9.5 Infectious-Related Dermatologic Conditions

9.5.1 Tinea Pedis

Tinea pedis is a common fungal infection primarily affecting the feet, characterized by its affinity for moist, warm environments that are endemic to athletic settings. Basketball athletes are particularly susceptible to tinea pedis due to prolonged foot enclosure in tight shoes, extensive sweating during gameplay, and exposure of feet to communal spaces like locker rooms and shower areas. Furthermore, the moist environment of basketball shoes, combined with constant foot compression and significant sweating, creates an ideal breeding ground for fungal proliferation. The pathophysiology of tinea pedis involves dermatophyte fungi, most commonly *Trichophyton rubrum*, which thrive in the dark, humid conditions typical of athletic footwear and locker room environments. Symptoms manifest as itching, burning sensations, dry and scaly skin, inflammation, and potential blister formation. Athletes may experience skin cracking, particularly between toes, with potential for secondary bacterial infections if left untreated [31]. The condition is fundamentally a superficial fungal infection of the skin, typically developing between toes or on the sole of the foot. Prevention and treatment strategies are multifaceted. Athletes should prioritize foot hygiene, properly wash and dry their socks, using antifungal powders and sprays, wearing moisture-wicking socks, and ensuring shoes are thoroughly dried between uses. Topical antifungal medications like clotrimazole, miconazole (Daktarin Cream made of miconazole nitrate), or terbinafine can effectively manage acute infections [32].

9.5.2 Tinea Manuum

Tinea Manuum is a fungal infection of the hands, due to repeated contact with contaminated surfaces. Basketballs can serve as transmission factors as multiple players repeatedly handle the same ball during a game or practice. The ball's contact with moisture from the player's hands, often due to sweat, creates a microenvironment on an unclean ball's surface that allows dermatophytes to survive and transfer between players. Furthermore, within basketball, there is frequent hand-to-hand contact and ensuing direct transmission during defensive plays, rebounds, and other situations. Finally, the locker room environments themselves can significantly contribute to infection risk. The moisture from showers, combined with insufficient ventilation, can maintain the humid conditions that promote fungal growth [33]. Preventative measures include good hygiene practices, such as proper hand washing and players using their own towels and equipment. The basketball should also be regularly disinfected to further mitigate the risk of dermatophyte proliferation. Treatment of tinea manuum is similar to tinea pedis, including topical antifungals such as miconazole and clotrimazole. In cases of systemic infection, oral medications such as terbinafine should be prescribed [34].

9.5.3 Onychomycosis

Onychomycosis is a fungal infection of the nail unit. As stated before, basketball players are especially vulnerable to sustaining trauma in their toes and nail bed. Basketball players perform frequent starts, stops, jumps, and quick directional changes. This can cause repeated trauma (tiny fissures and separations between the nail and nail bed) which creates entry points for dermatophytes to establish infection. Furthermore, basketball players often wear the same pair of shoes for extended periods of time. This prolonged exposure to a warm, moist environment increases the risk of fungal infection in the nail unit. Finally, locker rooms and shower facilities present other opportunities for the nail bed to be exposed to dermatophytes. Fungal organisms thrive on wet surfaces and walking barefoot in communal showers after sustaining trauma could potentially lead to onychomycosis. Even athletic socks can play a role in fungal infections. When socks become saturated with sweat, they can also maintain prolonged contact with toenails and extended periods of dampness can create an environment for fungi to thrive in [35–37]. The preventative measures as described in the tinea pedis section should also be applied to prevent onychomycosis, including drying feet after showering or playing, with special consideration given to spaces between toes. Players should also protect nail beds that sustained trauma by properly covering them and taking other preventative measures outlined in the subungual hematoma section. Treatment for onychomycosis usually includes oral antifungal drugs such as itraconazole. Providers can also prescribe antifungal nail polish like ciclopirox, or medicated nail cream such as efinaconazole [37].

9.6 Bacterial Infections

9.6.1 Impetigo

The close contact between players in the sport of basketball introduces the opportunity for the spread of impetigo. This bacterial infection is caused by gram-positive bacteria including *Staphylococcus aureus* or Group A *Streptococcus* (GAS) and can be further differentiated into two subtypes: nonbullous (the predominant form) and bullous [38]. Histologically, nonbullous impetigo is defined as infection that has reached just below the stratum corneum layer. Clinically, it often presents in previously traumatized skin, such as from abrasions or lacerations sustained during basketball gameplay. When these sites are impetiginized, they present with small vesicles or pustules with a characteristic oozing honey-colored crusting [39]. Often treatment can be achieved with topical antibiotics such as mupirocin and care to prevent further compromise to the epidermis that could potentially invite further impetiginization [40].

Bullous impetigo is almost always caused by *S. aureus* infection and can develop from untreated nonbullous impetigo. It is differentiated from nonbullous disease with deeper infection, occasionally presenting with deeper ulcerated infection known as ecthyma. Treatment is similar with topical antibiotics of lesions being complemented with systemic antibiotics as well [41]. With the increasing prevalence of antibiotic-resistant strains of organisms such as community-acquired methicillin-resistant *Staphylococcus aureus* (MRSA), considerations need to be made on preventing spread and optimizing treatment [42]. In the close quarters of a locker room and on the basketball court, skin-to-skin contact can cause rapid transmission. Similar to other contact sports, skin checks are recommended, both under the oversight of coaches and potentially even by referees officiating games [43].

9.6.2 Folliculitis

Another condition that basketball players may face is folliculitis (infection and inflammation of hair follicles). Aggravating factors include areas with more friction and recently shaved follicles. Clinical presentation of folliculitis includes the development of pruritic, erythematous papules and pustules around hair follicles. This condition may be relevant to basketball players in areas of frequent friction such as inner thighs, groin, distal lower extremities covered by tight clothing, and axilla. Clinical presentation is often sufficient for diagnosis, but performing a culture may be useful if the condition does not resolve with treatment. Most cases of folliculitis lead to spontaneous resolution. However, treatment may be required for more severe or resistant cases. When required, treatment can generally consist of topical mupirocin or clindamycin. Treatments vary based on the causative organism. For example, Staphylococcal folliculitis may be treated with Cephalexin or Azithromycin, while Staphylococcal folliculitis with suspicion of MRSA may be treated with oral Bactrim or clindamycin. For prevention, it is recommended that athletes not share towels and avoid shaving in high-friction areas [44].

9.6.3 Furuncles and Carbuncles

A furuncle is a boil or abscess formed within the hair follicle, and a carbuncle is a cluster of furuncles connected to each other beneath the skin, often resulting from infection by *Staphylococcus Aureus*. Furuncles and carbuncles present as tender, indurated, erythematous nodules, often with central pustules formed within hair follicles. Similar to folliculitis, diagnosis of furunculosis is based on clinical presentation; however, wound cultures can be performed to confirm etiology. Treatment of furuncles and carbuncles consists of incision and drainage, and prescription of trimethoprim-sulfamethoxazole. For bacterial infections, oral antibiotics, such as cephalexin or clindamycin, may also be recommended [44]. If the lesions are dry, athletes typically can return to play. It is recommended that players not return to play if the lesions are still moist or draining, even if the site is covered. Risk factors for furunculosis include contact with furuncles and prior skin injury. Therefore, methods to limit spread include avoiding direct contact with infected areas, avoiding sharing clothing or towels, and promptly implementing the proper treatment to infected athletes [45].

9.6.4 *Cellulitis*

Cellulitis is a bacterial infection of the subcutaneous tissue and deep dermis that is often accompanied by diffuse erythema, pain, warmth, and swelling. Clinical features may also include edematous and dilated skin lymphatics, leading to pear d'orange appearance, bulla formation, and linear erythematous streaks. In basketball players, cellulitis may occur due to lacerations or abrasions secondary to traumatic injury during falls or collisions. The majority of cases of cellulitis are nonculturable, but in 15% of culturable cases, most are attributed to *Streptococcus* and *Staphylococcus aureus*. Predisposing factors for cellulitis that basketball players may experience include cutaneous barrier disruption, the presence of bacterial colonization, fungal foot infections such as tinea pedis and onychomycosis, venous leg ulcers, and pressure ulcers [46].

Most cellulitis cases are diagnosed by physical exam and history alone, and tissue cultures performed with needle aspiration or biopsy often yield negative results. This may be due to a robust inflammatory response. Histologic features relevant to diagnosis include nonspecific dermal edema, diffuse and heavy neutrophil infiltration near blood vessels, and lymphatic dilation. Later stages of cellulitis may also include the presence of granulation tissue and lymphocytes. In cases of purulent cellulitis, where *S. aureus* is more likely, culture and sensitivity testing should always be performed to guide therapy. It is recommended that nonpurulent cellulitis without signs of systemic infections be treated with antistreptococcal antimicrobial agents and empirical antibiotic selection based on suspicion of MRSA and coverage narrowed according to culture results [46]. Severe cases of cellulitis, where additional surface layers of the skin become infected, may progress to erysipelas.

To prevent cellulitis, preventative measures for basketball players include regular foot examinations and treatment of underlying chronic dermatoses, including tinea pedis and onychomycosis. Intensive wound care for ulcerations and lacerations and maintenance of dry skin care at sites of injury may also reduce the incidence of cellulitis in athletes. Prophylactic antibiotics can also be considered for patients with recurrent cellulitis; however, potential allergy, drug resistance, and drug reactions must be considered with long-term antibiotic use [46].

9.7 Viral Infections

9.7.1 *Plantar Warts*

Plantar warts are hyperkeratotic, thick, endophytic lesions resulting from a local infection of human papillomavirus (HPV). Plantar warts are benign lesions that can be painful with applied pressure and result from the coalescence of plantar warts into large plaques [47]. HPV can be spread through direct contact with infected individuals or fomites. Therefore, athletes may be susceptible to these lesions if they walk barefoot in communal spaces such as locker rooms [48]. Basketball players also wear shoes and socks during play, potentially creating a warm, moist environment where the virus is able to thrive. Therefore, a potential preventative measure includes wearing foot coverings while in communal spaces and removing soiled athletic clothing immediately after use.

Diagnosis can be made visually or by paring down the hypertrophic epithelial component until thrombosed vessels that supply the wart tissue are detected in the dermis, often using a dermatoscope [47]. In order to rule out malignancy, diagnostic confirmation of human papillomavirus (HPV) includes polymerase chain reaction (PCR), excisional biopsy, and histopathological studies; however, these methods are often invasive and are not routinely used. Another reliable and less invasive option for definitive diagnosis is the wart-scraping method which involves DNA amplification of scrapings from the lesion surface [49]. Approximately two-thirds of HPV warts can resolve without treatment within two years of onset. There are also numerous effective treatment options, including cryotherapy using liquid nitrogen, propane, and diethyl ether directly applied to the lesion in two-, three-, or four-week intervals. Other treatments for warts include salicylic acid and zinc oxide [50].

9.7.2 Herpes Simplex Virus

Herpes Simplex Virus (HSV) is a virus that can be spread through direct contact with mucosal secretions or lesions of an individual with active primary or recurrent HSV infection [51]. Type 1 (HSV-1) is primarily transmitted through oral contact and results in vesicles in and around the mouth, while type 2 (HSV-2) is the leading cause of genital herpes and is a sexually transmitted infection. After initial infection, the HSV can become latent in neuronal cell bodies and can be reactivated, resulting in recurring eruptive lesions [52]. Symptoms of infection include the development of painful vesicles on the infected area, which may ulcerate and crust [51]. This may result in discomfort or pain during basketball sessions.

Diagnosis is clinical and based on the presence of multiple, round, superficial oral ulcerations, gingivitis, the presence of prior herpetic episodes, and reported exposure to HSV. Viral isolation in tissue cultures and HSV DNA PCR and serological assays may also be utilized to confirm the diagnosis [51]. Prolonged exposure to ultraviolet radiation increases the risk of reactivation of latent HSV; therefore, more frequent reactivation may occur in basketball players who use outdoor courts, which is especially relevant during warm summer months. Therefore, minimizing extreme sun exposure (especially in players who frequently practice outdoors), avoiding sunburns, and using sunscreen may be recommended to prevent recurrence [52]. Current management does not target viral eradication but rather suppression of recurrence and prevention of transmission. HSV will spontaneously resolve in immunocompetent individuals. When treatment is desired, antiviral agents include acyclovir or valacyclovir for most uncomplicated outpatient treatments. Acyclovir and related compounds are generally well tolerated despite long-term administration; however, the most frequent side effect is kidney toxicity. Acyclovir is available as a topical, oral, or IV medication [53].

9.7.3 Molluscum Contagiosum

Molluscum Contagiosum is a virus within the poxvirus family and causes localized cell proliferation. Clinical manifestations include clusters of firm, small, pruritic, umbilicated papules with a pearly surface. Dermatoscopy is the most common method of diagnosis; however, scraping or biopsy of lesions may be done to confirm the diagnosis [54]. Any cutaneous surface may be involved; however, favored sites include axillae, crural folds, popliteal, and antecubital fossae. Molluscum Contagiosum most commonly affects children and can be acquired through direct skin contact with infected individuals. Since basketball is a contact sport and involves sharing equipment, players are potentially at risk of infection via person-to-person contact [54].

On average, active molluscum contagiosum lesions resolve in 13.5 months, with 13% of cases not resolving within two years. Autoinoculation may be more likely in patients with atopic dermatitis due to a compromised skin barrier and underlying pruritis. Common in-office treatment options include cryotherapy, cantharidin application, and curettage [55]. If the lesions are pruritic, applying a topical steroid may be recommended to avoid scratching and potential viral spread from open or irritated lesions. In basketball, where close physical contact and shared equipment are integral to the sport, preventative measures to minimize transmission may include avoiding scratching the papules and sharing clothing or equipment [54].

9.8 Trauma-Related Dermatologic Conditions

Due to frequent physical contact, sudden movements, and falls on hard surfaces, basketball players may experience abrasions, lacerations, and bruising during gameplay.

9.8.1 Abrasions and Lacerations

Abrasions may result from "floor burns" if players fall or slide on the court surface. Basketball is both an indoor and outdoor sport, meaning that lacerations and abrasions can occur from various sources. Deep cuts or tears in skin resulting from collisions and falls, also known as lacerations, are another condition that basketball players may face. Outdoor asphalt courts may also lead to more severe abrasions and lacerations than indoor wood flooring due to the rough, abrasive texture of the surface. Histopathology of abrasions is rarely performed, but can be valuable in determining the stage of injury and can be correlated with the patient's history. Assessing the presence of extraneous material is crucial.

Abrasions are usually minor injuries and require no intervention and heal through primary intention; however, losing the protective epidermal layer leaves these lesions vulnerable to infection. Therefore, abrasions and lacerations should be cleansed and dressed to protect the area against reinjury. Debridement may also be necessary for extensive and deep abrasions, and in cases where the patient has no known allergies, topical antibiotic ointments may be prescribed [56]. Sleeves and protective pads worn on upper and lower extremities, particularly the knees and elbows, may be helpful in preventing these kinds of injuries during basketball gameplay.

9.8.2 *Contusions*

Direct ball trauma is a common source of facial abrasions and contusions, also known as bruises. Bruising may occur during basketball gameplay because of physical impact, collisions with other players, or falls. Common symptoms of contusions include discoloration of skin, swelling, and pain at the site of impact. Presentation of bruising varies with skin color, age, time from injury, and size of the original bruise. For example, bruises were significantly more black, red, and blue with increasing size. However, larger bruises became less red and more yellow at a faster rate. Additionally, one study comparing light, medium, and dark skin colors concluded that bruises on individuals with medium skin color were significantly more red and yellow than those of light or dark skin color. The authors also concluded that individuals with dark skin color had significantly darker bruises [57].

A potential preventive measure to avoid facial trauma is wearing a face mask during basketball gameplay. Additionally, one study justified adjusting the outer material of balls to a softer material since ball-to-face impact accounted for the majority of facial abrasions/contusions. However, this intervention may negatively impact gameplay and has previously received backlash from players [58]. Wearing well-fitting shoes that provide arch and ankle support may also provide stability and prevent contusions. Wearing knee and elbow pads also may prevent bruises from occurring. To control bleeding, pain, and inflammation from minor bruising, it is recommended that patients rest the injured area. Applying ice with cold packs several times daily, elevating the injured area, and wrapping the area to lightly compress and reduce swelling is also recommended [59].

9.9 Inflammatory Dermatologic Conditions

9.9.1 Irritant and Allergic Contact Dermatitis

Contact dermatitis is a very common dermatologic condition afflicting basketball players. Contact dermatitis comes in two main varieties: irritant and allergic. Irritant contact dermatitis (ICD), the more common type of dermatitis, is caused by direct skin injury due to an irritant and is not related to an immune response. Symptoms can include burning, pruritus, and pain. The injury manifests as dry, fissured skin and is typically found on the hands. The risk of irritant contact dermatitis is increased in athletes with atopic dermatitis. One particular manifestation of ICD specific to basketball is known as "basketball pebble fingers," which is a consequence of microtrauma secondary to abrasions in the fingers from the ball itself [1]. This happens commonly after long periods of play or return to play after a long period, particularly with balls designed for outdoor use (due to a more abrasive surface). This leads to fine abrasions, petechiae, and pain. This can affect performance, especially in regards to ball handling. Prevention of basketball pebble fingers and ICD includes applying topical emollients and avoiding balls with abrasive surfaces. Allergic contact dermatitis (ACD) is characterized by a type IV, or delayed-type, hypersensitivity response caused by repetitive exposure to allergens. The initial exposure to the sensitizer (the induction phase) occurs as a result of hapten-protein complex formation that eventually leads to form a T cell population specific to that antigen. Clinically, this manifests as erythematous, eczematous, or vesicular dermatitis at the site of exposure and pruritus.

Offending agents can often include rubber-containing balls/gear/shoes, nickel-containing jewelry, textile chemicals, fragrances, and other components of clothing and gear commonly worn by players. Ball-specific agents such as thiuram and mercaptobenzothiazole as well as knee pads containing formaldehyde resins, have been implicated in basketball-related ACD [60]. The diagnosis of allergic contact dermatitis is made based on history and physical exam. The definitive treatment for contact dermatitis is avoidance of the offending agent. Allergen patch testing can be useful when the cause is not apparent. Additionally, moisturizers and cool water soaks may be helpful in treating ACD when it does occur. Otherwise, ACD symptoms can be treated with antihistamines, topical steroids (<20% of body area affected) or oral steroids for more widespread disease. Topical immunomodulators like tacrolimus or even mycophenolate may be necessary for more severe disease. Again, it is important to remember that avoidance is key. Using uniform textiles free of latex and other offending agents and avoiding nickel-containing jewelry may help prevent ACD before it occurs. The American Contact Dermatitis Society's Contact Allergen Management Program is a helpful reference to avoid allergens [61].

9.9.2 Acne Mechanica

Acne vulgaris is the most prevalent reported skin condition in the United States [62]. Predisposing factors for acne vulgaris include genetics (in 80% of cases), hormonal changes, chemical contact, friction, and pressure [63]. While there are many conditions that may be predisposing towards acne vulgaris, acne mechanica refers to an acneiform eruption in areas of friction or pressure. Four main contributing factors include occlusion, heat, friction, and pressure. While the condition may not be as common in basketball players compared to hockey players, constant friction and occlusion of the skin can certainly lead to acne mechanica in basketball athletes. Equipment such as knee sleeves, elbow sleeves, headbands, and potentially tight jerseys may contribute to acne mechanica formation. This can be especially true in areas where sweat accumulates. Prevention measures can include wearing breathable cotton T-shirts, minimizing jersey pressure on the skin, and prompt bathing following sweating. What differentiates acne mechanica from typical acne vulgaris is that acne mechanica is primarily caused by mechanical causes (friction and pressure), whereas acne vulgaris has multiple predisposing factors. This is why interventions like topical antibiotics are less helpful for acne mechanica [64].

9.9.3 Atopic Dermatitis

Atopic dermatitis, also known as eczema, is the most common chronic skin condition and is yct anothcr inflammatory skin condition that can bc sccn in basketball athletes. This can be especially prevalent in places with pollution and low temperatures and/or humidity [65]. Although the causes of atopic dermatitis are not fully understood, family history and location in an area with low temperature and/or humidity play a role. The most common symptoms are itching and skin changes (including cracking and swelling). While ACD is caused by a type IV immune response, eczema pathophysiology is defined by a type II response. Diagnosis is clinical. While the exact causes of eczema are not clear, there are no specific preventative measures outside of avoiding potential triggers, which in the case of basketball players can include jersey/equipment materials and dry air inside gyms. Symptoms can be particularly bothersome for basketball athletes when the skin affected includes the hands. Eczema flare-ups can be treated with lifestyle changes, grip gloves, topical moisturizers, and steroids (systemically, if severe enough). Another preventative measure could be dribbling the ball more lightly. Some research also supports the potential of the use of vitamin D [66]. Additionally, monoclonal antibody therapies such as dupilumab and tralokinumab have become increasingly attractive treatment options for moderate-to-severe disease [67].

9.10 Miscellaneous Dermatologic Conditions

9.10.1 Xerosis

Xerosis results from inadequate hydrolipid composition within the skin, specifically the stratum corneum. Symptoms can include pain, pruritus, tightness, and burning sensations, with the limbs more commonly involved. Like eczema, xerosis of the hands (with ensuing symptoms and skin changes) can significantly affect basketball players' sports performance. Unfortunately for basketball athletes, areas with fewer sebaceous glands are more prone to xerosis, including the hands, forearms, and feet [68]. Contributing factors vary, from environmental factors and excessive skin cleansing to inflammatory disorders. It is important to discern whether patients have features associated with other dermatologic conditions, including atopic history, external triggers, medications, and medical history. Laboratory work up can be performed to assess for many possible associated contributing factors such as hypothyroidism but diagnosis is mostly clinical. Restoring skin moisturization and epidermal lipid composition is the focus of management. Options include skin creams, humidifiers, hydration, and petrolatum [69].

9.10.2 Solar Erythema

Solar erythema (commonly known as a sunburn) presents a challenge to outdoor basketball players. Therefore, sun protection and exercise outside peak hours of sunlight are recommended to prevent sunburns, premature aging, and skin cancer later in life. Sun protection may include sunglasses, hats, UV protective clothing, and remaining in shade by built or natural environments. Reapplication of sunscreen every 2–3 hours would also provide protection from solar erythema. Preventable measures can ultimately impact player performance and the long-term skin health of athletes [70].

References

1. Gottlieb R, Shalom A, Calleja-Gonzalez J. Physiology of basketball—field tests. Rev Article J Hum Kinet. 2021;77:159–67.
2. Emer J, Sivek R, Marciniak B. Sports dermatology: part 1 of 2 traumatic or mechanical injuries, inflammatory conditions, and exacerbations of pre-existing conditions. J Clin Aesthet Dermatol. 2015;8(4):31–43.
3. Nobles T, Syed HA, Miller RA. Intertrigo. Treasure Island (FL): StatPearls; 2024.
4. Raatma L. The curious, captivating, unusual history of sports. Capstone Press; 1 January 2012.
5. Romanelli M, Voegeli D, Colboc H, Bassetto F, Janowska A, Scarpa C, et al. The diagnosis, management and prevention of intertrigo in adults: a review. J Wound Care. 2023;32(7):411–20.

6. Verzi AE, Nasca MR, Dall'Oglio F, Cosentino C, Micali G. A novel treatment of intertrigo in athletes and overweight subjects. J Cosmet Dermatol. 2021;20 Suppl 1(Suppl 1):23–7.
7. Guerra KC, Toncar A, Krishnamurthy K. Miliaria. Treasure Island (FL): StatPearls; 2024.
8. Mowad CM, McGinley KJ, Foglia A, Leyden JJ. The role of extracellular polysaccharide substance produced by Staphylococcus epidermidis in Miliaria. J Am Acad Dermatol. 1995;33(5 Pt 1):729–33.
9. Gauer R, Meyers BK. Heat-related illnesses. Am Fam Physician. 2019;99(8):482–9.
10. Carter R 3rd, Garcia AM, Souhan BE. Patients presenting with miliaria while wearing flame resistant clothing in high ambient temperatures: a case series. J Med Case Rep. 2011;5:474.
11. Martins N, Ferreira IC, Barros L, Silva S, Henriques M. Candidiasis: predisposing factors, prevention, diagnosis and alternative treatment. Mycopathologia. 2014;177(5–6):223–40.
12. Arya NR, Rafiq NB. Candidiasis. Treasure Island (FL): StatPearls; 2024.
13. Pappas PG, Kauffman CA, Andes DR, Clancy CJ, Marr KA, Ostrosky-Zeichner L, et al. Clinical practice guideline for the management of candidiasis: 2016 update by the infectious diseases society of America. Clin Infect Dis. 2016;62(4):e1–50.
14. Taudorf EH, Jemec GBE, Hay RJ, Saunte DML. Cutaneous candidiasis—an evidence-based review of topical and systemic treatments to inform clinical practice. J Eur Acad Dermatol Venereol. 2019;33(10):1863–73.
15. Palaniappan V, Murthy AB, Karthikeyan K. Pitted keratolysis. Clin Exp Dermatol. 2023;48(9):978–83.
16. Bristow IR, Lee YL. Pitted keratolysis: a clinical review. J Am Podiatr Med Assoc. 2014;104(2):177–82.
17. Knapik JJ, Reynolds KL, Duplantis KL, Jones BH. Friction blisters. Pathophysiology, prevention and treatment. Sports Med. 1995;20(3):136–47.
18. Levine N. Friction blisters. Phys Sportsmed. 1982;10(3):84–92.
19. Freeman DB. Corns and calluses resulting from mechanical hyperkeratosis. Am Fam Physician. 2002;65(11):2277–80.
20. Hashmi F, Nester CJ, Wright CR, Lam S. The evaluation of three treatments for plantar callus: a three-armed randomised, comparative trial using biophysical outcome measures. Trials. 2016;17(1):251.
21. Elwell R. The management and treatment of hyperkeratosis. Br J Nurs. 2017 Apr 27;26(8):468–470.
22. Mailler EA, Adams BB. The Wear and Tear of 26.2 Dermatological injuries reported on marathon day. Br J Sports Med. 2004;38:498–501. https://doi.org/10.1136/bjsm.2004.011874.
23. Lin TK, Zhong L, Santiago JL. Anti-inflammatory and skin barrier repair effects of topical application of some plant oils. Int J Mol Sci. 2017;19(1):70.
24. Kockentiet B, Adams BB. Contact dermatitis in athletes. J Am Acad Dermatol. 2007;56(6):1048–55.
25. McMullen E, Gawkrodger DJ. Physical friction is under-recognized as an irritant that can cause or contribute to contact dermatitis. Br J Dermatol. 2006;154(1):154–6.
26. Litchman G, Nair PA, Atwater AR, Bhutta BS. Contact Dermatitis. Treasure Island (FL): StatPearls; 2024.
27. Thompson H. Shoe contact dermatitis: Dermatology Registrar; July 2022.
28. Akella A, Daniel AR, Gould MB, Mangal R, Ganti L. Subungual hematoma. Cureus. 2023;15(11):e48952.
29. Pingel C, McDowell C. Subungual Hematoma Drainage. Treasure Island (FL): StatPearls; 2024.
30. Aksović N, Bubanj S, Bjelica B, Kocić M, Lilić L, Zelenović M, Stanković D, Milanović F, Pajović L, Čaprić I, Milić V, Dobrescu T, Sufaru C. Sports Injuries in Basketball Players: A Systematic Review. Life (Basel). 2024 Jul 19;14(7):898. https://doi.org/10.3390/life14070898. PMID: 39063651; PMCID: PMC11278090.
31. Nigam PK, Syed HA, Saleh D. Tinea Pedis. Treasure Island (FL): StatPearls; 2024.
32. Leung AK, Barankin B, Lam JM, Leong KF, Hon KL. Tinea pedis: an updated review. Drugs Context. 2023:12.

33. Zinder SM, Basler RS, Foley J, Scarlata C, Vasily DB. National athletic trainers' association position statement: skin diseases. J Athl Train. 2010;45(4):411–28.
34. Chamorro, Monica J. "Tinea Manuum." StatPearls, StatPearls Publishing, 1 March 2024.
35. Daggett C, Brodell RT, Daniel CR, Jackson J. Onychomycosis in athletes. Am J Clin Dermatol. 2019;20(5):691–8.
36. Sabadin CS, Benvegnu SA, da Fontoura MM, Saggin LM, Tomimori J, Fischman O. Onychomycosis and tinea pedis in athletes from the State of Rio Grande Do Sul (Brazil): a cross-sectional study. Mycopathologia. 2011;171(3):183–9.
37. Bodman, Myron A., et al. "Onychomycosis." StatPearls, StatPearls Publishing, 9 January 2024.
38. Barton LL, Friedman AD. Impetigo: a reassessment of etiology and therapy. Pediatr Dermatol. 1987;4(3):185–8.
39. Edlich RF, Winters KL, Britt LD, Long WB. Bacterial diseases of the skin. J Long-Term Eff Med Implants. 2005;15(5):499–510.
40. Stulberg DL, Penrod MA, Blatny RA. Common bacterial skin infections. Am Fam Physician. 2002;66(1):119–24.
41. McLinn S. A bacteriologically controlled, randomized study comparing the efficacy of 2% mupirocin ointment (Bactroban) with oral erythromycin in the treatment of patients with impetigo. J Am Acad Dermatol. 1990;22(5 Pt 1):883–5.
42. Nardi NM, Schaefer TJ. Impetigo. In: StatPearls. Treasure Island (FL): StatPearls Publishing; July 31, 2023.
43. Bernard P. Management of common bacterial infections of the skin. Curr Opin Infect Dis. 2008;21(2):122–8.
44. Pujalte GGA, Costa LMC, Clapp AD, Presutti RJ, Sluzevich JC. More than skin deep: dermatologic conditions in athletes. Sports Health. 2023;15(1):74–85.
45. Adams BB. Dermatologic disorders of the athlete. Sports Med. 2002;32(5):309–21.
46. Raff AB, Kroshinsky D. Cellulitis: a review. JAMA. 2016;316(3):325–37.
47. Dina Esterowitz KEG, Cooper PH, Edlich RF. Plantar warts in the athlete. Am J Emerg Med. 1995;13(4):441–3.
48. Tyring S, Yen Moore A, Lupi O. Mucocutaneous manifestations of viral diseases: an illustrated guide to diagnosis and management. Milton, UK: Taylor & Francis Group; 2010.
49. Garcia-Oreja S, Alvaro-Afonso FJ, Sevillano-Fernandez D, Tardaguila-Garcia A, Lopez-Moral M, Lazaro-Martinez JL. A non-invasive method for diagnosing plantar warts caused by human papillomavirus (HPV). J Med Virol. 2022;94(6):2897–901.
50. Palmer WJ. Options for foot dermatoses. Dermatology Times. 2019;40(2):30,4.
51. Mahnaz Fatahzadeh RAS. Human herpes simplex virus infections: epidemiology, pathogenesis, symptomatology, diagnosis, and management. J Am Acad Dermatol. 2007;57(5):737–63.
52. Sfyri E, Tertipi N, Kefala V, Rallis E. Prevalence of plantar warts, genital warts, and herpetic infections in greek competitive swimmers. Viruses. 2024;16(11):1782.
53. Poole CL, James SH. Antiviral therapies for herpesviruses: current agents and new directions. Clin Ther. 2018;40(8):1282–98.
54. Schaffer JV, Berger EM. Molluscum Contagiosum. JAMA Dermatol. 2016;152(9):1072.
55. Oza VS. Molluscum Contagiosum therapeutics—new options may be around the corner. JAMA Dermatol. 2022;158(8):863–4.
56. Shrestha RKK, Ishaq H, Kanchan T. Abrasion. StatPearls: StatPearls Publishing; 2023.
57. Scafide KRN, Sheridan DJ, Campbell J, DeLeon VB, Hayat MJ. Evaluating change in bruise colorimetry and the effect of subject characteristics over time. Forensic Sci Med Pathol. 2013;9(3):367–76.
58. Othman S, Cohn JE, McKinnon B. On the court: a comprehensive analysis of basketball facial trauma. Craniomaxillofac Trauma Reconstr. 2019;12(4):266–70.
59. Wittstein JR. Muscle contusion (Bruise). Diseases and Conditions [Internet]. 2024 Dec 15, 2024. Available from: https://orthoinfo.aaos.org/en/diseases%2D%2Dconditions/muscle-contusion-bruise/#:~:text=Athletes%20in%20contact%20sports%20have,athlete%20away%20from%20the%20game.

60. Rodriguez-Serna M, Molinero J, Febrer I, Aliaga A. Persistant hand eczema in a child. Am J Contact Dermat. 2002;13(1):35–6. https://doi.org/10.1053/ajcd.2002.29383.
61. ACDS camp: American Contact Dermatitis Society (ACDS) [Internet]. American Contact Dermatitis Society; 2024 [cited 2024 Dec 30]. Available from: https://www.contactderm.org/resources/acds-camp.
62. Bickers DR, Lim HW, Margolis D, Weinstock MA, Goodman C, Faulkner E, et al. The burden of skin diseases: 2004 a joint project of the American Academy of Dermatology Association and the Society for Investigative Dermatology. J Am Acad Dermatol. 2006;55(3):490–500.
63. Bhate K, Williams HC. Epidemiology of acne vulgaris. Br J Dermatol. 2013;168(3):474–85.
64. Botros PA, Tsai G, Pujalte GG. Evaluation and management of acne. Prim Care. 2015;42(4):465–71.
65. Engebretsen KA, Johansen JD, Kezic S, Linneberg A, Thyssen JP. The effect of environmental humidity and temperature on skin barrier function and dermatitis. J Eur Acad Dermatol Venereol. 2016;30(2):223–49.
66. Kim MJ, Kim SN, Lee YW, Choe YB, Ahn KJ. Vitamin D status and efficacy of Vitamin D supplementation in atopic dermatitis: a systematic review and meta-analysis. Nutrients. 2016;8(12):789.
67. Halling AS, Loft N, Silverberg JI, Guttman-Yassky E, Thyssen JP. Real-world evidence of Dupilumab efficacy and risk of adverse events: a systematic review and meta-analysis. J Am Acad Dermatol. 2021;84(1):139–47.
68. Augustin M, Kirsten N, Körber A, Wilsmann-Theis D, Itschert G, Staubach-Renz P, Maul JT, Zander N. Prevalence, predictors and comorbidity of dry skin in the general population. J Eur Acad Dermatol Venereol. 2019;33(1):147–50.
69. Augustin M, Wilsmann-Theis D, Körber A, Kerscher M, Itschert G, Dippel M, et al. Diagnosis and treatment of xerosis cutis—a position paper. J Dtsch Dermatol Ges. 2019;17(Suppl 7):3–33.
70. Görig T, Apfelbacher C, Drewitz KP, Reimers AK, Breitbart EW, Diehl K. Sunburn and sun protection during recreational outdoor sport in summer: findings from the German general population aged 16–65 years. Photodermatol Photoimmunol Photomed. 2023;39(6):589–97.

Chapter 10
Dance & Gymnastics

Lauren Dender, Sophie Cilivio, Ryan Scheinkman, Stefania Radici, Rachel Cohen, Alexia Vignau, and Keyvan Nouri

10.1 Dance Introduction

Dance encompasses a broad range of activities but is generally related to any form of rhythmic movement. As a (typically) choreographed collection of actions, dance is a blend of athletic capabilities and artistic performance. Thus, dancers sustain injuries and suffer dermatologic complications unique to their athletic technique and particular movement styles. The variety of practiced dance styles can be attributed to its long-standing presence in our communities and cultural practices, dating back to approximately 8000 BCE [1]. Historically, dance has been deeply interwoven into the cultural fabric of rituals and communities. For example, the Chinese Lion dance originated in the Han dynasty and is still performed at Chinese New Year and cultural celebrations today [2]. Other forms, such as ballet, jazz, modern dance, and hip-hop are commonly practiced professionally as a performing art or competitive sport.

Professional dancers, such as those employed by ballet companies or as backup dancers for musicians, have an incredibly physically demanding trade. A recent analysis of the Occupational Information Network (O*NET) determined that dancers had the highest levels of job physicality out of all professions in the United States [3]. Dancers outperformed professional athletes, iron and steel workers, and firefighters, earning a 97 out of 100 for overall job physicality [3]. The physicality of professional dance can be attributed to the stamina, strength, flexibility, and coordination required to perform in shows multiple times a day or week [3]. For instance, Ballerinas at the Royal Ballet can dance in up to 113 performances per season and

L. Dender · S. Cilivio · R. Scheinkman (✉) · S. Radici · R. Cohen · A. Vignau · K. Nouri
Dr. Phillip Frost Department of Dermatology and Cutaneous Surgery, University of Miami, Miami, FL, USA
e-mail: ldender@med.miami.edu; scc147@med.miami.edu; scheinkman@med.miami.edu; sxr3896@miami.edu; rachelcohen@med.miami.edu; axv200@med.miami.edu; knouri@med.miami.edu

K. Nouri (ed.), *Sport-Related Skin Conditions*,
https://doi.org/10.1007/978-3-031-90444-8_10

average well over 20 hours of rehearsals a week on top of their performance schedules [4].

The physical demands of dance are explicitly demonstrated by the high degree of overuse injury seen within the sport. The Journal of Orthopaedic & Sports Physical Therapy published that an elite-level ballet company reported an average of 6.8 injuries per dancer during the 1-year period over which data was collected [5]. Beyond the physical demands, the environment of these professional companies or competitions instigates unique emotional pressures. Visible bruises and abrasions due to the partner work required for some pieces or performances are regular in dance. Additionally, the emotional triggers of portraying specific characters add another layer of intensity to the profession. For example, Kenneth MacMillan's 1978 ballet *Mayerling* portrays a young bride, Stephanie, who is violently assaulted on her wedding night by her husband [6]. The choreography in this piece involves Stephanie being grabbed and thrown violently during the partner work. *Mayerling* provides a specific, although not unique, example of dance's physical and emotional pressures due to the required physical and emotional contact between dance partners or other company members during the performance.

As demonstrated above, dancers rely on their bodies to achieve their performances. Different styles of dance, thus, have distinct demands on the dancer's anatomy. Ballet, a classical dance form, focuses on balance, gracefulness, and strength. Female-presenting dancers often wear pointe shoes. Pointe shoes are uniquely structured due to their solid toe box, which allows ballerinas to balance on the tip of their toes during rehearsal and performance [7]. The toe-box of pointe shoes results in the ballerina placing the entirety of their weight on their metatarsophalangeal heads, resulting in many of the pain and injuries often seen in ballet companies [7]. Modern/contemporary dance is frequently rehearsed and performed barefoot, focusing on a natural rooting into the ground and allowing for complete artistic expression in the feet. Countless hours barefoot during rehearsals can result in various conditions, including floor burns, calluses, and plantar warts [8]. Hip-hop is a unique dance category in that it is often performed in "street shoes" such as sneakers or even heels. These shoes may not be made with high intensity footwork in mind, potentially leading to painful injuries [9]. Due to the wide variety and particular demands of dance styles, a deeper dive into the dermatologic consequences of professional dance is warranted, as dance can exacerbate pre-existing skin disorders or cause them directly.

10.2 Dermatophyte Infections in Dance

Prolonged use of tightly fitting clothing, occlusive footwear, and exposure to excessive moisture or sweat are all factors inherent to the athletic artform of dance. These factors place dancers at an increased risk for acquiring fungal infections. Tinea pedis, or athletes foot, is a common fungal infection of the skin of the feet caused by dermatophyte species, namely: *Trichophyton rubrum, T mentagrophytes, T interdigitale,* and *Epidermophyton floccosum* [10]. Clinically, tinea pedis may present in a variety of ways, including interdigital tinea pedis, hyperkeratotic (moccasin-type), vesiculobullous or inflammatory, and ulcerative tinea pedis [11]. Interdigital tinea pedis typically presents with pruritic erosions or scales between the toes, with associated interdigital skin fissuring which may be painful to patients [10, 11]. Hyperkeratotic tinea pedis presents clinically as a diffuse, hyperkeratotic eruption in a "moccasin" distribution (involving the soles, medial, and lateral surfaces of the feet) with a variable degree of underlying erythema [11]. Vesiculobullous subtype of tinea pedis is a pruritic, potentially painful, vesicular or bullous eruption with underlying erythema most commonly occurring on the medial foot [11]. Ulcerative tinea pedis is a less common subtype that may present with interdigital erosions and ulcers that are usually associated with secondary bacterial infection [11].

Definitive diagnosis of tinea pedis can be made with a positive Potassium Hydroxide (KOH) preparation demonstrating segmented hyphae [10, 11]. Treatment of choice for most patients with tinea pedis includes the use of topical antifungal therapies (azoles, allylamines, butenafine, ciclopirox, and tolnaftate) that are generally applied once or twice daily for 4 weeks [10]. Patients with extensive infection or who have failed to respond to topical therapies may be treated with oral antifungal agents (e.g., terbinafine, itraconazole, griseofulvin). Due to the more extensive side effect profile associated with the systemic treatment route, including hepatotoxicity, cutaneous adverse reactions, and possible drug interactions, oral medications should be reserved for those who meet criteria and caution should be exercised when prescribing [11].

Tinea pedis may occur in conjunction with a variety of other dermatological conditions caused by superficial dermatophyte infections. Specifically, onychomycosis, a fungal infection of the nail, tends to occur in conjunction with tinea pedis and is commonly seen amongst dancers likely due to their occlusive footwear. Onychomycosis has a variety of subtypes. Distal subungual onychomycosis, the most common subtype, classically presents with a white, yellow or brown discoloration at the distal corner of the nailbed that may spread to involve the entire nail. Subungual hyperkeratosis and onycholysis may also be associated with the distal subungual subtype [12]. Additional subtypes of onychomycosis, although less common in the general population, are outlined in this chapter to detail the various clinical nail presentations for this condition that notoriously affects the dance world.

White superficial onychomycosis appears as dull, white spots on the surface of the nail plate that are soft and have a chalky scale when scraped lightly [12]. Another less common subtype, proximal subungual onychomycosis, affects the proximal aspect of the nail and extends distally. This specific subtype typically occurs in immunocompromised patients and has been utilized as a clinical marker for Acquired Immunodeficiency Syndrome (AIDS) secondary to HIV infection [12]. Infectious species reported to cause the proximal subungual form of onychomycosis includes *T ruburm, Fulsifarum spp., Candida albicans,* and *Aspergillus spp.* [12, 13]. Endonyx onychomycosis is identified as nail discoloration and nail splitting that occurs exclusively at the interior of the nail plate; there is no associated subungual hyperkeratosis [12]. Totally dystrophic onychomycosis is seen as a complete destruction of the nail bed with hyperkeratosis and nail ridging present. This presentation is typically the result of end-stage lateral distal subungual or proximal subungual onychomycoses [12]. While adequate patient history and physical exam findings may strongly suggest the diagnosis of onychomycosis, laboratory studies demonstrating an existing fungal nail infection confirms diagnosis. Diagnostic methods used include KOH preparations, polymerase chain reaction (PCR) testing, fungal cultures, and histopathologic examination of the nail. Treatment options include with topical antifungal creams, oral antifungal medication, and in some cases, a combination of both topical and systemic antifungal therapies. As discussed earlier in the treatment of tinea pedis, a thorough patient medical history and clinical image should be considered before prescribing oral antifungal agents [14]. In patients who are not candidates for oral antifungal therapies or who fail to respond to treatment with topical antifungal regimens, additional treatment options may include physical modalities such as lasers or surgical excision [14].

In the context of dermatophyte infections in the dancer, it is important to review the aspects of their daily routine in the sport to highlight areas where strategies may be implemented to reduce infection incidence and recurrence. The uniform of a ballet dancer typically includes the use of tights, a leotard, tightly slicked back hair into a bun with the use of hairsprays, hair ties, performance makeup, and bobby pins to secure the placement of a bun. Typically, as with other sports, these tools are carried in the dancer's bag along with their dance shoes and associated orthotic pads or support cushions used within their shoes. If a dancer who has tinea pedis keeps her dance shoes and toe pads in her bag, she is at risk of spreading fungal spores to other items in her dance bag (e.g., dance clothing, hairbrushes, hair ties, bobby pins, makeup brushes, etc.). As a result, dancers with untreated tinea pedis infection may be at risk for concurrent tinea infection including tinea mannum, tinea corporis, tinea curis, tinea capitis and tinea faceii. Proper patient/dancer education regarding tinea and prevention strategies should be implemented as preventative measures to avoid tinea infections in the dance world.

10.3 Trauma-Related Foot and Nail Conditions for Dance

Dancers across all genres of dance place an extraordinary amount of physical pressure and impact forces on their feet and toes, leaving them very susceptible to various conditions associated with repetitive nail trauma, blistering, bruising, and superficial skin tears. A survey was conducted on 112 professional ballet dancers to assessing pointe-shoe-related discomfort across different shoe brands revealed 100% of dancer participants reported toenail pain across all brands of pointe shoes (Fig. 10.1) [15]. Participants also reported pain in the heel, bunions (hallux valgus) and arches of the foot across all brands [15]. This study highlights the seemingly inescapable toenail pain and associated nail trauma ballet dancers endure.

Subungual hematoma, or collection of blood underneath the nail bed, is a common condition seen in dancers as a result of blunt trauma to the nail [16]. Clinically,

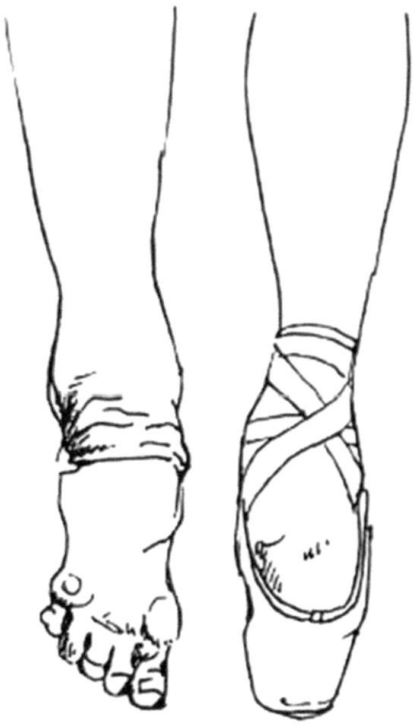

Fig. 10.1 Pointe-shoe-related Trauma

subungual hematomas present with significant "throbbing" pain and blue-to-black discoloration of the nail bed [16]. Treatment options for subungual hematoma includes trephination, a procedure where a medical provider places one or more holes into the nail plate as a means to evacuate the entrapped blood and associated pressure under the nail [16]. If there is existing nail avulsion (loss of the nail) or bleeding around the nail fold on initial evaluation, trephination is less likely to offer pain relief or any other clinical benefit [16]. In general, trephination is preferred over nail removal and nail bed repair in the case of painful subungual hematomas with intact nail folds [16]. Prior to treatment with trephination, medical providers should differentiate subungual hematoma from other nail conditions that may have a similar appearance, such as, subungual melanoma, junctional nevus, splinter hemorrhages, subungual keratoacanthoma and subungual epithelioma [16]. As these conditions also present with various pigment alterations of the nail, they are easily distinguished from subungual hematoma by patient history revealing prior nail trauma and associated nail pain present on physical exam [16].

A study evaluating work-related dermatoses of the feet in professional dancers found hyperkeratosis, onychomycosis, and subungual hematomas to be the most common dermatological conditions affecting the feet of the professional dancer [17]. Onychomycosis and subungual hematoma have been discussed previously in this chapter. Hyperkeratosis, or thickening of the keratinocyte layer in the stratum corneum, is a normal and common physiologic response of the skin to chronic excessive pressure or friction [18]. Chronic exposure to pressure and friction on the dancers' foot can lead to the physiologic hyperkeratosis and eventual development of callouses and corns on the feet. Callouses are a benign skin condition that presents with diffuse thickening of the stratum corneum in response to friction or pressure [18, 19]. Corns develop similarly to callouses; however, they differ in that there is a central hyperkeratotic "core" present and are often associated with pain [19]. Notably, corns typically develop at pressure points on the foot secondary to poorly-fitted shoes or an abnormal gait [19].

Corns and callouses are typically diagnosed via patient history and physical exam findings, however, it is important to differentiate these conditions clinically from plantar warts that, on close evaluation, will have several dark spots or punctate capillary thromboses. Treatment options for callouses and corns include prevention with the use of orthotic pads and properly-fitted shoes, and topical keratolytics such as salicylic acid or urea-based creams [19]. Debridement with a scalpel is an alternative treatment option that may provide rapid resolution of associated pain and discomfort [19].

Common remedies used by dancers pose risks to their overall health. A widely-used method to alleviate foot and toe pain/discomfort in ballet dancers is the off-label use of over-the-counter topical anesthetics containing lidocaine and benzocaine (e.g., Oragel) for direct application to the foot, toes, or other site of pain or injury [20]. Reports of soft-tissue infections being masked by off-lapel topical anesthetic use have been documented [20].

10.4 Bacterial Skin Infections in Dance

Dancers across all genres are prone to developing blisters and superficial skin tears from chronic use and friction with their footwear, or direct friction with the floor in some dance genres where footwear is not used (modern and contemporary dance). These trauma-related disruptions to the skin barrier place dancers at risk for developing secondary bacterial skin infections. The most common bacterial pathogens associated with superficial skin infections include *S. Aureus, S. pyogenes*, however, infection by other pathogens can also occur [21]. Dancers should be cautioned to look for signs of infection including pain, swelling, redness, and warmth, erythema or induration to the skin and should seek medical attention immediately if these signs of infection are present. Patients should be started on broad spectrum antibiotics and bacterial wound cultures should be taken to ensure proper antibiotic coverage of the causing pathogen [21].

When any form of skin tear, abrasion or de-roofing of a blister occurs, dancers should be cautioned to practice proper wound care hygiene to prevent the occurrence of a secondary skin infection. This can be achieved by advising dancers to cleaning their wound with gentle soap and water, covering the wound with Vaseline or Aquaphor and covering the site with a compressive dressing or Band-Aid to prevent introduction of bacteria to the wound. The compressive dressing should be changed once daily. Folliculitis, or inflammation of the hair follicle, is another dermatological condition with significant prevalence in the dance world due to their frequent exposure to sweat coupled with the compressive tights, leotards and other forms of spandex clothing worn by dancers. Bacterial folliculitis is most commonly a result of an infection with *S. aureus* or gram-negative species such as *P. aeruginosa* and presents clinically as follicular pustules and papules. In dancers there is an increased risk of folliculitis if compressive clothing is worn for extended amounts of time and the combined compressive effect of the clothing and moisture-filled environment from sweating results in occlusion of the hair follicle. Diagnosis is often achieved by thorough patient history and physical exam findings. Treatment of *S. aureus* folliculitis is not always necessary, with mild cases often resolving spontaneously [22]. Antimicrobial cleansers such as benzoyl peroxide may be helpful for the treatment of mild folliculitis and prevention of hair follicle occlusion, however, its efficacy has not been studied in clinical trials [22]. In cases of moderate or severe folliculitis, topical antibiotics such as mupirocin (3 times daily for 7 days) and clindamycin (2 times daily for 7–10 days) have been reported to effectively resolve disease [22].

10.5 Allergic and Irritant Contact Dermatitis Allergens in Dance

Dancers engage with various substances and materials in their daily rehearsals and performances that have the propensity to cause either allergic or irritant contact dermatitis. One such material is rosin. Rosin is a commercial colophony formulation manufactured from the sap of pine and spruce trees [23]. Colophony is a mixture of over 100 compounds, but the oxidation products and synthesized acids from modification are the primary allergens responsible for the adverse reactions seen [24]. Rosin has a wide range of uses, including for string instruments, but dancers use rosin on their shoes to create friction between the shoe and the floor [25]. Typically, dancers crush the rosin–purchased in small-rock forms–into a powder and then rub it into the toes and heels of their shoes [25].

The common acute allergic contact dermatitis reaction to rosin tends to occur within 1–3 days after exposure and is often confined to the area of contact with rosin [26]. However, due to the unique nature of dance, materials that have been in contact with one dancer or one area of an individual dancer's body can be spread to other areas of the body or dancers, resulting in reactions foreign to the site of original contact [26]. The reaction originates with an inflamed and itchy patch of skin and can progress to blistering and intense itchiness [26]. Chronic exposure to rosin, seen with professional dancers, can progress further, forming a thickened, lichenified area [26]. Dancers, despite tolerating rosin for years or decades without an adverse reaction, can experience allergic contact dermatitis as a result of rosin exposure [27]. Once a dancer encounters allergic contact dermatitis due to rosin, they have the allergy for life [27]. The development of this allergy can result in complex issues for dancers since, due to partner work and proximity to other company members, personal avoidance of rosin may not be enough to deter any unfavorable reactions.

Dancers are also uniquely predisposed to facial contact dermatitis due to the excessive use of cosmetics and hair products required for performances. Allergic and irritant contact dermatitis of the eyelids typically involves exposure to standard performance products such as makeup remover, mascara, makeup sponges, and eyelash curlers [28]. Water-based and waterproof mascara contain compounds that can irritate individuals, such as emulsifiers and volatile organic solvents [28]. As the irritating compounds vary by product, if a dancer experiences dermatitis due to one formulation of mascara, they may be able to use another formulation without any adverse effects [28]. While allergic or irritant contact dermatitis to eyeshadow is rare, individuals may experience dermatitis due to either pressed or cream eyeshadow. Similarly, they can switch to other eyeshadow formulations in hopes of better tolerating them [28]. Allergic dermatitis of the face commonly occurs due to either allergens applied directly to the face or allergens from hair products rinsed onto the face [28]. Thus, dancers who often have to apply heavy makeup or prosthetics to their faces or use harsh hair products, such as gels and hairsprays, to keep a desired style during their performance are uniquely susceptible to acquiring allergic contact dermatitis as a result [28]. Often, dancers must complete their makeup looks with false eyelashes or gemstones. Dancers glue these products to their faces using instant adhesives, which frequently include acrylates formed from polymerization of acrylic monomers [29]. Acrylates can be responsible for allergic contact dermatitis of the eyelid or other facial structures due to their use in false eyelash adhesive [29].

Adhesive tape is also widely used in the professional dance community. Many dancers, especially ballerinas who use pointe shoes, tape their feet to reduce friction and prevent blisters that can occur due to intense footwork or the specific shoe requirements of the performance. Tape-related foot dermatitis has been recorded in other professions, such as in military conscripts using medical tape in a similar manner to dancers [30]. While medical tape use is well-reported to cause irritant contact dermatitis, there is evidence that allergic contact dermatitis can also result from repeated use [30]. Medical tape contains many allergens, such as colophonium-associated materials, acrylates, and rubber additives [30]. The regular use of tape increases the risk of either allergic or irritant contact dermatitis, aggravated by the moisture and heat generated by exercise [30].

Dancers also commonly wear costumes for their performances. Neoprene is a widely used material for dance costumes and shoes due to its durability. However, contact with neoprene is reported to cause allergic contact dermatitis [31]. The accelerants used in neoprene production are known to be allergens [31]. Neoprene-associated contact dermatitis is rare but can potentially cause dancers much duress since company costumes are often shared and not made with individual specifications in mind [31]. Overall, dancers have ample profession-related contact with irritants and allergens that are well-reported to result in contact dermatitis. These substances are often unavoidable in the profession of dance and cannot be replaced with great ease. Treatments are characterized in earlier chapters (e.g. Chap. 4).

10.6 Hair Conditions in Dance

A dancer's hair can experience as much stress as their body. Dancers often need to tightly pull their hair out of their face, either to perform with their hair securely removed from their vision or due to costuming specifications (Fig. 10.2). This can increase the incidence of many hair-related disorders within the dance community. One such disorder within the dance community is that of traction alopecia. As a result of putting hair under tremendous tension, traction alopecia, specifically frontal traction alopecia, has been recorded at high levels in professional dancers (>20%) of one dance company [32].

Breakdancing explicitly puts dancers at risk for traction alopecia due to the "head-spin hole" formed from traction and scarring on the scalp [33]. Seborrheic dermatitis can be precipitated by sweating, hair spray, hair gel, and pomade, which are all common within the dance industry [34]. It is recommended that individuals with seborrheic dermatitis use the listed products minimally; however, this may not be feasible for dancers who have hair requirements for rehearsals and performances [34]. Prescription 2% ketoconazole shampoo has been shown to effectively clear seborrheic dermatitis and may also be used on a weekly basis as prophylaxis to prevent relapse in those prone to this condition [35].

10.7 Gymnastics Introduction

Gymnastics is a physically demanding sport requiring strength, flexibility, balance, and coordination. Athletes in this sport routinely perform complex maneuvers using various types of equipment such as mats, bars, beams, and vaults, often in close contact with one another and shared surfaces. Sweat creates a favorable

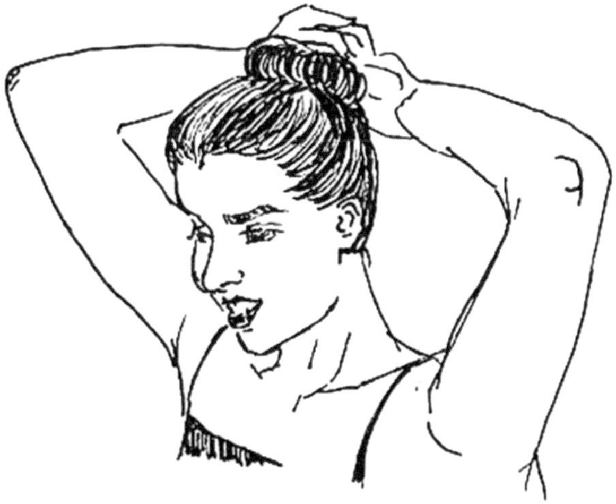

Fig. 10.2 Dancer Hair Style Producing Strain on Hair Follicles

environment for microbial proliferation on the skin that, when combined with physical stress, damages the body's exterior defenses, opening the door for pathogen invasion [36]. The nature of gymnastics, involving repetitive skin contact with equipment and communal spaces, increases the risk of developing various skin conditions. These shared surfaces are often reservoirs for microbes, creating an environment conducive to the transmission of infectious dermatological conditions.

The communal and often humid environment of gymnastic facilities, combined with frequent skin-to-surface contact, creates a high-risk setting for the transmission of infectious dermatological conditions. A study by Zhang et al. concluded that the surfaces of gymnastic equipment are potential dissemination pathways for highly dangerous pathogens as well as antimicrobial resistance, and the risks of indoor equipment are higher than outdoor equipment [36]. Pathogens, including fungi, bacteria, viruses, and parasites, thrive on surfaces such as mats and grips, allowing transmission through direct skin contact or indirectly through contaminated equipment. Locker rooms and gym equipment, characterized by moisture and high levels of skin contact, promote the growth and spread of these microorganisms. Gymnasts are particularly susceptible to infections due to the repetitive friction involved in training, which often leads to micro-abrasions that compromise the skin's natural protective barrier. Consequently, gymnasts face an elevated risk of developing both infectious and inflammatory skin conditions that can impact their health and performance. The correct diagnosis of sports dermatoses requires familiarity with their clinical characteristics. It is important for sports medicine healthcare providers to be able to recognize some of the common conditions so that appropriate treatment can be initiated and the spread of infectious agents reduced [37, 38].

10.8 Dermatophyte Infections in Gymnastics

Dermatophytosis of the feet, "athlete's foot," is the most common fungal disease [39]. Gymnasts are particularly at risk due to their frequent use of shared facilities and the sweaty conditions that result from repeated bare-footed practice. The repetitive friction from movements such as vaulting and tumbling can create micro-abrasions that compromise the skin's barrier, increasing susceptibility to infection. Athlete's foot typically presents with itching, scaling, and maceration between the toes and can spread to the soles and sides of the feet [39]. *Trichophyton rubrum* causes the majority of tinea pedis infections and typically produces a relatively non-inflammatory type of dermatophytosis characterized by dull erythema and pronounced silvery scaling that may involve the entire sole and sides of the foot, giving a moccasin or sandal appearance. *T. rubrum* thrives in warm, moist environments like gym locker rooms, communal showers, and mats. The infection spreads through direct contact with these contaminated surfaces. Hyperhidrosis is a predisposing factor for tinea infections. Because the disease often starts on the feet, the patient should be advised to dry the toes thoroughly after bathing. Dryness is essential to reduce the incidence of symptomatic reinfection [39]. Diagnostic tools and treatment options for tinea pedis and other dermatophyte infections are discussed in detail in earlier in this chapter.

To prevent infection or reoccurrence of disease, gymnasts should wear flip flops in communal showers, dry their feet thoroughly after practice, and use antifungal powders. The use of an antiseptic powder on the feet after bathing, particularly between the toes, is strongly advised for susceptible persons. Tolnaftate powder (Tinactin) or Zeasorb medicated powder is an excellent dusting powder for the feet. Plain talc, cornstarch, or rice powder may be dusted into socks and shoes to keep the feet dry. Periodic use of a topical antifungal agent may be required, especially when hot, sweat-inducing foot conditions cannot be avoided [39].

Onychomycosis or tinea unguium is a fungal infection of the nail bed, matrix, or plate that most often affects toenails rather than fingernails [40]. This condition frequently occurs in gymnasts due to repeated trauma to the nail beds during dismounts or landings. The constant pressure exerted on the feet increases the risk of fungal infections, particularly in toenails. Tinea unguium is more than a cosmetic problem, although people with this infection are often embarrassed about their nail disfigurement [40], and gymnasts perform their sport barefoot. Clinical presentation of onychomycosis, its clinical presentation, subtypes, diagnostic tools and treatment regimens is discussed in detail earlier in this chapter.

Tinea corporis includes all superficial dermatophyte infections of the skin other than those involving the scalp, beard, face, hands, feet, and groin. This form of ringworm is characterized by one or more circular, sharply circumscribed, slightly erythematous, dry, scaly, and sometimes hypopigmented patches. An advancing scaling edge is usually prominent. Progressive central clearing produces annular outlines that give them the name "ringworm." Although more common on the feet, lesions of tinea corporis can also form vesicles and bullae (bullous tinea) [39]. The fungus spreads by person-to-person contact or by touching contaminated surfaces [38], placing gymnasts at high risk. The fungus can live outside the host for an indeterminate time. Warm, moist environments increase the survival of this pathogen [38]. Gymnasts are particularly vulnerable to this infection due to the high levels of skin-to-surface contact with equipment and mats, which can harbor fungal spores for extended periods. Treatment of tinea is discussed earlier in this section.

Tinea versicolor, also called pityriasis versicolor, is caused by *Malassezia* spp. The major implicated species is *Malassezia globosa,* although *M. restricta, M. sympodialis, M. furfur, M. obtusa,* and *M. slooffiae* have also been implicated. Tinea versicolor typically presents as hypopigmented or hyperpigmented, coalescing scaly macules on the trunk and upper arms. Pink, atrophic, and trichrome variants exist and are more common during the summer months and favor oily areas of skin. In hypopigmented tinea versicolor, abnormally small and poorly melanized melanosomes are produced and are not transferred to keratinocytes properly. This becomes most conspicuous in dark-skinned people. This hypopigmentation may persist for weeks or months after the fungal disease is cured. UV exposure may speed the normalization of the pigment [39]. The lesions may be skin-colored, slightly hypopigmented, or slightly hyperpigmented, but all lesions on a person have a uniform color

[38]. This condition is more prevalent among athletes due to increased sweating, with gymnasts being particularly susceptible because of the humid conditions often found in gymnasiums. Treatment of tinea versicolor includes topical antifungals.

10.9 Parasitic Infectious Dermatoses

Gymnasts face an increased risk for developing pediculosis capitis (head lice) due to the regular physical contact during their practices and competitions, along with the sharing of items that touch the scalp. The close quarters in which gymnasts train, coupled with their communal activities, promote the spread of lice. Patients present with intense pruritus of the scalp and often have posterior cervical lymphadenopathy. Excoriations and small specks of louse dung are noted on the scalp, and secondary impetigo is common. Lice can often be detected, particularly during hair combing [39]. Topical pediculicides are considered first-line treatment for head lice. Manual removal of lice (known as wet combing) is used as an alternative treatment option to pediculicides, and oral therapy is used in the case of refractory conditions [41].

Sarcoptes scabiei, the itch mite, is an oval, ventrally flattened mite with dorsal spines. The fertilized female burrows into the stratum corneum and deposits her eggs. Scabies is characterized by pruritic papular lesions, excoriations, and burrows. Sites of predilection include the finger webs, wrists, axillae, areolae, umbilicus, lower abdomen, genitals, and buttocks. An imaginary circle intersecting the main sites of involvement—axillae, elbow flexures, wrists and hands, and crotch—has long been called the circle of Hebra. In adults, the scalp and face are usually spared [39]. Gymnasts are at risk due to close physical contact during training and competitions, and transmission is facilitated by the sharing of mats, grips, and other equipment. The mites prefer warm, moist environments, making gymnasiums an ideal setting for transmission. While treatment approach varies across different regions of the world, topical permethrin and oral ivermectin are the most common treatment options for scabies infection in the US [42].

10.10 Viral Infectious Dermatoses in Gymnastics

Infection with herpes simplex virus (HSV) is one of the most prevalent infections worldwide [38], with herpes simplex virus 1 (HSV-1) accounting for the majority of non-genital herpes infections [38]. HSV infections are particularly important because they are incurable and persist in the latent form for the lifetime of the individual [38]. Infection with HSV-1 is highly contagious to susceptible persons who come into direct contact with an infected individual with an active lesion [39]. It can also spread by respiratory droplets or exposure to mucocutaneous secretions of an asymptomatic person shedding virus without clinical disease. It has been shown that the majority of those with herpes simplex labialis (HSL) carry HSV-1 on their hands [37], placing gymnasts at a high risk of contraction. The virus can remain viable on skin, clothing, and plastic for brief periods of time, facilitating spread [37], through gyms, mats, and equipment. The incubation period is 2 to 20 days, with vesicles appearing within 3 to 5 days of direct skin-to-skin contact. They are usually located in the head but can occur in the extremities and trunk [38]. Lesions are frequently misdiagnosed as bacterial folliculitis [39]. The primary infection presents with burning, tingling, or stinging at the site. Vesicles rupture and, if confluent, can form erosive patches [38]. The virus is spread via skin-to-skin contact or from shared surfaces, especially when gymnasts have abrasions, which provide an entry point for the virus. Persons who present with active primary HSV infection may be treated with antiretroviral medications such as Acyclovir and Valacyclovir, which can shorten the length of HSV flare [43]. If patients begin antiretroviral therapy early after symptom onset (within 72 hours), treatment may lead to earlier healing of skin lesions, decreased pain and decreased duration of febrile symptoms if present [43].

Human papillomavirus (HPV) infections are a concern for athletes, as they can lead to warts on the hands and feet [44]. Gymnasts face the risk of developing warts from HPV due to direct skin contact with contaminated surfaces. Plantar warts, originating from HPV types 1, 2, 27, and 57, are particularly prevalent among gymnasts due to the friction experienced on the soles of their feet during landings while often performing barefoot. Infection with HPV is extremely common and most people will experience infection during their lifetime. Most HPV types cause specific types of warts and favor certain anatomic locations, such as plantar warts, common warts, and genital warts. HPVs 1, 2, 27, and 57 cause the vast majority of cutaneous (non-genital) warts. HPV-1 is associated with plantar warts in children younger than 12 years. HPV-2 is more common in hand warts. HPV-27 and HPV-57 are associated with common and plantar warts in adults (>21 years). External genital warts are caused by HPV-6/11 [39].

Verrucae vulgaris or "common warts", are skin lesions caused by human papilloma virus infections acquired from direct contact (e.g., person-to-person) or from the environment (e.g., showers, swimming pools). Wet or broken skin increases the chance of penetration [38]. Common warts are characterized by rough hyperkeratotic papules with papillomatous (cauliflower-like) projections and are typically located on the hands, favoring the fingers and palms [38, 39]. Lesions range in size from pinpoint to more than 1 cm, most averaging about 5 mm. They grow in size for weeks to months and usually present as elevated, rounded papules with a rough, grayish surface, which is so characteristic that it has given us the word "verrucous" [39]. In some cases, a single wart (mother wart) appears and grows slowly for a long time, and then suddenly many new warts erupt. On the surface of the wart, tiny black dots may be visible, representing thrombosed, dilated capillaries [38, 39]. Treatment options for verruca vulgaris include topical salicylic acid with liquid nitrogen cryotherapy [45]. Of note, patients should be educated on the risk for minor pain and possible hypopigmentation associated with cryotherapy treatment [45].

Human papillomaviruses 1, 2, 27, and 57 cause plantar warts. These warts generally appear at pressure points on the ball of the foot, especially over the mid-metatarsal area, but may be anywhere on the sole. Frequently, several lesions develop on one foot. Sometimes they are grouped, or several contiguous warts fuse so that they appear as one "mosaic" wart. The soft, pulpy cores are surrounded by a firm, horny ring. Plantar warts may be confused with corns or calluses, but warts have a soft, central core and black or bleeding points from the superficial capillaries when pared down; features that calluses lack [39].

Molluscum contagiosum virus (MCV), is a chronic, localized skin infection caused by the poxvirus that present as 2–5-millimeter, firm, skin colored, dome-shaped papules that can occur anywhere on the skin [46]. The lesions are often pruritic with a central dell or umbilication [38]. MCV is most easily transmitted by direct skin-to-skin contact, especially if the skin is wet [39]. Gymnasts face risk from the virus's transmission via skin-to-skin contact and contaminated surfaces. MCV is often a self-limited disease and there is debate over whether treatment intervention is warranted [46]. When treatment is preferred, first-line treatment options First line treatment options include liquid nitrogen cryotherapy, curettage, cantharidin, or podophyllotoxin [46].

10.11 Bacterial Infectious Diseases in Gymnastics

Impetigo is a very common and highly contagious bacterial infection that typically caused by either group A streptococcus (GAS) or *S. aureus* [37]. Skin infections can be either primary, with bacteria infecting normal skin, or secondary, with infection complicating minor skin trauma such as abrasions [37, 38]. Bacteria favor warm, moist conditions for growth and are spread by close contact with infected individuals, so this also makes gymnasts and other athletes highly susceptible to infection [37]. Impetigo presents with papules and pustules coalescing into an erythematous plaque with an overlying honey-colored crust, most commonly found on the face or extremities. The palms and soles are spared. A bullous variant with flaccid vesicles that quickly rupture may also be seen, often favoring the torso [38]. This condition is especially contagious among gymnasts, who may contract it through shared equipment or direct contact with infected teammates. The humid and sweaty environments in gym facilities further enhance bacterial proliferation.

Erysipelas is a serious skin infection caused by acute β-hemolytic group A streptococcal infection affecting the superficial dermal lymphatics. Gymnasts are particularly susceptible to erysipelas due to injuries that permit bacterial entry. Occasional cases caused by streptococci of group C or G are reported in adults. It is characterized by local redness, heat, swelling, and a highly characteristic raised, indurated border [38, 39]. The onset is often preceded by prodromal symptoms of malaise for several hours, which may be accompanied by a severe constitutional reaction with chills, high fever, headache, vomiting, and joint pains. The skin lesions may vary from transient hyperemia followed by slight desquamation to intense inflammation with vesicles or bullae. The eruption begins at any one point as an erythematous patch and spreads by peripheral extension. In the early stages, affected skin is bright red, hot to the touch, branny, and swollen. A distinctive feature of the inflammation is the advancing edge of the patch. This is raised and sharply demarcated and feels like a wall to the palpating finger. In some cases, vesicles or bullae that contain seropurulent fluid occur and may result in local gangrene [39]. Most cases of erysipelas can be managed with oral antibiotics in the outpatient setting; however, severe cases or immunocompromised status may require inpatient treatment with IV antibiotics and close monitorization. Antibiotic regimen should be targeted against β-hemolytic streptococcus, methicillin-sensitive staphylococcus aureus (MSSA) and in severe cases methicillin-resistant staphylococcus aureus (MRSA).

Gymnasts are exposed to a wide variety of materials and chemicals present in the gym that have the potential to cause skin irritation. Because gymnastics is a sport with a high amount of exposed skin contact, it can be expected that widespread skin problems may occur. One condition caused by gymnastics exposure is contact dermatitis, an inflammatory reaction that occurs when the athlete is in contact with a substance that damages the outer layer of the skin. The two variations of this condition are irritant contact dermatitis and allergic contact dermatitis. Irritant contact dermatitis is related to the quantity and concentration of the exposure to a nonspecific irritant [47]. For example, the friction generated when a gymnast's leg rubs against the balance beam or the chemical damage from using large amounts of adhesive tape used on the gymnast's joints to protect against injuries. Other irritants could include the spandex of the tight leotards, the carpets of the mats, and the fabric of the trampolines. On the other hand, allergic contact dermatitis is a type IV hypersensitivity (delayed) reaction in which an allergen triggers helper T-cells to release cytokines that activate macrophages to phagocytose the allergen. Allergic contact dermatitis in gymnastics may be due to the chalk used for better grip, sprays and gels used to keep hair out of the face, and latex in the mats.

Symptoms caused by contact dermatitis may range in color, severity, timing of development, and location. It could be an itchy rash appearing within hours or bumps and blisters appearing weeks later. It is worth noting that the reaction may appear leathery on darker skin colors while appearing dry, scaly on lighter skin colors [48]. In order to minimize exposure to the irritants or allergens, gymnasts may seek out alternative protections such as wearing tights to protect their legs when possible. A physician may recommend moisturizers to protect the dry skin and potentially a topical corticosteroid to reduce inflammation [48].

10.12 Hair Conditions in Gymnastics

Traction alopecia is a form of hair loss that may occur in people who frequently wear tight hairstyles [49]. This condition is especially difficult to avoid in gymnastics because there are policies regarding the hair of the gymnasts. For example, one rule states that hair must be "secured away from the face so as to not obscure her vision of the apparatus" [50]. Because this is policy, gymnasts can be penalized for hair malfunctions. For this reason, gymnasts tend to take advantage of reliable tight braids and buns that can keep the hair secure in place during flips and jumps. In order to avoid this type of hair loss, it is recommended to make the braids closest to the hairlines looser as to decrease tension on the strands [49].

Seborrheic dermatitis is a scaly rash that occurs in oily areas of the skin, primarily the scalp and face. It is primarily identified as white/yellow flakes and crusts attached to the scalp and hair. The hair styles and products used in gymnastics that may lead to weakened epidermal barrier integrity. This barrier is essential for guarding lower layers of skin from microorganisms and harmful agents. If damaged, a patient may be more susceptible to Seborrheic dermatitis [51]. Treatment for this condition may include topical antifungals and anti-inflammatory medications as well as maintaining scalp help [51]. Telogen effluvium is a condition in which hair in the resting (telogen) phase is excessively shed due to metabolic stress, hormones, or medications [52]. The constant high stress involved in gymnastics can cause or contribute to the excessive hair loss seen in telogen effluvium. The best treatment in the case of sports, however, is reducing the stressor.

10.13 General Skin Reactions in Gymnastics

Although there is limited research in gymnasts, acne mechanica is a flare-up of acne in areas of the body with high skin friction. Symptoms can start as rough bumps and eventually transform into pimples or acne cysts [53]. This condition has the potential to affect almost all sports due to close contact with heavy equipment, padding and helmets, and fast movements accompanied by heat. Acne mechanica is present in gymnastics due to friction between the tight leotards and the skin, as well as in between the thighs when running for floor and vault routines. Treatment may include face washing with benzoyl peroxide or salicylic acid and/or prescribed antibiotics [54].

Miliaria, sometimes referred to as “heat rash”, is a condition that occurs when the sweat glands become blocked with debris and bacteria causing the sweat to divert flow to the dermis and epidermis [55]. The three different types of Miliaria are differentiated by the depth of the ductal occlusion: crystalline in the stratum corneum, rubra in the sub corneal layers of the epidermis, and profunda in the dermal-epidermal junction [55]. Breathable clothing may be recommended for patients experiencing Miliaria, however, this may not be achievable in many sports. Most gymnastic leotards are tight-fitting and made of spandex and nylon prioritizing durability and stretch over breathability. This puts gymnasts at higher risk of Miliaria. Although most cases of Miliaria resolve on their own, some severe cases may cause anhidrosis, permanently damaging thermal regulation. If a gymnast notices Miliaria, he or she should stay in air conditioning, avoid creams which block sweat glands, and stay hydrated [55].

Hyperhidrosis is a condition characterized by excessive sweating primarily in the palms, hands, underarms, and face. Physicians use a starch-iodine test or a vapometer to measure the amount of sweat. Drying topical creams are the first line of defense, then followed by anticholinergics. Primary hyperhidrosis is inherited while secondary hyperhidrosis is caused by a different concurrent disease process, including but not limited to: gout, diabetes, menopause, neurological syndromes, etc. [56]. Excessive sweating can become a surprisingly large problem in sports, especially performance/audience-based activities. Sweating in the palms and hands can worsen a gymnast's grip, making certain activities more challenging and dangerous. Sweating more than others, especially in noticeable areas such as the face, can make a gymnast feel embarrassed and add extra stress to the sport.

Cholinergic urticaria is a skin condition consisting of hives produced as an immune reaction to increased body temperature and sweating. This differs from "heat rash" due to the presence of elevated skin bumps. The etiology of this condition is not yet determined, however, there are studies hypothesizing a relation to histamine and an allergy to sweat [57]. Fortunately for gymnasts, their uniforms do not trap in too much heat and their gymnasium facilities are often air conditioned. Nevertheless, any athlete involved in high exertion sports may experience cholinergic urticaria after sweating. Provocation tests are done by increasing the patient's body temperature (either via exercise or a heated bath) in order to rule out other causes of hives [57]. Once the diagnosis is confirmed, the physician may treat the patient with various anti-allergic medications.

10.14 Worsening of Existing Dermatological Conditions in Gymnasts

The amount of skin an athlete has exposed to the world is greatly dependent on the sport he or she chooses. Hockey and football players may never think about an audience judging their skin, while gymnasts, ballerinas, and swimmers may have an added level of anxiety associated with sport-associated skin conditions. Six-time Olympic medalist and gymnast Suni Lee has commented in various news sources explaining the difficulty of performing her sport while facing eczema flare-ups. Lee said while on a dermatology panel, "Being on a competition floor, having so many eyes on you and just trying not to be worried about if people are looking at my skin, or itching myself, because the more that I itch myself, the flakier it's going to get, the drier it's going to get" [58]. It can be debilitating to incur a distracting skin condition while simultaneously focusing on a sport. Furthermore, removing or reducing the stressor is oftentimes not an available option when policies, such as the type of uniform or equipment materials, are strict. For this reason, sport-related skin conditions should not be overlooked, and more creative solutions must be researched for cures. These conditions are summarized in Table 10.1.

Calluses belong to the hyperkeratosis group of skin conditions, which are described as thickened regions of increased keratin in the outermost layer of the skin. These skin formations are commonly caused by long term physical or

Table 10.1 Worsening of existing dermatological conditions in gymnasts

Disease/ condition	Symptoms and physical exam findings	Treatment recommendations
Calluses	Thickened regions of skin in palms of hands	Topical corticosteroids
Abrasion	Superficial damage to epithelium	Clean and protect wound
Laceration	Cuts that penetrate through the superficial layers of the skin	Anesthetizing, cleaning, and suturing the wound.
Friction burns	1st degree burns only affecting the outer layers of skin	Reduce friction and wear protective gear/clothing
Blisters	Fluid-filled vesicles and bullae	Sterile drainage in severe presentations
Piezogenic papules	Painless, skin-colored papules that come and go with application of pressure	Cushioned shoes
Tache/talon noir	Black discolorations	Cushioned shoes
Ecchymosis (bruise)	Various discolorations, occasionally tender or swollen	Rest, ice, and elevation

chemical injury, however they can also be related to nutritional deficits or drug side-effects [59]. For gymnasts, calluses are most prevalent in the palms of the hands due to high friction with the bars. The calluses should be tough enough to protect the skin in times of frequent rubbing, but smooth enough to slide around the bar with ease. It is similar to the fingertips of a guitarist or violinist: you want the calluses to provide strength to the skin region, but not alter the sound of the music. Topical management of the calluses with corticosteroids may be recommended to avoid scarring [59].

An abrasion is superficial damage to the epithelium that can be caused by a variety of injuries. Abrasions are primarily accidental, often occurring from falling or bumping into an object, and vary in severity. Linear abrasions, or scratches, can be due to something sharp such as a papercut. A grazed abrasion may be due to skin dragging across a surface, such as a skid mark on a knee after tripping. A patterned abrasion has a mark on the skin that matches the object that caused injury, such as the nail markings from a cat scratch [60, 61]. Most abrasions heal on their own without any scarring or medical treatment necessary. However, it is important to clean and protect the wound as it is at higher risk of infection while lacking a protective epithelial barrier [61]. Gymnasts may experience abrasions on their arms and elbows when rubbing against carpeted surfaces, on their hands when changing positions on bars or rings, or simply from accidentally bumping into equipment in the gymnasium. Abrasions are minor injuries common in many sports and should not be seen as a deterrent to exercise.

Unlike abrasions, lacerations are cuts that penetrate deeper through the superficial layers of skin. They can be very serious injuries needing immediate medical treatment. Treatment includes anesthetizing, cleaning, and suturing the wound in order to reduce risk of infection and scar formation. If that patient is not up to date on his or her tetanus vaccine, it is important to administer immunoglobulin treatment and a vaccine [62]. Lacerations are much less common than abrasions and are less uncommon in gymnastics due to their correlation with blunt trauma. Gymnasts may experience a laceration if they were to land a jump or a flip on a sharp object or hit a sharp piece of equipment.

Friction burns are similar to abrasions, but with the added component of heat. They are commonly minor injuries that cause first degree burns only affecting the outer layers of skin. However, friction burns can become more severe in the cases of motorcycle vehicle accidents or exercise treadmill falls. The greater the velocity over the object and the rougher the surface, the worse the friction burn. Primary preventative measures include covering the skin and wearing protective gear including knee or elbow pads [63]. Gymnasts may find it especially helpful to wear these pads when learning new skills or performing floor routines.

Blisters are fluid-filled vesicles and bullae that can appear anywhere on the body due to repetitive friction causing a separation between the epidermal and dermal layers of skin. Blisters are commonly formed on the feet and hands where there is frequent rubbing and friction motion. They can feel highly sensitive with a sensation of "burning or stinging" [64]. Minor blisters go away on their own, however, severe blisters may need to be treated with sterile drainage and monitoring. Even minor blisters can be quite irritating and distracting. It may make a gymnast favor one hand or foot over the other, or even lead them to skipping practice altogether.

Piezogenic papules are small herniations of adipose tissue through the dermis of the skin. They appear as painless, skin-colored papules that come and go with application of pressure. There have yet to be direct links to genetics or syndromes to explain why this condition occurs in some more than others. In the case of gymnasts, it would make sense that excessive pressure due to the force of landing could cause small tears in which adipose tissue can seep through [65]. Gymnasts put this force in their wrists and feet, putting them at increased risk for piezogenic papules in these areas.

Tache noir (black palm) and Talon noir (black heel) are asymptomatic dermatological conditions in the hands and feet that occur due to repetitive microtrauma or shear force. The stress on these body parts causes damage to the papillary blood vessels leading to a black discoloration of the skin [66]. Both tache noir and talon noir can occur in gymnasts due to the shear landing force they incur from propelling off vaults, swinging between uneven bars, flipping off of hard balance beams, etc. Fortunately, these black spots do not affect sports performance and can resolve on their own within weeks. Gymnasts should wear cushioned shoes when outside of the gym to avoid extra stress on the heels.

Ecchymosis, more commonly known as a bruise, is a discoloration caused by leaking blood vessels without any breakage of the skin barrier. The pooling of blood can appear in a variety of colors from yellow to purple to black. The bruise can be tender to touch and can also swell to a raised bump. Platelets in the blood are responsible for stopping the leakage of the vessel, so patients with platelet disorders or patients on blood thinners may be more prone to blood leakage and bruises upon injury [67]. Athletes of all kinds experience ecchymoses, especially those in contact sports. Gymnasts may incur ecchymoses upon hitting a hard object such as the beam or floor. Bruises will heal on their own over several weeks, but rest, ice and elevation of the injured area may allow for a faster recovery. If a patient bruises easily or experiences frequent bruising without significant inciting trauma, patient should receive further evaluation for possible platelet disorder or other hematological abnormalities [67].

References

1. Mathpal Y. Prehistoric painting of Bhimbetka. Abhinav Publications; 1984.
2. WECA UK Lion Dance – History. 2024.
3. Routhier S. Top 20 most physically demanding jobs in America. 2022.
4. Shaw JW, Mattiussi AM, Brown DD, Williams S, Springham M, Pedlar CR, et al. Rehearsal and performance volume in professional ballet: a five-season cohort study. J Dance Med Sci. 2023;27(1):3–12.
5. Allen N, Nevill A, Brooks J, Koutedakis Y, Wyon M. Ballet injuries: injury incidence and severity over 1 year. J Orthop Sports Phys Ther. 2012;42(9):781–A1.
6. Cappelle L. Bringing consent to ballet, one intimacy workshop at a time. The New York Times. 2022 2022/04/13.
7. Stretanski MF. Classical Ballet. Am J Phys Med Rehabil. 2002;81(5):392–3.
8. Saal RC, Edwards JF, Whitlock SM, Byrd RC. Dermatologic conditions in dancers: a state-wide survey. Arch Dermatol Res. 2023;316(1):54.
9. Mikkelsen P, Jarvis D, Kulig K. Heeled shoes increase knee work demand during repeated hopping in dancers. Med Probl Perform Art. 2018;33(4):243–50.
10. Nigam PK, Syed HA, Saleh D. Tinea Pedis. In: StatPearls. Treasure Island (FL): StatPearls Publishing Copyright © 2024, StatPearls Publishing LLC; 2024.
11. Goldstein A, Goldstein B. Dermatophyte (tinea) infections. 2024 October 25th, 2024. In: UpToDate [Internet]. Waltham, MA: UpToDate, Inc. Available from: https://www.uptodate.com/contents/dermatophyte-tinea-infections.
12. Goldstein A, Bhatia N. Onychomycosis: epidemiology, clinical features and diagnosis. 2023 October 25th, 2024. In: UpToDate [Internet]. Waltham, MA: UpToDate, Inc. Available from: https://www.uptodate.com/contents/onychomycosis-epidemiology-clinical-features-and-diagnosis?search=onychomycosis&source=search_result&selectedTitle=2%7E55&usage_type=default&display_rank=2#H1952057527.
13. Hay RJ, Baran R. Onychomycosis: a proposed revision of the clinical classification. J Am Acad Dermatol. 2011;65(6):1219–27.
14. Goldstein A, Bhatia N. Onychomycosis: management. 2022 October 26th, 2024. In: UpToDate [Internet]. Waltham, MA: UpToDate Inc. Available from: https://www.uptodate.com/contents/onychomycosis-management?search=onychomycosis%20treatment&source=search_result&selectedTitle=1%7E55&usage_type=default&display_rank=1#H782570158.
15. Buckner BJ. Comprehensive evaluation of the ballet pointe shoe according on professional ballet dancers [M.S.]. United States – North Carolina: North Carolina State University; 2019.
16. Fastle RK, Bothner J. Subungual Hematoma 2023 [updated 2023/08/21. Available from: https://www.uptodate.com/contents/subungual-hematoma?search=subungual%20hematoma&source=search_result&selectedTitle=1%7E25&usage_type=default&display_rank=1#H3424400.
17. Zahn R, Schmidt M, Wallner A, Fischer T, Ohlendorf D, Wanke EM. Work-related dermatoses of the feet in professional dancers: a pilot study. Med Probl Perform Art. 2023;38(1):16–22.
18. Freeman DB. Corns and calluses resulting from mechanical hyperkeratosis. Am Fam Physician. 2002;65(11):2277–80.

19. Goldstein AO. Overview of benign lesions of the skin 2024 [updated 2024/04/12. Available from: https://www.uptodate.com/contents/overview-of-benign-lesions-of-the-skin?search=corns%20skin%20callus%20treatment&source=search_result&selectedTitle=1%7E129&usage_type=default&display_rank=1#H1101420580.
20. Marks A. 7 Habits Your Podiatrist Wishes You Would Quit 2018 [updated 2018/02/22. Available from: https://www.dancemagazine.com/foot-care-mistakes/#gsc.tab=0.
21. Spelman D, Baddour LM. Acute cellulitis and erysipelas in adults: treatment 2023 [updated 2023/12/15. Available from: https://www.uptodate.com/contents/acute-cellulitis-and-erysipelas-in-adults-treatment?search=erysipelas%20treatment%20adult&source=search_result&selectedTitle=1%7E37&usage_type=default&display_rank=1#H924541965.
22. Jackson JD, Rosen T, Ofori AO. Infectious folliculitis 2023 [updated 2023/01/04. Available from: https://www.uptodate.com/contents/infectious-folliculitis?search=folliculitis&source=search_result&selectedTitle=1%7E112&usage_type=default&display_rank=1#H604478868.
23. Ngan V, Coulson I. Rosin and colophony contact allergy: dermnetnz.org; 2002 [updated 2002. Available from: https://dermnetnz.org/topics/rosin-allergy.
24. Downs AMR, Sansom JE. Colophony allergy: a review. Contact Derm. 1999;41(6):305–10.
25. Chien JA. Ballet myth busters: San Francisco Ballet; 2021 [Available from: https://www.sfballet.org/discover/backstage/ballet-myth-busters-5/.
26. Fisher AA, Rietschel RL, Fowler JF. Fisher's contact dermatitis. Hamilton: Bc Decker Inc; 2008.
27. Fathi R, Dugdale DC, Conaway B. Contact dermatitis information: Mount Sinai Health System; 2023 [updated 2023. Available from: https://www.mountsinai.org/health-library/diseases-conditions/contact-dermatitis.
28. Zirwas MJ. Contact dermatitis to cosmetics. Clin Rev Allergy Immunol. 2018;56(1):119–28.
29. Kim YJ, Chung JK. Bilateral eyelid contact dermatitis and toxic conjunctivitis due to acrylate-containing glue. Ann Dermatol. 2014;26(4):543–4.
30. Hamnerius N, Dahlin J, Bruze M, Nilsson K, Sukakul T, Svedman C. Colophonium-related allergic contact dermatitis caused by medical adhesive tape used to prevent skin lesions in soldiers. Acta Derm Venereol. 2023;103:adv18428.
31. Stern EB, Callinan N, Hank M, Lewis EJ, Schousboe JT, Ytterberg SR. Neoprene splinting: dermatological issues. Am J Occup Ther. 1998;52(7):573–8.
32. Wanke EM, Zimmermann OL, Schmidt M, Ohlendorf D, Wallner A, Fischer T. Skin health in dance focusing on professional dance and Latin American formation dance during periods of different training loads. Appl Sci. 2022;12(22):11485.
33. Hall M, Lim H, Kim S, Fulda KG, Surve SA. A cross-sectional study comparing traumatic alopecia among b-boys and b-girls to other dance styles and its impact on dance performance and health. J Dance Med Sci. 2023;27:13–9.
34. Ludmann P. Seborrheic dermatitis: tips for managing: www.aad.org; 2022 [Available from: https://www.aad.org/public/diseases/a-z/seborrheic-dermatitis-self-care.
35. Peter RU, Richarz-Barthauer U. Successful treatment and prophylaxis of scalp seborrhoeic dermatitis and dandruff with 2% ketoconazole shampoo: results of a multicentre, double-blind, placebo-controlled trial. Br J Dermatol. 1995;132(3):441–5.
36. Zhang M, Ma Y, Xu H, Wang M, Li L. Surfaces of gymnastic equipment as reservoirs of microbial pathogens with potential for transmission of bacterial infection and antimicrobial resistance. Front Microbiol. 2023;14:1182594.
37. Pecci M, Comeau D, Chawla V. Skin conditions in the athlete. Am J Sports Med. 2009;37(2):406–18.
38. Pujalte GGA, Costa LMC, Clapp AD, Presutti RJ, Sluzevich JC. More than skin deep: dermatologic conditions in athletes. Sports Health. 2023;15(1):74–85.
39. James WD, Treat JR, Rosenbach MA, Neuhaus IM. Andrews' Diseases of the skin. Elsevier; 2020.
40. Rodgers P, Bassler M. Treating onychomycosis. Am Fam Physician. 2001;63(4):663–72.

41. Goldstein AO, Goldstein BG. Pediculosis capitis 2024 [Available from: https://www.uptodate.com/contents/pediculosis-capitis?search=head%20lice&source=search_result&selectedTitle=1%7E23&usage_type=default&display_rank=1#H88337.
42. Goldstein BG, Goldstein AO. Scabies: management 2022 [updated 2022/10/31. Available from: https://www.uptodate.com/contents/scabies-management?search=scabies%20treatment&source=search_result&selectedTitle=1%7E88&usage_type=default&display_rank=1#H3053413688.
43. Wald A, Johnston C. Treatment and prevention of herpes simplex virus type 1 in immunocompetent adolescents and adults 2024 [updated 2024/07/15. Available from: https://www.uptodate.com/contents/treatment-and-prevention-of-herpes-simplex-virus-type-1-in-immunocompetent-adolescents-and-adults?search=hsv%201%20treatment&source=search_result&selectedTitle=1%7E123&usage_type=default&display_rank=1#H16.
44. Adams BB. Dermatologic disorders of the athlete. Sports Med. 2002;32(5):309–21.
45. Goldstein BG, Goldstein AO, Morris-Jones R. Cutaneous warts (common, plantar, and flat warts) 2023 [updated 2023/07/27. Available from: https://www.uptodate.com/contents/cutaneous-warts-common-plantar-and-flat-warts?search=verruca%20vulgaris%20treatment&source=search_result&selectedTitle=1%7E62&usage_type=default&display_rank=1#H23.
46. Isaacs SN. Molluscum contagiosum 2024 [updated 2024/01/10. Available from: https://www.uptodate.com/contents/molluscum-contagiosum?search=molluscum%20contagiosum&source=search_result&selectedTitle=1%7E62&usage_type=default&display_rank=1#H2178689971.
47. Litchman G, Nair PA, Atwater AR, et al. Contact dermatitis. Updated 2023 Sep 4 ed. Treasure Island (FL): StatPearls Publishing; 2024.
48. Contact Dermatitis: National Health Service; 2024 [Available from: https://www.nhs.uk/conditions/contact-dermatitis/.
49. Ludmann P, Schleehauf B. Hairstyles and Hair Loss 2024 [updated 2024/11/06. Available from: https://www.aad.org/public/diseases/hair-loss/causes/hairstyles.
50. USA gymnastics women's program rules and policies 2022–2023. USA Gymnastics; 2022.
51. Borda LJ, Wikramanayake TC. Seborrheic dermatitis and dandruff: a comprehensive review. J Clin Investig Dermatol. 2015;3(2)
52. Hughes EC, Syed HA, Saleh D. Telogen Effluvium. Updated 2024 May 1 ed. Treasure Island (FL): StatPearls Publishing; 2024.
53. Sports Equipment and Acne: American Academy of Dermatology Association; 2024 [Available from: https://www.aad.org/public/diseases/acne/causes/sports-equipment.
54. Decker A, Graber EM. Over-the-counter acne treatments: a review. J Clin Aesthet Dermatol. 2012;5(5):32–40.
55. Guerra KC, Toncar A, Krishnamurthy K. Miliaria. Updated 2024 Sep 1 ed. Treasure Island (FL): StatPearls Publishing; 2024.
56. Excessive Sweating: Johns Hopkins Medicine; 2024 [Available from: https://www.hopkinsmedicine.org/health/conditions-and-diseases/excessive-sweating#:~:text=What%20is%20hyperhidrosis%3F,order%20to%20avoid%20touching%20others.
57. Fukunaga A, Oda Y, Imamura S, Mizuno M, Fukumoto T, Washio K. Cholinergic Urticaria: subtype classification and clinical approach. Am J Clin Dermatol. 2023;24(1):41–54.
58. Lee S. Olympian Suni Lee Speaks on AD Panel. In: Block J, Golant A, Genovese M, editors. National Eczema Association. DermWire News, Practical Dermatology: Practical Dermatology; 2024.
59. Farci F, Mahabal GD. Hyperkeratosis. Updated 2023 Sep 4 ed. Treasure Island (FL): StatPearls Publishing; 2024.
60. Clinic C. Abrasion. Cleveland Clinic; 2024 [Available from: https://my.clevelandclinic.org/health/diseases/25079-abrasion.
61. Shrestha R, Krishan K, Ishaq H, et al. Abrasion. Updated 2023 Aug 17 ed. Treasure Island (FL): StatPearls Publishing; 2024.

62. Newman RK, Mahdy H. Laceration. Updated 2022 Oct 8 ed. Treasure Island (FL): StatPearls Publishing; 2024.
63. Agrawal A, Raibagkar SC, Vora HJ. Friction burns: epidemiology and prevention. Ann Burns Fire Disasters. 2008;21(1):3–6.
64. Bishop J. Blister Critical Care Nursing Clinics of North America 2004 [Available from: https://www.sciencedirect.com/topics/medicine-and-dentistry/blister.
65. Brown F, Cook C. Piezogenic Pedal Papule. Updated 2023 Aug 16 ed. Treasure Island (FL): StatPearls Publishing; 2024.
66. Choudhury S, Mandal A. Talon noir: a case report and literature review. Cureus. 2023;15(3):e35905.
67. Kraut EH, Fenton J. Easy Bruising 2024 [updated 2024/04/30. Available from: https://www.uptodate.com/contents/easy-bruising#H428230970.

Chapter 11
Martial Arts, Wrestling, and Weightlifting Sports

Ricardo Cooke, Hannah Metheny, Rahul Aggarwal, Ryan Scheinkman, Alexia Vignau, Rachel Cohen, Philippe Jean-Pierre, and Keyvan Nouri

11.1 Introduction

Olympic weightlifting, powerlifting, CrossFit, strongman competitions, and bodybuilding are all fundamentally grounded in weightlifting [1–5]. In ancient Greece, Olympic weightlifting was initially practiced by lifting heavy stones and other weights to demonstrate strength. In 1896, this lifting form was formalized into Olympic weightlifting and became part of the first modern Olympic games [6]. Powerlifting was born in the United States through twentieth-century local, national, and international strength competitions overseen by the Amateur Athletic Union (AAU). Powerlifting became formalized with the establishment of the International Powerlifting Federation (IPF) in 1972 [7]. The origins of CrossFit can be traced to Greg Glassman's work in developing fitness regimens for law enforcement and military personnel in the 1990s. It was officially founded in 2000 by Glassman, and the CrossFit Games have been held annually since 2007 [4]. Strongman competitions developed from feats of strength performed by ancient and modern cultures and were formalized by the first strongman competition, the 1977 World Strongest Man contest [8]. Eugen Sandow is considered the "father of bodybuilding," as he popularized the art of physique development and organized the first physique competition in 1901. Joe Weider founded the Mr. Olympia event in 1946 [9, 10].

Ricardo Cooke and Hannah Metheny contributed equally with all other contributors.

R. Cooke · H. Metheny · R. Aggarwal · R. Scheinkman (✉) · A. Vignau · R. Cohen
P. Jean-Pierre · K. Nouri
Dr. Phillip Frost Department of Dermatology and Cutaneous Surgery, University of Miami, Miami, FL, USA
e-mail: rbc87@med.miami.edu; hannah.metheny@med.miami.edu; rxa1273@med.miami.edu; scheinkman@med.miami.edu; axv200@med.miami.edu; rachelcohen@med.miami.edu; philanator@med.miami.edu; knouri@med.miami.edu

K. Nouri (ed.), *Sport-Related Skin Conditions*,
https://doi.org/10.1007/978-3-031-90444-8_11

Each sport necessitates a unique skill set. Olympic lifting requires explosive power and precise technique to perform the snatch and clean and jerk lifts [1]. On the other hand, powerlifting demands a showcase of maximal strength to excel at the deadlift, bench press, and squat lifts [2]. CrossFit combines high-intensity conditioning with gymnastics and weightlifting movements [3]. Strongman events force athletes to complete feats of strength, such as vehicle pulls and atlas stone lifts, to test their raw power [4]. Lastly, athletes develop maximal muscle mass through intense training and strict diet regimes to develop the physiques emphasized in bodybuilding [5]. Dermatological conditions among weightlifting athletes arise from exposure to unique equipment, environmental factors, and training demands. Weightlifters face increased risks of friction-induced lesions from both the explosive power required for the sport and from direct contact with equipment like metal barbells, bumper plates, and wooden lifting platforms. For example, weightlifting athletes may develop acne mechanica from direct contact with plastic on weightlifting benches or wearing a weightlifting belt [11]. These athletes are also at an increased risk for pressure-related conditions. The intense grip required to hold a heavy load on the weightlifting bar can lead to the development of calluses and corns on the hands [12].

CrossFit is a sport of a high intensity and diverse nature that can lead to a greater variety of skin issues, including acne mechanica from equipment like pull-up bars, gymnastic grips, and plyo boxes. These athletes are also at a higher risk of heat and sweat-related conditions like intertrigo due to the combination of weightlifting, gymnastics, and high-intensity conditioning performed in crowded gym environments [4]. Strongman athletes may endure trauma from demonstrations of strength involving implements like atlas stones, car deadlifts, and farmer's walk implements and are therefore at increased risk for contusions, abrasions, and athlete's nodules. Training outdoors exposes these athletes to environmental risk factors as well [3]. Finally, intense training and strict dietary regimes required of bodybuilders can predispose them to friction-based skin problems from equipment like dumbbells, resistance bands, and exercise machines. They may be highly susceptible to infectious disease in a shared gym environment, training in minimal clothing [5]. A greater understanding of these disorders contributes to optimizing athlete health and performance through preventative strategies and specialized management. For example, the American Academy of Dermatology offers recommendations to prevent skin conditions in athletes and skin infections at the gym rooted in hygiene [13, 14].

Wrestling and martial arts are ancient forms of combat sports that have evolved into many diverse competitive disciplines practiced worldwide. These sports combine elements of physical conditioning, technical skills, and strategic thinking. Wrestling and martial arts can present unique dermatologic challenges due to their intensive physical contact nature [15]. Around 8.5% of all adverse events in wrestling are attributed to skin infections [16]. Wrestling, one of humanity's oldest forms of organized sport, dates back to prehistoric times and remains prominent in amateur and professional settings. Modern wrestling encompasses several distinct styles, including freestyle, Greco-Roman, and collegiate wrestling, each with specific rules governing permitted techniques and contact areas [17]. Martial arts have similarly diverse origins and manifestations. Eastern traditions such as karate, originating from Okinawa, Japan, emphasize striking techniques using hands and feet. Taekwondo, developed in Korea, focuses predominantly on kicking techniques and rapid footwork [18]. Brazilian Jiu-Jitsu emphasizes ground fighting and submission techniques, while Mixed Martial Arts (MMA) combines elements from various combat disciplines into a comprehensive fighting system [19].

The nature of martial arts creates multiple pathways for dermatologic conditions to develop. First, direct physical contact in these sports can cause many pathologies and symptoms. Striking actions can generate trauma, which results in contusions, abrasions, and lacerations. Grappling techniques involve prolonged skin-skin contact, which facilitates the transmission of bacterial and fungal infections. Joint Locks and Submissions can cause friction burns and pressure-related skin injuries [20]. There are also environmental factors surrounding wrestling and martial arts that harbor pathogenic organisms and can serve as vectors for disease transmission. This includes shared protective gear (headgear, gloves, shin guards), practice mats, and other athletic surfaces. Facilities such as humid locker room environments, shared shower facilities, and equipment storage areas are conducive to fungal growth [21].

Furthermore, combat sports such as wrestling and martial arts present unique risks for transmission of bodily fluids through cuts and abrasions, saliva contact during close combat, and sweat exchange during extended contact periods [22]. These various exposure routes create an environment conducive to the development and transmission of multiple dermatologic conditions, ranging from infectious diseases to traumatic injuries. Understanding these risk factors is crucial for improved treatment of combat sports athletes and for developing effective preventive strategies [23].

11.2 Dermatophytic Conditions

Tinea (colloquially referred to as ringworm) refers to an infection caused by fungi (dermatophytes) that infect skin, hair, and nails [23]. Weightlifters are prone to these infections from shared equipment, locker room use, and possibly skin-to-skin contact [24]. When the infection appears on the feet, this is known as Tinea Pedis or "athlete's foot." Tinea Pedis presents most commonly within the toe-web spaces as an erythematous plaque or on the soles of the feet and appears scaly [25]. When the infection is present on the hands, it is termed Tinea Manuum. Treatment for Tinea Pedis and Tinea Manuum includes topical antifungals for a few days, and the spread of infection can be limited by treating infected persons as soon as possible [25]. Ensuring that lifters, martial artists, and wrestlers properly sanitize equipment after use can decrease infections. Tinea Cruris, or jock itch, and Tinea Corporis, occur when the dermatophytes infect the groin and body, respectively. Like other dermatophyte infections, these appear as well-demarcated scaly plaques [25]. Treatment is similar to Tinea Pedis in that topical antifungals are used and prevented by treating affected individuals as soon as possible [25]. Tinea Corporis, in particular, is so common in wrestlers that it was given the unique name of Tinea Gladiatorum due to an outbreak in 1992–1993 from a high school wrestling team with the disease potentially linked to wrestling mats used [16, 24, 26].

Onychomycosis or Tinea Unguium describes a dermatophyte infection of the nails, while Tinea Capitis or Scalp Ringworms describes a dermatophyte infection of the scalp. These athletes are susceptible to these infections, like other Tinea infections, due to locker room use, shared equipment, and skin-to-skin contact. Onychomycosis can affect the nail bed, matrix, or plate and can spread secondary to a Tinea Pedis or Manuum infection. Presentation involves yellowing or discoloration of the nails [27]. Tinea Capitis appears similar to other Tinea infections with a well-demarcated scaly plaque [24]. Onychomycosis and Tinea Capitis both require oral antifungals. Prevention includes proper hygiene and limiting the spread of preexisting Tinea infections.

Tinea versicolor refers to an infection caused by Malassezia species. Athletes are susceptible to this infection due to excessive sweating and contact with equipment. The presentation presents itself as hypo- or hyperpigmented, coalescing scaly macules. These appear on the trunk and upper arms [27]. Oily skin and warm climates also play a role. Treatment consists of antifungals, but the infection may reappear. Prevention includes showering after participating in the sport and sanitizing equipment before [27].

11.3 Parasitic Infectious Dermatosis

Pediculosis Capitis, or head lice, can affect those involved in weightlifting sports. These athletes typically get infected via sharing clothing and through skin-to-skin contact. Affected individuals can present with intense pruritus of the scalp and possible posterior cervical lymphadenopathy [27]. While combing, the lice may be identified on the scalp. Treatment involves direct killing or removal of the lice and ova. The most commonly used treatment is permethrin, but other treatments exist, such as ivermectin and malathion [27]. Prevention involves limiting the use of shared clothing and limiting the spread of infection by effectively treating individuals before resuming sports. Pediculosis Corporis occurs when body lice lay eggs in the seams of clothing [27]. Sharing clothing helps transmit the infection along with skin-to-skin contact. Patients with this disease generally present with generalized itching, erythematous blue and copper-colored macules, wheals, and lichenification. Treatment involves using permethrin or malathion to treat or wash clothing [20]. Prevention includes limiting the sharing of clothing. The mite Sarcoptes scabiei causes scabies. Athletes such as wrestlers can contract scabies through prolonged physical contact or sharing contaminated clothing. The presentation includes pruritic papular lesions, excoriations, and burrows. The infection can be present in areas such as the finger webs, wrists, and lower abdomen [27]. The most common treatment consists of permethrin or benzyl benzoate [27]. Prevention or limiting the spread of infection includes limiting skin-to-skin contact and sharing clothing.

11.4 Viral Infectious Dermatosis

Verruca refers to an infection of the skin by the HPV virus. Infection is widespread, and most individuals will experience it eventually. Transmission can occur in lifters primarily through contaminated surfaces and equipment. Warts can present in many forms, including verruca vulgaris, also known as common warts, and verruca plan taris, or plantar warts. Common warts are usually found on the hands, primarily the fingers and palms. They present as elevated, rounded papules with a rough, grayish surface [27]. Plantar warts appear on the soles, but mainly at pressure points on the ball of the foot. They can present as single or grouped soft puppy cores surrounded by a firm, horny ring. Bleeding is also possible at the pressure points [27]. There are several treatment options for both common and plantar warts. These include cryotherapy, topical salicylic acid, silver nitrate, cantharone, and surgical ablation [27]. Sanitizing equipment and shared spaces can reduce the instances of infection. Molluscum contagiosum refers to infection by the pox virus. Due to wet skin, lifters are especially prone to infection by the virus [27]. These lesions can present as tiny, firm, fleshed-colored, dome-shaped papules with central umbilication. Infections usually resolve within a year but can be treated with curettage or topical medications [24]. The spread of infection can be limited by covering the site of infection or limiting skin-to-skin contact when lesions are visible. Herpes Gladiatorum, also known as mat herpes, is a skin infection caused by the Herpes Simplex Virus Type 1 (HSV-1), which presents as a vesicular rash with HSV representing the most commonly reported cutaneous infection in wrestlers [20, 27]. Marital artists such as mixed-martial arts fighters are also prone to this infection. Prevention includes the use of antiviral therapy during training and competitions by wrestlers with a history of orolabial herpes [27].

11.5 Bacterial Infectious Dermatosis

Impetigo is a bacterial skin infection caused primarily by Group A. Streptococci and Staphylococcus aureus [26, 27]. Lifting athletes are susceptible due to the use of shared equipment as well as the heat and humidity of the facilities. The infection can be classified as primary, when the bacteria infect normal skin, or secondary, with infection complicating minor skin trauma such as abrasions [26]. There are three common variants of impetigo: bullous, nonbullous, and ecthyma. Nonbullous impetigo presents as papules, eventually progressing to vesicles and pustules with surrounding erythema. With bullous impetigo, the vesicles enlarge to form bullae with clear yellow fluid, eventually rupturing and leaving a thin, brown crust.

Ecthyma presents as punched-out, ulcerated lesions with a raised yellow crust [26]. Treatment consists of a course of antibiotics, which can be topical, such as mupirocin, or oral, such as augmentin [28]. Impetigo can be prevented or reduced by washing hands and cleaning machines before use.

Erysipelas, like impetigo, is a bacterial skin infection primarily caused by GAS and S. aureus [26]. These athletes are susceptible to a prior infection with impetigo, abrasions, or a break in the skin barrier [26]. With erysipelas, the superficial skin, as well as the upper dermis, are affected. The infection presents as erythema, edema, warmth, and possibly systemic symptoms such as a fever [26]. A characteristic raised, indurated border is also present [27]. The bacteria can also spread via the equipment used. Like impetigo, treatment consists of antibiotics and can be prevented or reduced by washing hands and cleaning machines before use. Cellulitis arises when the subcutaneous tissue is involved in a bacterial skin infection, primarily by GAS and S. aureus. Prior infection by GAS or S. aureus, as well as abrasions and cuts, put weightlifters at risk [26]. Presentation of the lesion includes mild local erythema, tenderness, malaise, and possibly fever or chills [27]. Like impetigo, treatment consists of antibiotics and can be prevented or reduced by washing hands and cleaning machines before use.

Carbuncles, furuncles, and abscesses arise, most commonly due to S. aureus [26]. Lifters can primarily acquire these infections in areas of friction or abrasions [26]. Skin abscesses involve the dermis and deeper skin tissues. They arise from pus within these tissues. A furuncle (boil) arises from an infected hair follicle. A carbuncle originates from a group of furuncles. Abscesses present as painful, tender nodules with erythema. The nodules may have a raised central pustule surrounded by a ring of erythema. Treatment involves incision of the abscess. If the athlete is immunocompromised, antibiotics such as those used in cellulitis may be used [26]. Like other infections by S. aureus, the likelihood of disease can be reduced with hand washing and cleaning equipment before use. Folliculitis is a superficial infection of hair follicles. These athletes are susceptible due to skin-to-skin contact and abrasions. Sharing soaps or sponges, as well as the use of whirlpools and hot tubs, puts athletes at risk for Pseudomonas folliculitis [26]. The most common cause is S. aureus, but Pseudomonas can also cause it. Folliculitis presents as a group of erythematous papules or pustules, typically appearing in areas of occlusive barriers and can be pruritic or painful. Treatment involves using antibiotics to fight S. aureus or Pseudomonas [27]. Pseudomonas folliculitis may be self-limited [26]. Prevention includes proper hygiene and cleaning pools.

11.6 Friction and Pressure-Related Dermatological Conditions

Abrasions are superficial injuries that are usually maintained at the level of the epidermis (Fig. 11.1). The most common mechanism of injury involves friction or blunt trauma. This usually occurs in weightlifting due to contact with barbells or other equipment. Wrestlers and martial artists can obtain abrasions from equipment and through physical contact with other participants and the ground. Abrasions are usually minor wounds that heal without scarring unless the dermis is involved. Treatment usually begins with water irrigation and typically does not require extensive medical therapy [29]. Prevention can be done by wearing protective clothing, such as longer socks, when powerlifters perform deadlifts. Within the world of martial arts, MMA fighters, in particular, experience lacerations at an astounding rate. Lacerations are the most common injury type sustained by MMA fighters. The face is the most common area affected, followed by the wrist/hands [30]. This is understood as the nature of the sport, which consists of striking the opponent to cause damage. This should explain why lacerations exist in other types of martial arts, such as karate and boxing. Lacerations are treated based on the severity, from minimal intervention to possible hospitalization. Injuries are prevented or minimized by stopping the sport when indicated [30].

Acne mechanica represents acneiform folliculitis present in sports. Triggers include friction, pressure, and heat [24]. As such, lifting sports involve a significant amount of pressure from equipment such as lifting suits or tight shoes. Clinically,

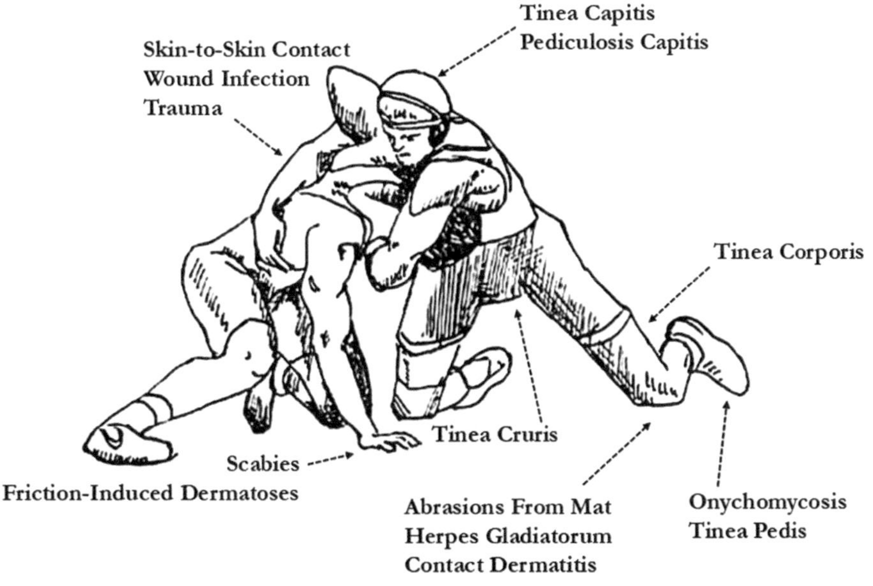

Fig. 11.1 Partial representation of wrestling dermatoses

this condition presents as red papules, pustules, and nodules. Usually, the lesions are located in the distribution of protective equipment. Treatment includes benzoyl peroxide, topical and systemic steroids, and topical retinoids. Prevention methods include moisture-wicking clothes or absorbent cotton shirts under equipment and proper hygiene following physical activity [24].

Blisters can plague those involved in sports involving significant friction or pressure. Although more common in marathon runners, weightlifters can experience blisters due to excessively tight attire, particularly in shoes [24]. Lifting heavy weights can also result in blisters on the hands. Blisters typically appear as clear or hemorrhagic vesicles that can be tender. Blisters larger than one centimeter are referred to as bullae [26]. Small blisters can resolve spontaneously, but more prominent blisters can be treated with needle compression followed by petrolatum. Friction is minimized with an adhesion bandage or secondary skin product [24].

Hyperkeratosis is defined as the thickening of the outer layer of the skin. In athletes, this can present as calluses and corns. A callus is a nonpenetrating circumscribed hyperkeratosis formed due to pressure. Within athletes, they can form on the palms and soles, especially within weightlifters. Weightlifting can result in calluses forming on the distal palm at the metacarpal head. Prolonged gripping can be an inciting factor [31]. Weightlifters are also susceptible to forming tache noir, black palm, that forms due to punctate hemorrhages caused by increased pressure in athletes' hands, presenting as a black discoloration of the affected area [32]. Corns are a type of thickening usually caused by tight shoes. Repeated friction or pressure of the skin that overlies the bony prominences may lead to the thickening of the skin and, consequently, corn formation [33]. Calluses may be beneficial to athletes but can be treated and prevented using padding to reduce pressure or keratolytics to relieve painful calluses. This can be achieved with the use of lifting gloves. Corns can spontaneously regress once the stimulus is removed and prevented from wearing properly sized shoes [27].

11.7 Environmental and Equipment Induced Dermatoses

Contact dermatitis is classified as an inflammatory reaction due to contact with a substance. This can further be classified into irritant and allergic contact dermatitis, both prevalent in athletes as hypersensitivity reactions with further inciting factors including trauma, heat, and moisture [24]. Trauma in weightlifting can occur from contact with sports equipment or machines. Frequent contact with metal bars against the lifter's skin causes friction that may result in erythema, abrasion, and lichenification. The chalk used to improve grip strength has been documented as inducing contact dermatitis [34]. Allergic contact dermatitis may also develop from contact with nickel and palladium in the weights or bars [34]. The acute presentation includes erythema, crusting, and scaling vesicles. Once subacute, pruritus, scaling, and ill-defined patches and plaques appear. Chronic dermatitis appears as acanthosis and possible lichenification. Treatment involves the removal of the causative agent, and topical steroids can be used acutely. Avoiding triggers, as well as moisturizers, can decrease occurrences [24].

Miliaria is a common skin condition resulting from the blockage of eccrine sweat glands and ducts. As such, sweating is the most common risk factor. Other factors, such as hot and humid climates, also play a part [35]. Due to the stress of lifting sports such as Strongman or CrossFit, sweating is expected. Intense training, tight clothing, and locker rooms, all contribute to these risk factors. The clinical presentation depends on the type of miliaria present. Three main types are distinguished based on the specific depth in which the eccrine ducts are blocked [27, 35]. Miliaria crystallina presents as small, clear, superficial vesicles without an inflammatory reaction and triggered by increased perspiration or when clothing prevents heat and moisture dissipation. Miliaria rubra appears as pruritic pustules and is preceded by another dermatitis that has caused injury, destruction, or blockage of the sweat glands, such as contact dermatitis, lichen simplex chronicus, or intertrigo. Miliaria profunda is characterized by nonpruritic, flesh-colored, deep-seated, whitish papules and usually follows miliaria rubra in the tropic. All three types are generally self-limiting and prevented with avoidance of the triggers [27].

Intertrigo is described as a superficial inflammatory dermatitis. It is discussed here as most occurrences usually occur during hot and humid weather within obese individuals. Strongmen and heavyweight lifters can potentially meet the criteria, especially when combined with the sweaty environment of the contact sport. To better grasp their size, NFL linemen seem to be one of the most prominent athletes at 140 kg or 308 lb. However, on average, they weigh 13 kg less than the average strongman competitor [36]. Intertrigo is usually located where two skin surfaces are close to one another, such as the creases of the neck, axillae, inguinal, perineal, and intergluteal areas. Heat, friction, and moisture all result in the skin folds becoming erythematous, macerated, and secondarily affected by bacteria. Bacterial pathogens include streptococci, staphylococci, Pseudomonas, or Corynebacterium species. Treatment is aimed at eliminating maceration using local antibiotics or fungicides as well as separating the skin folds, possibly with gauze. Low-potency topical corticosteroids or tacrolimus can also be added to reduce inflammation [27].

References

1. Storey A, Smith HK. Unique aspects of competitive weightlifting: performance, training and physiology. Sports Med. 2012;42(9):769–90.
2. Haff GG, Triplett NT, editors. Essentials of strength training and conditioning. 4th ed. Champaign, IL: Human Kinetics; 2016. https://doi.org/10.1096/fj.201600529R.
3. Winwood PW, Hume PA, Cronin JB, Keogh JW. Retrospective injury epidemiology of strongman athletes. J Strength Cond Res. 2014;28(1):28–42.
4. Glassman G. The CrossFit training guide. CrossFit J. 2010;100:1–115.
5. Spendlove J, et al. Dietary intake of competitive bodybuilders. Sports Med. 2015;45(7):1041–63.
6. Stone MH, Pierce KC, Sands WA, Stone ME. Weightlifting: a brief overview. Strength Cond J. 2007;29(5):24–31.

7. Warpeha J. A history of powerlifting in the United States: 50 years after York [Internet]. 2015 Sep 4. Available from: [cited 2024 Oct 29].
8. Kind A, Veit W, Helms E, Heffernan C. What is Strength? SRXIV 2024; https://doi.org/10.51224/SRXIV.467.
9. Chapman DL. Sandow the magnificent: Eugen Sandow and the beginnings of bodybuilding. Urbana and Chicago: University of Illinois Press; 1994.
10. Schwarzenegger A, Hall DK. Arnold: the education of a bodybuilder. New York: Simon & Schuster; 1977.
11. American Academy of Dermatology. Sports equipment and acne mechanica [Internet]. Available from: https://www.aad.org/public/diseases/acne/causes/sports-equipment"\l ":~:text=You%20get%20this%20type%20of,of%20athletes%20get%20acne%20mechanica" \t "_new. [cited 2024 Nov 2].
12. Bender TW. Cutaneous manifestations of disease in athletes. J Am Acad Dermatol. 2017;76(6):1053–65.
13. American Academy of Dermatology. Preventing athletic skin infections. [Internet] Available from: [cited 2024 Nov 2].
14. American Academy of Dermatology. Prevent skin infections at the gym [Internet]. Available from: [cited 2024 Nov 2.]
15. Lystad RP, et al. Injury incidence, severity and profile in Olympic combat sports: a comparative analysis of 7712 athlete exposures from three consecutive Olympic Games. Br J Sports Med. 2021;55(19):1077–83.
16. Williams C, et al. Notes from the field: outbreak of skin lesions among high school wrestlers--Arizona, 2014. MMWR Morb Mortal Wkly Rep. 2015;64(20):559–60.
17. Wrestling. Encyclopædia Britannica Inc. 2020.
18. Bu B, et al. Effects of martial arts on health status: a systematic review. J Evid Based Med. 2010;3(4):205–19.
19. Ji M. Analysis of injury types for mixed martial arts athletes. J Phys Ther Sci. 2016;28(5):1544–6.
20. Wilson EK, et al. Cutaneous infections in wrestlers. Sports Health. 2013;5(5):423–37. https://doi.org/10.1177/1941738113481179.
21. Zinder SM, et al. National athletic trainers' association position statement: skin diseases. J Athl Train. 2010;45(4):411–28.
22. Dorman JM. Contagious diseases in competitive sport: what are the risks? J Am Coll Heal. 2000;49(3):105–9.
23. Pujalte GGA, et al. More than skin deep: dermatologic conditions in athletes. Sports Health. 2023;15(1):74–85.
24. Pecci M, Comeau D, Chawla V. Skin conditions in the athlete. Am J Sports Med. 2009;37(2):406–18.
25. Rodgers P, Bassler M. Treating onychomycosis. Am Fam Physician. 2001;63(4):663–72–77–8.
26. Beller M, Gessner BD. An outbreak of tinea Corporis gladiatorum on a high school wrestling team. J Am Acad Dermatol. 1994;31(2 Pt 1):197–201.
27. James WD, Elston D, Treat JR, Rosenbach MA, Neuhaus IM. Andrews' diseases of the skin. 13th ed. Elsevier; 2020.
28. Hartman-Adams H, Banvard C, Juckett G. Impetigo: diagnosis and treatment. Am Fam Physician. 2014;90(4):229–35.
29. Shrestha R, et al. Abrasion. In: StatPearls. Treasure Island (FL): StatPearls Publishing Copyright © 2024, StatPearls Publishing LLC.; 2024.
30. Jensen AR, et al. Injuries sustained by the mixed martial arts athlete. Sports Health. 2017;9(1):64–9.
31. Stricklin SM, et al. Clues from hands Part 1: personal details about patients revealed by hand examination. Mo Med. 2014;111(4):349–51.
32. Freiman A, Barankin B, Elpern DJ. Sports dermatology part 1: common dermatoses. CMAJ. 2004;171(8):851–3.

33. Al Aboud AM, Yarrarapu SNS. Corns. In: StatPearls. Treasure Island (FL): StatPearls Publishing Copyright © 2024, StatPearls Publishing LLC.; 2024.
34. Kockentiet B, Adams BB. Contact dermatitis in athletes. J Am Acad Dermatol. 2007;56(6):1048–55.
35. Guerra KC, Toncar A, Krishnamurthy K. Miliaria. In: StatPearls. Treasure Island (FL): StatPearls Publishing Copyright © 2024, StatPearls Publishing LLC.; 2024.
36. Kraemer WJ, et al. Body composition in elite strongman competitors. J Strength Cond Res. 2020;34(12):3326–30.

Chapter 12
Cycling

Stefania Radici, Carlos Lange Nava, Ryan Scheinkman, and Keyvan Nouri

12.1 Introduction

Cycling and biking sports encompass a diverse range of disciplines, including road cycling, mountain biking, track cycling, and recreational biking. These activities appeal to individuals of all ages and skill levels, from elite athletes competing in prestigious events like the Tour de France to casual enthusiasts biking for exercise, transportation, or leisure. While the specific demands of these disciplines vary based on terrain, equipment, and competitive intensity, they all share fundamental principles such as reliance on pedaling mechanics, balance on a saddle seat, and specialized gear. The global rise in popularity of cycling as a means of exercise, transportation, and sport highlights its numerous physical benefits, including enhanced cardiovascular health, improved endurance, and strengthened musculature. However, this surge in participation has also brought increased recognition of the unique dermatological challenges faced by cyclists. Prolonged mechanical friction, sustained pressure, environmental exposure, and sweat retention contribute to a wide range of skin conditions that can significantly impact both performance and quality of life.

Physicians, particularly dermatologists treating these patients, play a crucial role in recognizing, preventing, and managing these cycling-related dermatoses. Cyclists frequently experience a variety of mechanical skin conditions due to extended contact with equipment such as saddles, handlebars, helmets, and footwear. Common issues include saddle sores, characterized by ischemic or friction-induced dermatitis in the perineal region, as well as calluses and blisters on the hands and feet caused

S. Radici · C. L. Nava · R. Scheinkman (✉) · K. Nouri
Dr. Phillip Frost Department of Dermatology and Cutaneous Surgery, University of Miami, Miami, FL, USA
e-mail: sxr3896@miami.edu; cxl1033@med.miami.edu; scheinkman@med.miami.edu; knouri@med.miami.edu

K. Nouri (ed.), *Sport-Related Skin Conditions*,
https://doi.org/10.1007/978-3-031-90444-8_12

by repetitive gripping and pressure. These conditions often impair an athlete's ability to train and compete.

Environmental exposure adds another dimension to the dermatological risks associated with cycling. Outdoor cyclists are frequently subjected to ultraviolet (UV) radiation, wind, and fluctuating weather conditions. These factors significantly increase the risk of sunburn, chronic photodamage, and long-term skin cancers such as melanoma and squamous cell carcinoma. Despite these risks, sun-protective measures such as the regular application of broad-spectrum sunscreen, wearing UPF-rated clothing, and using helmets with integrated visors are often underutilized. Raising awareness and educating athletes on effective sun protection strategies remain critical to mitigating these risks.

Cyclists are also prone to dermatological conditions exacerbated by heat and humidity. Extended physical exertion in hot weather amplifies sweat production, creating occlusive environments under helmets, gloves, and cycling shoes. These conditions increase the likelihood of dermatoses such as acne mechanica, intertrigo, and tinea pedis. The combination of sweat, friction, and synthetic materials found in cycling gear also elevates the risk of contact dermatitis from irritants or allergens present in gloves, chamois pads, or shoe linings. The allergic and irritant contact dermatitis caused by exposure to cycling gear materials and topical agents is a significant concern for both competitive and recreational riders.

Unique to cycling are the dermatological conditions affecting the genital and perineal regions due to prolonged saddle contact. This can lead to conditions like perineal nodular induration, vulvar lymphedema, and scrotal dermatoses, which are not only physically debilitating but also underdiagnosed due to the stigma surrounding these topics. Physicians must approach these conditions with sensitivity and a thorough understanding of their pathophysiology to provide effective care.

Mitigating these risks requires a multidisciplinary approach involving dermatologists, sports medicine physicians, and cycling specialists. Protective strategies such as ergonomic adjustments, the use of moisture-wicking and UV-protective clothing, proper hygiene practices, and early diagnosis and treatment are essential in managing these conditions. By proactively addressing these challenges, physicians can help cyclists maintain optimal performance, prevent long-term complications, and enjoy the sport with confidence.

12.2 Friction and Pressure-Related Dermatoses

12.2.1 Intertrigo

Intertrigo, commonly known as "chafing," occurs due to skin-to-skin friction combined with increased heat and humidity, leading to maceration and recurrent inflammation, which are hallmark features of this condition [1]. Intertrigo typically appears as a bright red, sometimes eroded patch [2] and most frequently affects areas such as the inguinal region, submammary folds, and gluteal clefts, where friction and moisture are exacerbated [3]. Although primarily caused by mechanical skin friction, intertrigo can be complicated by secondary infections, with Candida being the most common pathogen. Gram-positive and gram-negative bacterial infections are also possible but less frequent [2]. Cyclists are especially vulnerable to intertrigo due to the repetitive pedaling motion, which increases friction and heat in susceptible areas. This risk is heightened during prolonged rides, particularly at high speeds, where mechanical stress and sweat accumulation create an environment conducive to the development of intertrigo. Additional risk factors include hyperhidrosis, poor hygiene, closed-toed or ill-fitting shoes, and tight-fitting clothes that retain moisture [2].

Treatment typically involves topical or oral antibiotic or antifungal coverage or topical anti-inflammatories (i.e. corticosteroid creams or calcineurin inhibitors) in the absence of secondary infections [2]. For Candida-associated cases, treatment includes topical antifungal therapies, including azoles or Nystatin, applied twice daily for 2–4 weeks [4]. If painful or itchy lesions are present, antifungal-corticosteroid combinations can be utilized for symptomatic relief [4]. Preventive and therapeutic strategies emphasize measures to keep the skin dry and minimize friction, which is critical in managing and reducing the recurrence of intertrigo [2, 4]. The use of light, non-constricting, moisture-wicking fabrics like cotton or polyester is recommended, while nylon and other synthetic fibers should be avoided as they can exacerbate symptoms [2]. Miconazole powder can be used on flare-prone areas, but it is not effective with active disease [2]. Additional recommendations include showering immediately after training, drying off completely, and wearing clean, dry clothing [2].

12.2.2 Acne Mechanica and Acne Keloidalis Nuchae

Acne mechanica refers to acneiform eruptions caused by mechanical pressures, friction, rubbing, squeezing, or stretching of the skin [5, 6]. These eruptions are typically characterized by red papules, pustules, and nodules that typically arise in areas subjected to repeated sweating, occlusion, friction, and pressure, such as beneath protective equipment [2, 7]. Commonly affected areas include the chin, forehead, jawline, neck, and shoulders [7]. Cyclists, much like athletes in sports like American football, are particularly susceptible to developing papules and pustules in areas occluded by tight garments and padding that are integral to their gear [5]. Similar patterns are observed in athletes of other sports—football and hockey players often develop rashes under pads, helmets, or chinstraps, while golfers may experience lesions in a pattern corresponding to their bag straps and equestrians under chinstraps [2]. Cyclists face comparable risks due to their use of helmets, chinstraps, and tight protective clothing. Notably, this condition can occur even in the absence of underlying acne vulgaris [8]. Unlike acne vulgaris, which has a multifactorial etiology, acne mechanica is directly associated with mechanical stress, making conventional antibiotic treatments less effective [5].

Treatment for acne mechanica typically includes benzoyl peroxide, topical and systemic antibiotics, and topical retinoids, such as tretinoin cream [2]. For severe and refractory cases, systemic isotretinoin can be used; however, there is a risk of myopathy and tendinitis [2]. Preventative strategies focus on wearing moisture-wicking fabrics or clean, absorbent cotton clothing under sports gear. Additionally, diligent skin cleansing following intense physical activity is essential for managing and preventing further outbreaks [2].

A more severe related condition, acne keloidalis nuchae, is characterized by chronic fibrotic folliculitis and perifolliculitis in the neck and occipital scalp [7]. The condition is not limited to athletes but may be seen more frequently in those wearing helmets, which contributes to friction and occlusion within the affected area [9]. This condition can lead to hypertrophic scars or keloid formation, highlighting the importance of early intervention and management [7, 9]. Treatment for acne keloidalis nuchae includes topical and intralesional corticosteroids, topical antibiotics, topical retinoids, and electrosurgical excision [9].

12.2.3 Corns and Calluses (Hyperkeratosis)

Hyperkeratosis, the thickening of the skin, develops as a natural protective response to repeated mechanical trauma. This can occur due to poorly fitting footwear, anatomical deformities, or repetitive physical activities, leading to the formation of corns and calluses. While corns are more sharply defined and narrowly based, calluses are broad-based areas of thickened, hyperkeratotic papules or plaques. These formations typically appear in high-friction areas such as the hands and feet and are usually painless [10, 11]. Risk factors for developing corns and calluses include bony protuberances, abnormal biomechanical foot function, poorly fitting shoes, and repetitive trauma, such as that caused by athletic activities [10]. The cycle of friction, pressure, and skin thickening continues until a corn or callus forms [10]. In many cases, treatment is unnecessary as these protective layers help prevent blisters [11]. However, treatment may be sought for cosmetic or symptomatic relief. Common therapeutic options include keratolytic agents like salicylic acid or urea and mechanical debridement [9, 11]. Treatment should aim to relieve symptoms while addressing the underlying biomechanical causes. Paring down the thickened skin or removing the central core of a corn can provide immediate relief [10]. Results can be maintained by periodically filing calluses after soaking the skin in warm water. Topical agents such as salicylic acid or urea are effective to further soften hardened skin [10]. Other clinical approaches include curettage and cryotherapy. The use of soft cushions, such as silicone sheets can reduce friction and enhance comfort. Preventative measures include wearing properly fitted footwear and utilizing orthotic devices to correct biomechanical irregularities [10].

12.2.4 *Friction Blisters*

Friction blisters are fluid-filled bullae that result from repetitive frictional stress, often in moist environments and are typically accompanied by pain and tenderness [9, 11]. These lesions are normally filled with clear fluid that is similar in composition to plasma; however, they can be hemorrhagic, most frequently occurring on high-pressure areas of the feet, such as the tips of the toes, the balls of the feet, and the posterior heel where mechanical stress is highest [9, 11]. Blisters are very common, affecting amateur and professional athletes alike, and most often develop on volar surfaces where a thick stratum corneum exists that serves as the blister roof [9].

For painful blisters, careful drainage can be performed using a sterile #11 blade to create a small incision at the blister's periphery [11, 12]. This preserves the blister roof, which acts as a biological dressing to protect underlying tissue [9, 12]. The drained area should then be dressed with antiseptic, petroleum jelly, and a clean bandage to promote healing and reduce the risk of infection [9, 11]. Antibiotic ointment is required only rarely unless indications of infection are present [12]. Synthetic dressings, though more costly, adhere firmly to the affected area and provide outstanding protection [12]. Prevention involves minimizing friction and moisture, including avoiding any irregular surfaces that may rub on the skin, such as wrinkles in garments or seams in equipment [9]. Using acrylic socks has been shown to be more effective at preventing blisters than cotton socks [11]. Proper fitting footwear and moisture-wicking materials are also key preventative measures [12].

12.3 Genital and Perineal Dermatoses

Cycling poses several health risks for both male and female athletes, particularly affecting the genital and perineal regions. The repetitive pressure, friction, and trauma associated with prolonged saddle contact can result in a range of dermatological complications.

12.3.1 *Saddle Sores (Ischial Dermatosis)*

Cyclists frequently experience saddle sores, a common issue among both novice and competitive riders, regardless of gender. These lesions arise from prolonged contact with the bicycle saddle and are caused by a combination of mechanical and physiological factors, including friction, pressure, heat, moisture, and bacterial proliferation in the saddle area [13, 14]. Cyclists who engage in frequent or long-distance riding are at heightened risk [14]. Saddle sores can range from mild discomfort to significant pain and restricted mobility, potentially reducing participation in cycling and impacting performance, especially in competitive settings [13].

Saddle sores can advance from chafing and folliculitis to abrasions, abscesses, and soft tissue infections [13]. Saddle sores can develop into perinodular indurations (PNIs), which are discussed subsequently [14]. Female cyclists, particularly competitive ones, are more susceptible to additional saddle-related complications, including genital trauma, vulvar diseases, sexual dysfunction, and genitourinary infections [13]. The sensitivity and stigma associated with this region of the body mean that saddle sores can cause embarrassment and can deter athletes from discussing the issue openly with healthcare providers and support staff [14], complicating timely diagnosis and treatment.

Treatment begins with rest, which is often frustrating for cyclists, especially competitive athletes. Additional interventions include the application of heat or cold therapy, topical treatments containing steroidal, antifungal, or antibacterial agents, and wearing loose, breathable clothing to minimize irritation [13]. In cases where saddle sores escalate in size or severity, corticosteroids may be administered through creams or injections. However, caution is advised, as prolonged use of steroids can cause skin atrophy and exacerbate pressure-related issues over time. Surgical excision is considered a last resort for large or refractory lesions [14]. Preventative measures are essential to mitigate the risk of saddle sores. These include optimizing saddle design, adjusting the cyclist's riding position, and selecting high-quality cycling shorts with well-fitted chamois [13]. The use of chamois cream as a lubricant to minimize friction, along with maintaining good personal hygiene and grooming in the perineal area, is highly recommended [14]. Consistent care, such as cleaning and drying the area after cycling sessions, is crucial.

12.3.2 Perineal Nodular Induration (PNI)/Ischiatic Hygroma ("Cyclist's Nodule")

Perineal nodular induration, also known as ischiatic hygroma, is a pseudoneoplastic lesion resulting from repetitive microtrauma caused by friction and vibration between the bicycle saddle and the ischial tuberosities [15, 16]. This ongoing mechanical stress impacts the superficial perineal fascia, forming a nodular mass that can range significantly in size and cause considerable pain or discomfort under sustained saddle pressure [15]. In some cases, labial nodules measuring up to 60 mm in diameter have been documented [16]. In male cyclists, PNI commonly appears as a nodular mass near the median raphe, posterior to the scrotum. Its distinct morphology has led to colloquial terms such as "cyclist's nodule" or "cyclist's third testicle" [15]. Although the condition is predominantly reported in men, it can also occur in women. Due to anatomical differences, PNI in female cyclists is likely underdiagnosed and often confused with other mesenchymal lesions in the vulvar region [15]. Cases of PNI in women have been misdiagnosed as lipomas or even referred to oncology centers under suspicion of malignancy [15]. Advanced diagnostic imaging, such as MRIs and even biopsies, are sometimes unnecessarily pursued. Awareness of this condition among healthcare providers can enable accurate diagnosis through a thorough history and physical examination, circumventing costly diagnostic workups [15].

PNI is characterized as a reactive fibroblastic and myofibroblastic pseudotumor, emphasizing the importance of distinguishing it from neoplasms or other pathological growths [8]. Healthcare providers should maintain a high index of suspicion for PNI in cyclists presenting with groin pain and palpable nodular masses, particularly in those with a history of prolonged or frequent saddle use [8]. Effective treatment primarily involves ergonomic modifications to the bicycle saddle to minimize friction and pressure on the perineal region. Surgical excision may be warranted to provide relief in cases where symptoms persist or the nodules cause significant discomfort [8].

12.3.3 Vulvar Lymphedema and Labial Hypertrophy ("Bicyclist's Vulva")

"Bicyclist's vulva" is an emerging term that refers to chronic swelling and hypertrophy of the labium majus, predominantly observed in female high-level cycling competitors [15, 16]. This condition may present as unilateral or bilateral enlargement of the labia and is strongly associated with prolonged and intense cycling activities [15, 16]. Vulvar lymphedema is thought to result from a combination of repetitive microtrauma, chronic inflammation, and localized lymphatic obstruction in the inguinal area, exacerbated by the cyclist's characteristic curved posture [15]. Labial hypertrophy, a closely related condition, is believed to develop due to chronic saddle pressure on the vulvoperineal region. This pressure can compromise lymphatic circulation, leading to edema, persistent tissue thickening, and hypertrophy [15, 16]. Labial hypertrophy is often associated with concurrent conditions such as folliculitis, skin infections, or intravulval hematomas, and the structural changes it induces tend to persist even after these secondary conditions resolve [16]. The nonspecific symptoms of vulvar lymphedema and the often unilateral presentation of labial hypertrophy contribute to under-recognition by dermatologists and gynecologists [15, 16]. Bilateral labial hypertrophy, in particular, is thought to be underdiagnosed, as symmetrical tissue enlargement is more challenging to identify clinically [16]. Both conditions are generally painless but may cause discomfort, particularly during cycling. They can also affect saddle selection, as poorly designed saddles with inadequate central cut-outs may exacerbate symptoms by increasing pressure and friction on the vulvoperineal area [16]. Optimizing bicycle fit is critical in preventing both conditions. Key measures include adjusting the saddle to minimize pressure and friction, selecting saddles with well-designed central cut-outs, and ensuring proper bike ergonomics [15, 16]. Reducing training intensity and duration may also help mitigate the risk of developing these conditions [16]. Conservative treatment strategies focus on managing symptoms and reducing inflammation. Applying ice packs immediately after cycling sessions can alleviate swelling, while elevating the legs post-ride improves lymphatic drainage and decreases localized edema [15]. For labial hypertrophy, addressing the structural tissue changes may involve additional ergonomic adjustments or surgical consultation in severe cases.

12.3.4 Perineal Folliculitis

Perineal folliculitis is a frequently encountered condition among male and female cyclists that occurs centrally at the perineum [16]. It arises due to inflammation of hair follicles, primarily triggered by the combination of friction and prolonged occlusion caused by tight cycling shorts and sustained contact with the saddle [16]. The repetitive mechanical stress, heat, and sweat accumulation exacerbate the condition, making it particularly prevalent in long-distance or competitive cyclists. Cyclists are advised to wear breathable, moisture-wicking clothing to reduce moisture buildup and friction in the perineal region. Proper hygiene practices are crucial, including regular cleaning and ensuring the area remains dry. Pubic hair removal also increases the risk of folliculitis. Riders who use a razor to remove hair increase their risk significantly. Limiting hair removal is the best option for riders to avoid this condition [16]. It's also worth noting that applying cycling-specific chamois cream directly to the skin significantly reduces the incidence of folliculitis [16].

12.3.5 Scrotal Dermatoses

Male cyclists frequently experience scrotal irritation and related dermatoses, primarily attributed to prolonged friction and occlusion. While the exact mechanism remains unclear, repeated microtrauma has been proposed as a potential causative factor [17]. A study by Nashan et al. reported that the prevalence of scrotal abnormalities in on-road cyclists is comparable to that in infertile men, reaching approximately 40%. This finding warrants further scientific investigation, particularly given the association between bicycling and erectile dysfunction, which has been observed in up to 19% of cyclists, as reported in multiple studies [17]. Ultrasound (US) evaluations have revealed distinct patterns of abnormalities in cyclists. Among mountain bikers, testicular and extratesticular calcifications were identified in up to 84% of cases, often attributed to torsion of the appendix testis, inflammation of the tunica vaginalis, or hematomas [17]. In contrast, on-road cyclists demonstrated a higher prevalence of hydroceles, spermatoceles, and varicoceles, occurring in up to 28% of cases [17]. These findings highlight the potential for cycling-related trauma to contribute to scrotal pathologies. Sweat accumulation and the use of synthetic materials in cycling gear may further aggravate these conditions. Preventive measures, including the use of padded cycling shorts, properly fitted saddles, and shock-absorbing suspension systems, are essential to mitigate these risks and protect scrotal health [17].

12.4 Infectious-Related Dermatoses

12.4.1 Bacterial Infections

Impetigo is a skin infection commonly caused by *Streptococcus pyogenes* (GAS) or *Staphylococcus aureus* bacteria that is transmissible [18]. It can occur as a primary infection on previously healthy skin or as a secondary infection, complicating minor skin trauma such as abrasions [2, 11, 18]. Impetigo typically presents with papules and pustules that coalesce into erythematous plaques covered by a characteristic honey-colored crust [2, 11]. Lesions are most commonly observed on the face, extremities, and areas prone to friction or minor trauma, while the palms and soles are generally unaffected [2]. A bullous form of impetigo, featuring flaccid vesicles that rupture quickly, may also occur and is commonly localized to the torso [2]. Cyclists are particularly prone to impetigo due to frequent skin injuries caused by falls, prolonged contact with equipment, and repetitive friction from cycling gear. Warm, moist conditions inside helmets, gloves, or cycling shoes, coupled with sweat accumulation, further promote bacterial growth, making athletes particularly vulnerable to this condition [18]. The risk is especially significant when equipment is shared or inadequately cleaned between uses.

For mild cases, removing the overlying crust and applying topical mupirocin is usually sufficient. Severe infections may require systemic antibiotics such as first-generation cephalosporins or macrolides [11]. If methicillin-resistant *Staphylococcus aureus* (MRSA) is identified through culture, antibiotic treatment should be adjusted accordingly [11]. Despite increased educational efforts promoting awareness about appropriate hygiene, the incidence of MRSA infections continues to be high among athletes [9].

Cyclists should avoid direct skin-to-skin contact with infected individuals and refrain from sharing unwashed gear, towels, or clothing. Proper cleaning and sanitization of helmets, gloves, and other cycling equipment are critical for reducing bacterial transmission. Open wounds should be promptly cleaned and dressed with dry bandages, with twice-daily application of mupirocin or triple antibiotic ointments until the wounds are fully closed [11]. Athletes should not resume group rides or competitions until lesions are completely dry, as covering lesions alone does not eliminate the risk of transmission [2].

Folliculitis is a dermatological condition due to infection and inflammation of hair follicles [2, 11, 19]. The condition is most commonly caused by *Staphylococcus aureus*, although other pathogens may occasionally be involved [11]. Staphylococcal folliculitis can affect any hair-bearing region, but the trunk and extremities are particularly susceptible. Other frequently affected areas include the thighs, axillae, and pubic region, which are often subject to friction or occlusion [19]. Cyclists are especially prone to folliculitis in regions of prolonged contact and friction, such as the groin, thighs, and areas under cycling shorts. Predisposing factors for folliculitis include recently shaved follicles and regions exposed to increased friction, both of which can exacerbate irritation and susceptibility to infection [2]. The condition typically presents with erythematous papules and pustules centered around hair follicles [2, 11]. In some cases, the condition may progress to form nonhealing crusted sores, which can appear anywhere on the skin except the palms and soles [2]. While folliculitis is often mildly pruritic, it can also be painful, particularly in occluded areas like the axillary folds [11].

For methicillin-susceptible *S. aureus* (MSSA), oral antibiotics such as cephalosporins or macrolides are effective. For methicillin-resistant *S. aureus* (MRSA), treatment with doxycycline or sulfamethoxazole/trimethoprim is recommended [11]. Antibiotic therapy should continue for a minimum of 72 hours, after which new lesions should stop forming after 48 hours, adhering to a "48-hour/72-hour" rule before returning to cycling or other activities [2]. For medium- and low-risk contact sports, the lesions should be dry, not oozing, and may be covered with bandages [2]. Secondary infections, indicated by worsening erythema, edema, pain, or active drainage, may require further medical attention [2]. Cyclists can minimize the risk of folliculitis by keeping their cycling gear, particularly shorts and helmets, clean and avoiding shared towels or unwashed equipment. Showering promptly after cycling with antibacterial soap is also recommended. For athletes using hot tubs post-ride, ensuring the tub is regularly sanitized can help prevent folliculitis [11].

A furuncle is an acute, tender, circumscribed staphylococcal abscess originating from a hair follicle, often culminating in central suppuration [19]. When multiple furuncles converge to form interconnected lesions with separate heads, they are referred to as carbuncles [2, 19]. These lesions often develop due to autoinoculation, where bacteria spread from one site to another [19]. They commonly occur in occluded areas in the folds of the skin yet can appear in areas of repeated trauma between equipment and skin, which results in friction [11]. Commonly affected areas include the nape of the neck, axillae, and perineum, although lesions can develop on any hair-bearing site subjected to mechanical stress [19]. Factors that compromise the skin barrier, such as irritation, hyperhidrosis, dermatitis, shaving, or other forms of trauma, create entry points for *Staphylococcus aureus*, the common causative agent [19]. Deep skin invasion can result in furuncles, with methicillin-resistant *S. aureus* (MRSA) being a frequent pathogen [19]. While some lesions resolve without rupture, most progress to central necrosis and rupture, releasing purulent, necrotic material [19].

Treatment should be instituted promptly. This therapy is similar to that for impetigo and consists of topical and oral antibiotics (mupirocin twice daily and dicloxacillin 500 mg three times daily) and frequent warm soaks [12]. For small or mild cases, warm compresses and topical antibiotics, such as mupirocin, are typically sufficient. Oral antibiotics like dicloxacillin (500 mg three times daily) may also be prescribed for more symptomatic cases [12]. Larger abscesses or severely symptomatic lesions often require incision and drainage. In cases of very large abscesses, a surgical drain may be necessary to prevent premature incision closure and recurrence [11]. For MRSA infections, incision and drainage are essential, and antibiot ics effective against MRSA, such as doxycycline or trimethoprim/sulfamethoxazole, should be considered [11]. Cyclists can minimize the risk of furuncles and carbuncles by cleaning open wounds with antibacterial soap and keeping them covered with topical antibiotics to prevent deeper infections [11]. Ensuring cycling gear is clean and dry and wearing moisture-wicking materials can also reduce risk. Cyclists should only return to riding once lesions are completely dry. If lesions remain moist or draining, return to activity is not recommended, even if the affected area is covered [2].

12.4.2 Fungal Infections

Tinea corporis involves superficial dermatophyte infections of the skin, excluding the scalp, beard, face, hands, feet, and groin [19]. It is characterized by circular, sharply defined, slightly erythematous, dry, and scaly patches that may sometimes appear hypopigmented [12, 19]. The lesions often feature a distinct advancing scaling edge and central clearing, resulting in the annular or ring-like shape that gives the condition its common name, "ringworm" [12, 19]. Warm, moist environments significantly enhance the survival and propagation of the causative dermatophytes [19] such as those created by prolonged use of tight or sweat-retaining cycling gear.

To confirm the diagnosis, microscopic visualization of the hyphae using potassium hydroxide obtained from a culture of affected area can be performed [12]. Treatment involves topical antifungal creams for localized infections and oral antifungal agents for widespread or refractory cases [12]. One study suggested that 100% of athletes treated with weekly fluconazole (100 mg) had negative cultures after 3 weeks; unfortunately, the optimal duration of therapy remains undefined [12]. Cyclists should avoid sharing helmets, gloves, or other equipment and refrain from close contact with others if the lesions are active and cannot be covered [12].

Tinea cruris, also known as "jock itch," is a superficial fungal infection that predominantly affects men, often involving the upper and inner thighs [19]. It is particularly common during warm and humid conditions. The infection initially presents as a small, erythematous, scaling, or vesicular patch that expands peripherally over time [19]. A distinctive feature is the central clearing of lesions, which creates a curved, well-defined border, often with vesicles or pustules along the edges [19]. The infection may spread downward along the thighs and backward to the perineum or anus, although the scrotum is seldom involved [19].

Diagnosis can be confirmed with microscopic examination in the same manner as other tinea infections [11, 12]. Treatment includes topical antifungal creams for mild cases, while oral antifungal agents like terbinafine or fluconazole are prescribed for more severe infections [11]. Cyclists, especially those riding in hot or humid climates, should wear moisture-wicking shorts and practice good hygiene to minimize the risk of developing tinea cruris.

Tinea pedis, commonly referred to as "athlete's foot," is the most prevalent fungal infection affecting the feet [12, 19]. The majority of cases are caused by *Trichophyton rubrum* [12, 19], which typically induces a non-inflammatory dermatophytosis [19]. Cyclists, who often wear closed, non-breathable footwear for extended periods, are particularly susceptible to this condition. Tinea pedis is characterized by dull erythema and prominent silvery scaling, which can involve the entire sole and sides of the foot, creating a moccasin- or sandal-like appearance [19]. Clinically, tinea pedis is marked by itching, scaling, and maceration, primarily between the toes, and in some cases confined to a small patch near a fungus-infected toenail or localized between the toes [19].

Diagnosis is confirmed using potassium hydroxide (KOH) examination of skin scrapings or fungal culture [11, 12]. Treatment includes topical antifungal creams for mild cases and oral antifungal agents, such as terbinafine or fluconazole, for severe or resistant infections [11]. Cyclists can reduce the risk of tinea pedis by using synthetic, moisture-wicking socks, ensuring their cycling shoes are dry, and wearing sandals in communal areas like locker rooms and showers [12].

Onychomycosis is a fungal infection that involves the nail bed, matrix, or plate, with toenails more frequently affected than fingernails [20]. The constant pressure on the feet heightens the risk of fungal infections, especially in toenails. Continuous pressure and trauma to the feet further increase the likelihood of these infections. Cyclists are particularly susceptible due to the constant pressure and repetitive trauma exerted on the feet during long rides, especially in tight, non-breathable cycling shoes. This persistent pressure, combined with sweat and moisture accumulation, creates an ideal environment for fungal infections to thrive. The most common subtype, distal subungual onychomycosis, is caused by *Trichophyton rubrum* and accounts for up to 30% of superficial fungal infections [19, 20]. This form may present distally or laterally and is commonly associated with concurrent tinea pedis [20]. The fungus often spreads from the plantar surfaces of the feet [21]. Another subtype, white superficial onychomycosis, constitutes 10% of cases and is predominantly caused by *T. mentagrophytes*. This variant presents as well-defined opaque "white islands" on the nail plate, which coalesce over time, resulting in a rough, soft, and crumbly nail texture [20, 21]. Proximal subungual onychomycosis, although rare in healthy individuals, may develop secondary to local trauma [20], a common occurrence in cyclists due to repetitive impacts or poorly fitting footwear.

Onychomycosis presents many challenges for treatment due to the growth properties of the nail plate [22]. Newer antifugal agents, like fluconazole, itraconazole, and terbinafine, offer high cure rates and good safety profiles compared to older antifungals (e.g. ketoconazole and griseofulvin) [22]. Systemic treatments like oral itraconazole and oral terbinafine offer superior treatment [22]. Preventative strategies for cyclists include wearing moisture-wicking socks, ensuring proper shoe fit, and allowing shoes to fully dry between rides. Regular foot hygiene and avoiding barefoot walking in communal areas such as locker rooms can further reduce the risk of onychomycosis.

12.4.3 *Viral Infections*

Herpes simplex virus (HSV) infection has a high global prevalence, with herpes simplex virus 1 (HSV-1) accounting for the majority of non-genital herpes infections [2, 18]. Grouped vesicles on an erythematous base characterize HSV infection, although early lesions may exhibit no vesicles, and late lesions may demonstrate only erosions [11, 12]. Typically, the lesions are located on the head, neck, and upper extremities [12] but can occur in any area of skin that comes into contact with an actively infected, moist rash of another individual [11]. Infection with HSV-1 is highly contagious to susceptible persons who come into direct contact with an infected individual with an active lesion [19]. HSV infections are significant due to their incurable nature and the virus's ability to persist in a latent form throughout an individual's lifetime [18]. HSV-1 travels to the sensory dorsal root ganglion, where latency is established. Reactivation episodes can occur, and stress, cold, fever, and corticosteroids can trigger reactivation [2].

Oral antiviral therapy can reduce the duration and severity of the infection and help limit transmission when initiated early, particularly during the prodromal phase or within the first 48 hours of recurrence [2]. Antiviral agents, especially valaciclovir (1 g twice daily) and famciclovir (250 mg three times daily) are effective for treating HSV infection [12]. To prevent transmission, athletes should not share equipment or towels [12]. Preventative strategies should also include avoiding skin-to-skin contact with infected individuals, particularly when lesions are active [11].

Human papillomavirus (HPV) infection poses a particular concern to athletes when it causes warts on the hands and feet [12]. Warts are verrucous, well-defined, occasionally painful, papules and plaques usually present on the soles and hands [12]. Plantar warts, caused by specific HPV strains, such as types 1, 2, 27, and 57, are commonly seen in areas of pressure on the soles, such as the mid-metatarsal region or the ball of the foot [12]. For cyclists, prolonged pressure and repetitive friction from cycling shoes can exacerbate the risk of developing plantar warts, especially in poorly ventilated or moist footwear. These warts often present as verrucous, well-defined, occasionally painful papules or plaques [12]. It is not unusual for multiple lesions to appear on a single foot; sometimes, these warts coalesce into a larger "mosaic" wart. Plantar warts are characterized by soft, pulpy cores surrounded by firm, keratinized rings and can be distinguished from corns or calluses by the presence of a central, soft core and visible black or bleeding points from superficial capillaries when pared down—features absent in calluses [12, 19].

Treatment options include various destructive and non-destructive methods, such as cryotherapy with liquid nitrogen, laser therapy, curettage, salicylic acid, cantharidin, and trichloroacetic acid [2]. Topical medications such as imiquimod, 5-fluorouracil, and squaric acid diphenylcyclopropenone are also available. For generalized lesions, oral medications such as cimetidine or zinc sulfate may be effective [2]. Clinicians typically destroy warts using various methods such as cryosurgery, salicylic-acid, and cantharidin; however, the associated pain and tme required for healing make these treatments less desirable for cyclists [12]. A newer topical agent, imiquimod, offers an immunomodulatory effect and may be highly effective without causing the discomfort often associated with destructive treatments [12]. This can be particularly beneficial for cyclists who cannot afford to miss training or competition. To prevent both the transmission and acquisition of the virus, athletes should practice proper foot hygiene and wear sandals in locker rooms and communal showers [12].

12.5 Environmental Exposure Dermatoses

Cycling, particularly outdoors, exposes athletes to various environmental hazards that can significantly affect skin health. Prolonged exposure to the sun, wind, heat, and cold introduces distinct dermatological challenges. Preventative measures are critical for reducing the risk of both acute and chronic skin conditions. Athletes involved in outdoor sports should consistently use water-resistant sunscreens, wear sun-protective clothing, and schedule training sessions during periods of lower sun exposure. Regular consultations with a dermatologist are also advised to monitor and manage potential skin concerns [23].

12.5.1 Sun-Related Dermatoses

Participation in outdoor sports is associated with increased exposure to UV radiation [9]. Outdoor cycling entails considerable exposure to UV radiation, making cyclists especially vulnerable to sun-induced skin conditions. UV radiation remains a primary risk factor for the development of skin cancer, highlighting the importance of preventative strategies for athletes engaged in high-exposure activities [7, 23].

Young adults participating in outdoor aerobic activities, such as cycling, are more prone to experiencing sunburns [9]. Physical exertion increases sweating, which can enhance the skin's photosensitivity and heighten the risk of UV-induced damage, including sunburn [24]. Cyclists are particularly susceptible to sunburn due to prolonged outdoor exposure, especially during peak UV intensity hours. This risk is compounded by inconsistent adherence to UV protection measures, such as irregular sunscreen application [9]. Reflective surfaces like water and snow further intensify UV exposure, reflecting up to 85–95% of ultraviolet rays, which can exacerbate sunburn risks for cyclists during wet or snowy conditions [9]. These factors emphasize the critical importance of effective protective strategies, including sunscreen application and avoiding outdoor activities during high-risk periods.

Treatment for sunburn includes cooling the skin with compresses or cool baths, using oral non-steroidal anti-inflammatory drugs (NSAIDs) to manage pain and inflammation, and applying bland emollients to soothe the affected area [9]. Preventive measures focus on sun safety through minimizing direct exposure, wearing photoprotective clothing, hats, and sunglasses, and applying sunscreen to all exposed skin [9]. Proper sunscreen application in sufficient quantities, along with frequent reapplication—particularly after sweating—is essential to reducing the risk of sunburn [9].

Solar urticaria is a photosensitivity disorder characterized by the rapid onset of itching, burning sensations, and erythematous wheals in sun-exposed areas, typically occurring within minutes of exposure to natural sunlight [11]. Diagnosis is relies on physical examination, which reveals urticaria on exposed skin, combined with a history of symptoms occurring shortly after sun exposure [11]. This condition is most frequently observed during late spring and early summer when UV radiation levels are highest. For cyclists, the risk of solar urticaria can be particularly pronounce due to prolonged sun exposure during periods of outdoor rides and competitions. Effective management strategies include the use of antihistamines to alleviate itching and burning sensations, wearing sun-protective clothing and avoidance of peak sunlight hours [11].

Repeated and prolonged exposure to UV-A radiation significantly contributes to photodamage, amplifying the harmful effects of UV-B radiation and elevating the risk of skin cancer [24]. Chronic UV exposure can lead to visible signs of aging, including wrinkles, reduced skin elasticity, and pigmentation changes [24]. Cyclists, due to their outdoor training and competition, face an elevated risk of chronic photodamage, emphasizing the necessity of sun safety measures like broad-spectrum sunscreen, protective gear, and scheduling rides during lower UV index periods to minimize long-term skin damage.

Actinic keratosis (AK) is precipitated primarily by solar irradiation, most frequently occurring on common sun-exposed areas such as the face, scalp, neck, hands, and forearms, accounting for approximately 75% of cases [25, 26]. Cyclists, who often spend extended periods outdoors, are particularly at risk for developing AK due to prolonged UV radiation exposure. These precancerous lesions pose a significant risk of progression to squamous cell carcinoma (SCC) if left untreated [26], with rates of malignant transformation ranging from 0.025% to 16% [25]. The risk of progression to SCC increases substantially in individuals with multiple AK lesions. For example, the risk is four times higher in patients with 6–20 lesions and 11 times higher in those with more than 20 lesions [25].

Three distinct dermoscopic patterns are commonly associated with non-pigmented AK [25]. The first pattern exhibits a red pseudo-network with discrete white scales. The second, known as the "strawberry pattern," is characterized by an erythematous background. The third pattern displays enlarged follicular openings filled with keratotic plugs set against a scaly, white-to-yellow background [25]. Early detection of AK, often presenting as rough, scaly patches on sun-exposed skin, is critical in preventing progression to SCC. Apart from the concern of SCC development, AKs are often present in a field of cancerization (FC), where multiple subclinical lesions coexist in a background of sun-damaged skin [26].

Treatment options for AK can be categorized into lesion-directed and field-directed approaches. Lesion-directed therapies include cryotherapy, laser therapy, surgical excision or shave biopsy, and curettage, targeting specific atypical keratinocytes within individual lesions [25]. In contrast, field-directed treatments address broader areas of chronically sun-damaged skin, also referred to as “field cancerization” [25, 26]. These treatments include 5-fluorouracil (5-FU), diclofenac 3% gel, chemical peeling, imiquimod, and photodynamic therapy (PDT) [25, 26]. Both treatment modalities aim to remove atypical keratinocytes and reduce the overall risk of progression to more severe conditions [25]. Preventive strategies play a crucial role in minimizing the risk of AK among cyclists. Regular use of broad-spectrum sunscreen, wearing sun-protective clothing, and utilizing helmets with integrated visors are essential measures for reducing UV exposure. These protective behaviors, combined with early detection and appropriate treatment, are key to managing AK and preventing its progression to SCC in cyclists.

Ultraviolet radiation is the most significant environmental risk factor for skin cancer [24, 27]. Cyclists and athletes involved in outdoor sports are particularly vulnerable due to high cumulative UV exposure, especially in endurance activities. Factors such as altitude-related increases in UV intensity and reflections from surfaces like snow or water during certain cycling events further amplify this risk [24, 27]. Athletes practicing outdoor sports often experience substantial UV exposure due to prolonged training and competition schedules that coincide with peak UV intensity hours [24, 27]. Outdoor sports rarely allow for shade, and activities during the summer months between 11:00 am and 3:00 pm should be avoided to minimize UV-related harm [24]. Endurance athletes, in particular, have been found to exhibit a higher frequency of risk factors for cutaneous melanoma, such as increased numbers of melanocytic nevi and solar lentigines, making them more susceptible to melanoma development [24]. Additionally, the immunosuppressive effects of intense physical activity may further elevate the risk of skin cancers in outdoor athletes. While regular, low-impact exercise is beneficial for overall health, excessive high-intensity training can impair immune function due to repetitive tissue trauma. This trauma shifts cytokine profiles towards a T-helper 2 lymphocytic response, suppressing cell-mediated immunity. Coupled with UV-induced immunosuppression, this creates a favorable environment for tumor initiation and promotion in cyclists and other endurance athletes [24]. Preventative measures are essential for cyclists and include consistent use of broad-spectrum sunscreen, wearing ultraviolet protective factor-rated (UPF-rated) clothing, and scheduling rides during lower UV-intensity periods to mitigate these risks.

12.5.2 Weather-Related Dermatoses

Cold urticaria may develop after prolonged exposure to cold wind or low outside temperatures during long cycling rides. This condition is characterized by the appearance of urticarial wheals, ranging from small to large, in areas exposed to the cold, particularly when combined with contact with cold water [11]. In some cases, the presentation can also be generalized. Cyclists are particularly susceptible during colder months and rainy seasons, as being drenched while riding in the rain increases exposure to triggering conditions.

Management strategies include the application of ice to soothe the affected skin for about 5 minutes if urticaria wheals are present [11]. Additionally, oral antihistamines are often effective in alleviating inflammation and reducing associated itching, providing symptomatic relief [11]. Cyclists should consider wearing insulated, moisture-resistant clothing to minimize cold exposure and prevent episodes of cold urticaria during and after rides.

Cyclists are particularly vulnerable to windburn due to prolonged exposure to high-speed winds during outdoor rides. Despite its name, windburn it not a true burn but rather a form of skin irritation caused by the wind stripping away the outer protective oil layer of the skin [28]. Windburn presents as erythema, dryness, irritation, and sometimes a burning sensation on exposed skin. This condition is especially exacerbated during colder months when the skin's natural barrier is already weakened by dry air and lower humidity levels, leading to chapping, flaking, cracking, and, in severe cases, bleeding [28]. Cracks and small breaks in the skin can create openings for infectious agents, raising the risk of infection [28].

Research on windburn remains limited, and it is not well recognized in medical literature, highlighting the need for further investigation into this condition. However, effective treatments and preventative measures can significantly alleviate and reduce the occurrence of windburn. To soothe affected skin, emollient moisturizers containing mineral oil or petroleum are recommended, as they form a protective layer to retain moisture. For lip protection, products with petroleum or dimethicone as a primary ingredient are particularly beneficial [28]. Avoidance of alcohol-based products is crucial, as they can further dry and damage the skin's natural barrier [28]. After outdoor exposure, gradual re-warming of the skin is advised, as sudden temperature changes can exacerbate skin damage [28]. Preventative strategies include the use of wind-resistant clothing, such as face masks or balaclavas, which act as a physical shield against harsh winds. Applying protective balms or moisturizers prior to rides helps maintain skin hydration and minimizes irritation [28].

Cycling in cold weather increases the risk of frostbite and chilblains, especially in areas such as the fingers, toes, and face that are exposed or poorly insulated. Frostbite develops when skin temperatures fall below approximately −2 °C (28 °F), leading to erythema, edema, numbness, and eventually marked hyperemia and pain [10]. Chilblains, also known as pernio, are painful, inflamed lesions caused by repeated exposure to cold, damp, non-freezing conditions. These lesions typically present as erythematous to blue-violet macules, papules, or nodules, often symmetrically distributed on the distal toes and fingers and less frequently on the heels, nose, and ears. Deep pernio may appear as blue–erythrocyanotic plaques on the thighs, calves, or buttocks. Symptoms include itching, burning, or pain, with onset usually within 24 hours of cold exposure. Lesions generally resolve within 1–3 weeks [10]. Preventative measures include wearing insulated gloves, face masks, and thermal cycling gear to maintain adequate warmth. Frostbite treatment involves rapid rewarming in a warm water bath [10, 12]. For chilblains, a double-blind, placebo-controlled trial demonstrated the efficacy of nifedipine (20–60 mg daily). While medium- to high-potency topical corticosteroids are frequently prescribed, supporting evidence for their effectiveness remains limited [10].

Miliaria, commonly known as heat rash, results from the obstruction of eccrine sweat glands, causing a rash characterized by sweat-filled vesicles to form under the skin [29]. This condition, also referred to as "prickly heat" or "sweat rash," and is particularly prevalent in warm, humid climates, and is exacerbated during the summer months [29]. Cyclists training in such environments are highly susceptible, as the combination of prolonged exertion and tight, non-breathable cycling gear promotes sweat retention and duct blockage. The obstruction can be further aggravated by bacterial biofilms, such as those formed by *Staphylococcus epidermidis* [29]. A case study highlighted the role of heat-retentive, chemically treated protective clothing, in combination with heat retention from perspiration-soaked clothing in hot environments, in the development of maliaria-like rashes [30]. The presence of miliaria was found to be more concentrated in areas in contact with clothes and equipment [30]. Contributing factors include excessive sweating caused by high temperature and humidity, as well as the pooling of sweat on the skin's surface under occlusive gear. Notably, miliaria can also develop in low humid conditions as long as occlusive skin conditions are present, as the pooling of sweet on the skin results in overhydration of the stratum corneum, causing blockage of sweat ducts [30]. Additionally, natural skin bacteria, including Staphylococcus epidermidis and Staphylococcus aureus, are implicated in the pathogenesis of miliaria [30].

Miliaria is classified into three types based on the depth of sweat gland obstruction. Miliaria crystallina, the mildest form, presents as superficial, water-like vesicles and typically resolves quickly without inflammation [29]. Miliaria rubra, the most common type, is characterized by itchy, painful red papules and vesicles that appear in areas of friction and sweat accumulation, often accompanied by inflammation [29]. When bacterial infection occurs, pustules form, leading to a variant known as *miliaria pustulosa* [29]. The least common and most severe form, miliaria profunda, involves deeper sweat gland obstruction and presents as firm, flesh-colored papules [29]. This form is typically observed in individuals with recurrent episodes of miliaria rubra [29]. Cyclists are particularly prone to miliaria rubra and pustulosa in areas exposed to friction and sweat, such as the trunk and under cycling gear. Progression from miliaria to heat exhaustion and collapse is possible if the affected individual is not removed from the hot or occlusive environment while treatment for miliaria is underway [30].

Treatment aims to alleviate inflammation and prevent bacterial superinfection. Mild corticosteroids, such as 0.1% triamcinolone cream, are effective for reducing inflammation, while topical antibiotics like clindamycin are used for pustular cases [29]. Miliaria crystallina is self-limiting and typically resolves without intervention [29]. Preventative measures include wearing loose, moisture-wicking clothing to enhance ventilation, staying hydrated, and avoiding prolonged heat exposure [29, 30]. Maintaining proper hygiene, regular exfoliation, and limiting the use of occlusive gear can reduce the risk of miliaria [29, 30], ensuring greater comfort and skin health for cyclists.

Cyclists are particularly susceptible to xerosis (dry skin) and eczematous dermatitis due to prolonged exposure to environmental conditions and the physical demands of the sport. Cyclists are frequently exposed to harsh environmental factors such as wind, sun, and repetitive friction caused by cycling gear, which can contribute to developing these conditions. Xerosis is characterized by dehydrated skin that may exhibit light-to-severe flaking, scaling, fine lines, cracks, and erythema [31, 32]. Environmental factors, including prolonged UV radiation exposure, cold temperatures, frequent bathing after rides, and the use of harsh soaps, are common causes of xerosis [31, 32]. The plantar area of the foot is especially vulnerable to xerosis due to its reliance on sweat secretions for hydration [32], which can be disrupted by the confined environment of cycling shoes, leading to additional moisture loss and irritation.

Cyclists with xerosis may be at an increased risk for hand eczema, particularly if underlying atopic dermatitis (AD) is present [31]. Xerosis is also recognized as a symptom of dermatitis, often accompanied by inflammation and pain [32]. Studies have identified a positive association between generalized xerosis and eczematous conditions like AD, hand eczema, and contact sensitization in adults [31]. The relationship with contact sensitization may be linked to the frequent use of topical products containing allergens applied to treat xerotic or inflamed skin [31]. AD, a chronic inflammatory skin condition, is characterized by severe pruritus, xerosis, and visible eczematous skin lesions [33]. While genetic predisposition plays a role, the rising prevalence of AD may be attributed to increased exposure to various environmental stressors such as UV radiation, harsh climatic conditions, and pollution [33] frequently encountered during outdoor cycling.

To prevent and manage xerosis, it is essential to maintain the skin's epidermal barrier function, which protects underlying tissues from infection and damage [32]. Cyclists should regularly use emollients and moisturizers to restore hydration and prevent water loss [32]. Prevention strategies include using non-abrasive, moisture-wicking cycling apparel, avoiding prolonged exposure to harsh weather, and using soap-free cleansers for post-ride bathing.

For eczematous dermatitis, including AD, treatment often involves liberal use of emollients combined with topical corticosteroids to manage flare-ups [34]. Corticosteroids should be applied twice daily during active lesions, typically for 2 weeks or less, based on clinical improvement [34]. Combinatorial therapy of topical calcineurin inhibitors and corticosteroids are indicated for this condition [34].

12.6 Allergic and Irritant Contact Dermatoses

Contact dermatitis is a prevalent condition in sports, often triggered by exposure to irritants or allergens. It is categorized as either irritant contact dermatitis (ICD), accounting for approximately 80% of cases, or allergic contact dermatitis (ACD), which comprises the remaining 20% [11]. In cycling sports, this condition can result from prolonged contact with materials such as bike saddles, gloves, helmets, or clothing treated with dyes or chemical agents. Cyclists with contact dermatitis typically present with erythematous, scaling, and lichenified rashes, which are frequently pruritic but may also cause a burning sensation, particularly in ICD [11]. Blistering can occur in severe reactions. A thorough history and physical examination are essential for diagnosis, focusing on the materials and substances in contact with the affected area. Patch testing may be necessary to confirm specific allergens or irritants [11].

Contact dermatitis is often facilitated and exacerbated in sports by sweating into equipment, repetitive wetting, repeated drying, friction, and various chemicals that are used in different sports settings [11, 12]. Cyclists may develop contact dermatitis due to exposure to specific allergens or irritants found in their equipment, such as helmets, gloves, cycling shoes, or topical medications applied to the skin. Topical benzocaine and lanolin, which are used in many topical medications and creams, have been reported to be one of the most common causes of ACD in sports [11, 12]. The clinical features of ACD often include itching, scaling, erythema, vesiculation, fissuring, hyperkeratosis, and lichenification [33]. Prolonged friction, sweat accumulation, and synthetic materials in cycling gear can exacerbate the risk of irritant or allergic contact dermatitis. Cyclists wearing rubber or synthetic materials in helmets, gloves, and shoes may develop ICD due to prolonged exposure to irritants, especially when sweating increases skin permeability. Rubber chemicals are a well-documented cause of contact dermatitis, which has been reported in athletes who had close contact with rubber in their sports equipment and developed eczematous skin lesions [35]. Cycling shoes, particularly insoles with rubber components, are a common source of irritant dermatitis, as they are in close contact with sweat-soaked skin [11, 12]. Materials such as rubber, neoprene, and benzoyl peroxide, commonly used in goggles, sunglasses, and eye shields, can induce ACD, particularly around the face and eyes [11]. Similarly, topical agents like benzocaine and lanolin, frequently used to treat blisters or irritation, can trigger ACD on the feet and other areas exposed to these substances [11].

The cornerstone of treatment for both ICD and ACD is identifying and avoiding known triggers [9]. Medium- to high-potency topical corticosteroids, applied twice daily, are effective for managing symptoms on the body [11]. For sensitive areas like the face, groin, or axilla, mild-potency corticosteroids (e.g., hydrocortisone 2.5%) or calcineurin inhibitors (pimecrolimus, tacrolimus) are recommended to minimize the risk of hypopigmentation and skin thinning [11]. Preventive strategies for cyclists include using well-ventilated, moisture-wicking gear to minimize sweat accumulation and friction, as well as ensuring proper hygiene and promptly cleaning exposed skin after cycling. Identifying and avoiding allergens in topical creams and cycling equipment is essential. Regular maintenance of cycling gear, such as washing helmets and gloves, can further reduce the risk of contact dermatitis [11].

References

1. Verzì AE, Nasca MR, Dall'Oglio F, Cosentino C, Micali G. A novel treatment of intertrigo in athletes and overweight subjects. J Cosmet Dermatol. 2021;20 Suppl 1(Suppl 1):23–7.
2. Pujalte GGA, Costa LMC, Clapp AD, Presutti RJ, Sluzevich JC. More than skin deep: dermatologic conditions in athletes. Sports Health. 2023;15(1):74–85.
3. Everink IHJ, Kottner J, van Haastregt JCM, Halfens R, Schols J. Skin areas, clinical severity, duration and risk factors of intertrigo: a secondary data analysis. J Tissue Viability. 2021;30(1):102–7.
4. Metin A, Dilek N, Bilgili SG. Recurrent candidal intertrigo: challenges and solutions. Clin Cosmet Investig Dermatol. 2018;11:175–85.
5. Mazhar M, Simpson M, Marathe K. Inner thigh friction as a cause of acne mechanica. Pediatr Dermatol. 2019;36(4):546–7.
6. Mills OH Jr, Kligman A. Acne mechanica. Arch Dermatol. 1975;111(4):481–3.
7. Liebich C, Wergin VV, Schubert I, Von Bruehl ML, Marquart C, Halle M, et al. Dermatoses in competitive athletes. Deutsche Zeitschrift f¸r Sportmedizin. 2021;71(1):5–12.
8. Strauss RM, Harrington CI. Stump acne: a new variant of acne mechanica and a cause of immobility. Br J Dermatol. 2001;144(3):647–8.
9. Cruz SA, Stein SL. A review of sports-related dermatologic conditions. Transl Sports Med. 2020;3(4):300–8.
10. Sarah Hannam MLS. Disorders due to physical agents. In: Dermatology. 5th ed. Elsevier.
11. Carr PC, MD, Cropley TG, MD. Sports dermatology: skin diseases in athletes. Clin Sports Med. 2019;38(4):597–618.
12. Adams BB. Dermatologic disorders of the athlete. Sports Med. 2002;32(5):309–21.
13. Bury K, Leavy JE, O'Connor A, Jancey J. Prevalence, prevention and treatment of saddle sores among female competitive cyclists: a scoping review: protocol. Methods Protoc. 2020;3(1):4.
14. Napier D, Heron N. Getting to the bottom of saddle sores: a scoping review of the definition, prevalence, management and prevention of saddle sores in cycling. Int J Environ Res Public Health. 2022;19(13):8073.
15. Norman M, Vitale K. "Bumpy" ride for the female cyclist: a rare case of perineal nodular induration, the ischial hygroma. Int J Surg Case Rep. 2020;73:277–80.
16. Steffanoni C. We Need to Talk About Women's Bike Fit Issues 2024 [Available from: https://www.alignedsportstherapy.com.au/post/saddle-pain-when-cycling.
17. Mitterberger M, Pinggera GM, Neuwirt H, Colleselli D, Pelzer A, Bartsch G, et al. Do mountain bikers have a higher risk of scrotal disorders than on-road cyclists? Clin J Sport Med. 2008;18(1):49–54.
18. Pecci M, Comeau D, Chawla V. Skin conditions in the athlete. Am J Sports Med. 2009;37(2):406–18.
19. William D, James MD, Treat JR, Rosenbach MA, Neuhaus IM. Andrews' diseases of the skin. 13th ed. Elsevier; 2020.
20. Rodgers P, Bassler M. Treating onychomycosis. Am Fam Physician. 2001;63(4):663–72, 77–8.
21. Baran R, de Berker DAR, Holzberg M, Thomas L. Baran and Dawber's diseases of the nails and their management. Somerset: John Wiley & Sons, Incorporated; 2012.
22. Elewski BE. Onychomycosis: pathogenesis, diagnosis, and management. Clin Microbiol Rev. 1998;11(3):415–29.
23. De Luca JF, Adams BB, Yosipovitch G. Skin manifestations of athletes competing in the summer olympics. Sports Med. 2012;42(5):399–413.
24. Moehrle M. Outdoor sports and skin cancer. Clin Dermatol. 2008;26(1):12–5.
25. Dianzani C, Conforti C, Giuffrida R, Corneli P, di Meo N, Farinazzo E, et al. Current therapies for actinic keratosis. Int J Dermatol. 2020;59(6):677–84.
26. Bernal Masferrer L, Gracia Cazaña T, Bernad Alonso I, Álvarez-Salafranca M, Almenara Blasco M, Gallego Rentero M, et al. Topical immunotherapy for actinic keratosis and field cancerization. Cancers (Basel). 2024;16(6):1133.

27. Moehrle M, Heinrich L, Schmid A, Garbe C. Extreme UV exposure of professional cyclists. Dermatology. 2000;201(1):44–5.
28. Bowen K. Protecting yourself from windburn. Truck News. 2006;26(3):34.
29. Guerra KC, Toncar A, Krishnamurthy K. Miliaria. In: StatPearls. Treasure Island (FL): StatPearls Publishing Copyright © 2024, StatPearls Publishing LLC; 2024.
30. Carter R 3rd, Garcia AM, Souhan BE. Patients presenting with miliaria while wearing flame resistant clothing in high ambient temperatures: a case series. J Med Case Rep. 2011;5:474.
31. Thyssen JP, Johansen JD, Zachariae C, Menné T, Linneberg A. Xerosis is associated with atopic dermatitis, hand eczema and contact sensitization independent of filaggrin gene mutations. Acta Derm Venereol. 2013;93(4):406–10.
32. Parker J, Scharfbillig R, Jones S. Moisturisers for the treatment of foot xerosis: a systematic review. J Foot Ankle Res. 2017;10:9.
33. Kim K. Influences of environmental chemicals on atopic dermatitis. Toxicol Res. 2015;31(2):89–96.
34. Frazier W, Bhardwaj N. Atopic dermatitis: diagnosis and treatment. Am Fam Physician. 2020;101(10):590–8.
35. Moritz K, Sesztak-Greinecker G, Wantke F, Götz M, Jarisch R, Hemmer W. Allergic contact dermatitis due to rubber in sports equipment. Contact Derm. 2007;57(2):131–2.

Index

K. Nouri (ed.), *Sport-Related Skin Conditions*,
https://doi.org/10.1007/978-3-031-90444-8

MIX
Papier aus verantwortungsvollen Quellen
Paper from responsible sources
FSC® C105338

If you have any concerns about our products, you can contact us on
ProductSafety@springernature.com

In case Publisher is established outside the EU, the EU authorized representative is:
Springer Nature Customer Service Center GmbH
Europaplatz 3, 69115 Heidelberg, Germany

Printed by Libri Plureos GmbH
in Hamburg, Germany